HISTONE DEACETYLASES

CANCER DRUG DISCOVERY AND DEVELOPMENT

BEVERLY A. TEICHER, SERIES EDITOR

HISTONE DEACETYLASES

TRANSCRIPTIONAL REGULATION AND OTHER CELLULAR FUNCTIONS

Edited by

ERIC VERDIN, MD

Gladstone Institute of Virology and Immunology
University of California, San Francisco, CA

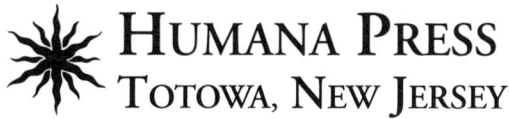
HUMANA PRESS
TOTOWA, NEW JERSEY

© 2006 Humana Press Inc.
999 Riverview Drive, Suite 208
Totowa, New Jersey 07512

www.humanapress.com

This publication is printed on acid-free paper. ∞

ANSI Z39.48-1984 (American National Standards Institute) Permanence of Paper for Printed Library Materials.

Cover design by Patricia F. Cleary.

Cover illustration: The acetyl-lysine binding site of Sir2 proteins (Fig. 3A, Chap. 9; *see* complete caption on pp. 208–209 and discussion on pp. 206–207).

For additional copies, pricing for bulk purchases, and/or information about other Humana titles, contact Humana at the above address or at any of the following numbers: Tel.: 973-256-1699; Fax: 973-256-8341; E-mail: humana@humanapr.com or visit our Website at www.humanapress.com

eISBN 1-59745-024-3

Printed in the United States of America. 10 9 8 7 6 5 4 3 2 1

Library of Congress Cataloging-in-Publication Data

Histone deacetylases : transcriptional regulation and other cellular functions / edited by Eric Verdin.
    p. ; cm. -- (Cancer drug discovery and development)
    Includes bibliographical references and index.
    ISBN 1-58829-499-4 (alk. paper)
    1. Histone deacetylase. 2. Cell cycle. 3. Enzymes. 4. Cancer --Chemotherapy. I. Verdin, Eric. II. Series.
[DNLM: 1. Histone Deacetylases--physiology. 2. Cell Cycle--drug effects. 3. Enzyme Repression--physiology. 4. Histone Deacetylases--antagonists & inhibitors. 5. Neoplasms--drug therapy. 6. Sirtuins--physiology. QU 136 H673 2006]
    QP552.H5H55 2006
    616.99'4061--dc22
                                                                                      2005031537

PREFACE

Forty years ago, Vince Allfrey discovered the reversible acetylation of histone proteins and proposed that this posttranslational modification could regulate gene expression *(1)*. The role of histone acetylation in transcriptional regulation remained controversial until 1996, when two papers reported the identification of the first acetyltransferase, GCN5 *(2)* and the first histone deacetylase, HDAC1 *(3)*. The realization that these enzymes were homologous to previously identified yeast transcriptional regulators established histone acetylation as a key regulatory mechanism for gene expression.

These discoveries have triggered a wave of interest in histone posttranslational modifications and have led to the discovery of 18 potential human histone deacetylases in the past eight years. Human histone deacetylases are divided into three families, Class I (HDAC1, -2, -3, and -8) and Class II HDACs (HDAC4, -5, -6, -7, 9, -10, and -11), are homologous to the yeast histone deacetylases Rpd3 and Hda1, respectively, and share some degree of sequence homology. In contrast, the Class III histone deacetylases are homologous to the yeast protein Sir2 and use NAD as a cofactor. The human class III HDACs are called sirtuins (SIRT1–7). In many cases, these deacetylases target nonhistone proteins for deacetylation, suggesting that their biological activities go beyond gene regulation. Despite the youth of this research field, the first inhibitors of histone deacetylases are in clinical trials as novel anticancer agents.

The purpose of *Histone Deacetylases: Transcriptional Regulation and Other Cellular Functions* is to summarize this rapidly evolving field. Much has been learned about these proteins, including the identification of the enzymes, the elucidation of their enzymatic mechanisms of action, and the identification of their substrates and partners. Structures have been solved for a number of enzymes, alone or in complex with small-molecule inhibitors. Several HDAC genes have been knocked out in mice and their biological roles have been defined. Despite these impressive advances, our knowledge is still fragmentary and much remains to be done.

We hope that this book will serve as a landmark survey of what has been accomplished in these first eight years. We also hope that we have successfully outlined for our readers a clear agenda of what needs to be done in the next few years to define fully the role of HDACs in biology and in disease.

Eric Verdin, MD

1. Allfrey VG, Faulkner R, Mirsky AE. Acetylation and methylation of histones and their possible role in the regulation of RNA synthesis. Proc Natl Acad Sci USA 1964;51:786–794.

2. Brownell JE, Zhou J, Ranalli T, et al. *Tetrahymena* histone acetyltransferase A: a homolog to yeast Gcn5p linking histone acetylation to gene activation. Cell 1996;84:843–851.

3. Taunton J, Hassig CA, Schreiber SL. A mammalian histone deacetylase related to the yeast transcriptional regulator Rpd3p. Science 1996;272:408–411.

CONTENTS

IV. Histone Deacetylase Inhibitors

CONTRIBUTORS

NIDHI AHUJA, PhD • *Gladstone Institutes, University of California, San Francisco, CA*

PETER ATADJA, PhD • *Department of Oncology, Novartis Institutes for Biomedical Research, Cambridge, MA*

MARGIE T. BORRA, PhD • *Department of Biomolecular Chemistry, University of Wisconsin, Madison, Madison, WI*

VINCENT CASTRONOVO, MD, PhD • *Biologie Générale et Cellulaire, Labo de Recherche sur les Métastases, University of Liège, Liège, Belgium*

DALIA COHEN, PhD • *Department of Functional Genomics, Novartis Institutes for Biomedical Research, Cambridge, MA*

JOHN M. DENU, PhD • *Department of Biomolecular Chemistry, University of Wisconsin, Madison, Madison, WI*

ROY A. FRYE, MD, PhD • *Department of Pathology, University of Pittsburgh, Pittsburgh, PA*

BRIAN GABRIELLI, PhD • *Epithelial Pathobiology Group, Centre for Immunology and Cancer Research, University of Queensland Department of Medicine, Princess Alexandra Hospital, Brisbane, Queensland, Australia*

MEIER HSU • *Department of Oncology, Novartis Institutes for Biomedical Research, Cambridge, MA*

AKIHIRO ITO, PhD • *Chemical Genetics Laboratory, RIKEN, Saitama, Japan*

HERBERT G. KASLER, PhD • *Gladstone Institute of Virology and Immunology, University of California, San Francisco, CA*

PAUL KWON • *Department of Oncology, Novartis Institutes for Biomedical Research, Cambridge, MA*

RONEN MARMORSTEIN, PhD • *Professor, Gene Expression and Regulation Program, The Wistar Institute, Philadelphia, PA*

BRETT MARSHALL • *Gladstone Institute of Virology and Immunology, University of California, San Francisco, CA*

J. ANDREW MCKEE, MD • *Department of Pharmacology and Cancer Biology, Duke University, Durham, NC*

TIMOTHY A. MCKINSEY, PhD • *Myogen, Inc, Westminster, CO*

DOMINIQUE MEUNIER, PhD • *Max F. Perutz Laboratories, Vienna Biocenter, University of Vienna, Vienna, Austria*

NORIKAZU NISHINO, PhD • *Graduate School of Life Science and Systems Engineering, Kyushu Institute of Technology, Kitakyushu, Japan; CREST Research Project, Japan Science and Technology Agency*

BRIAN J. NORTH, PhD • *Gladstone Institute of Virology and Immunology, University of California, San Francisco, CA*

ERIC N. OLSON, PhD • *Department of Molecular Biology, University of Texas Southwestern Medical Center at Dallas, Dallas, TX*

DANNY REINBERG, PhD • *Division of Nucleic Acids Enzymology, Department of Biochemistry, Robert Wood Johnson Medical School, University of Medicine and Dentistry of New Jersey, Piscataway, NJ*

MICHAEL SCHER, PhD • *Division of Nucleic Acids Enzymology, Department of Biochemistry, Robert Wood Johnson Medical School, University of Medicine and Dentistry of New Jersey, Piscataway, NJ*

BJOERN SCHWER, MD • *Gladstone Institute of Virology and Immunology, University of California, San Francisco, CA*

CHRISTIAN SEISER, PhD • *Max F. Perutz Laboratories, Vienna Biocenter, University of Vienna, Vienna, Austria*

EDWARD SETO, PhD • *Cancer Biology, H. Lee Moffitt Cancer Center, Tampa, FL*

ALEJANDRO VAQUERO, PhD • *Division of Nucleic Acids Enzymology, Department of Biochemistry, Robert Wood Johnson Medical School, University of Medicine and Dentistry of NJ, Piscataway, NJ*

ERIC VERDIN, MD • *Gladstone Institute of Virology and Immunology, University of California, San Francisco, CA*

DAVID WALTREGNY, MD, PhD • *Biologie Générale et Cellulaire, Labo de Recherche sur les Métastases, University of Liège, Liège, Belgium*

TSO-PANG YAO, PhD • *Department of Pharmacology and Cancer Biology, Duke University, Durham, NC*

MINORU YOSHIDA, PhD • *Chemical Genetics Laboratory, RIKEN, Saitama, Japan; CREST Research Project, Japan Science and Technology Agency*

KEHAO ZHAO, PhD • *Gene Expression and Regulation Program, The Wistar Institute, Philadelphia, PA*

COLOR PLATES

I

CLASS I HISTONE DEACETYLASES

1 Histone Deacetylase 1

Dominique Meunier, PhD *and Christian Seiser, PhD*

SUMMARY

HDAC1 was the first histone deacetylase identified in mammals and is considered the prototype of this large family of enzymes. Transcriptional repression mediated by HDAC1 plays a crucial role in the regulation of a variety of biological processes, including cell cycle progression, proliferation, and differentiation. Interestingly, HDAC1 can also influence other cellular activities, such as DNA replication and chromosome segregation, via mechanisms that do not involve transcriptional repression. In addition, HDAC1 is essential for embryonic development

From: *Cancer Drug Discovery and Development*
Histone Deacetylases: Transcriptional Regulation and Other Cellular Functions
Edited by: E. Verdin © Humana Press Inc., Totowa, NJ

Acronyms and Abbreviations

BRCA1	Breast cancer 1 gene
CoREST	Corepressor of RE1 silencing transcription factor
EED	Embryonic ectoderm development protein
EZH2	Enhancer of zeste homolog 2 (*Drosophila*)
HAT	Histone acetyltransferase
HDA-1	Histone deacetylase 1 (Yeast)
MAD	MAX dimerization protein
MAX	MYC-associated factor X
MBD3	Methyl-CpG-binding domain protein 3
MDM2	Mouse double minute 2
Mi-2-alpha, (CHD3)	Dermatomyositis-specific autoantigen 2 alpha, also called chromodomain helicase DNA-binding protein 3
Mi-2-beta, (CHD4)	Dermatomyositis-specific autoantigen 2 beta, also called chromodomain helicase DNA-binding protein 4
MTA1, MTA2	Metastasis-associated gene 1, metastasis-associated gene 2
MYC	Myelocytomatosis oncogene
NF-Y	Nuclear transcription factor Y
P/CAF	p300/CBP-associated factor
RPD3	Reduced potassium dependency 3
SAP18	SIN3-associated polypeptide, 18 KDa
SAP30	SIN3-associated polypeptide, 30 KDa
SIN3	SWI-independent 3
SP1, SP3	Specific protein 1, specific protein 3
YY1	Ying yang 1

and appears to play a critical role in cellular defense against viral infection. Finally, increasing evidence points toward the importance of HDAC1 in tumor formation and/or progression, and cumulative observations indicate that the enzyme is a crucial target for HDAC inhibitors in cancer therapy.

Key Words: Histone deacetylase 1, HDAC1, transcriptional repression, biological function, cell cycle regulation, proliferation, differentiation, replication, mitosis, development, cancer, chromatin.

HISTONE DEACETYLASE 1: A BRIEF HISTORY

Histone deacetylase 1 (HDAC1) was the first protein found to possess histone deacetylase activity in mammals. Taking advantage of the recent discovery of trapoxin, a potent inhibitor of HDAC activity *(1,2)*, Taunton and colleagues *(3)* isolated HDAC1 from a human T-cell line using a trapoxin-based affinity matrix. HDAC1 was subsequently identified as a growth factor-inducible enzyme with HDAC activity in mouse T-cells *(4)*. Sequence analyses revealed that both the human and mouse HDAC1 proteins are highly homologous to the *Saccharomyces cerevisiae* RPD3 protein *(3–5)*, a known transcriptional regulator *(6)*. Although mouse HDAC1 failed to complement the yeast *rpd3Δ* deletion *(4)*, extensive investigations since then have clearly demonstrated the crucial role played by HDAC1 in the transcriptional repression of a variety of mammalian genes involved in cell cycle progression, proliferation, differentiation, development and cancer.

EVOLUTIONARY CONSERVATION OF HDAC1

The mammalian HDAC1 protein belongs to an ancient family of enzymes highly conserved throughout eukaryotic and prokaryotic evolution. Eukaryotic HDACs have been divided into three classes—I, II and III—based on sequence similarity *(7,8)*. HDAC1, together with HDAC2, HDAC3, and HDAC8, belongs to the RPD3-like class I of HDACs. A recent phylogenetic analysis has revealed that class I can be further divided into an HDAC1/HDAC2 and an HDAC3 subclass *(9)*. The HDAC1/HDAC2 subclass consists of the vertebrate HDAC1 and HDAC2 proteins, the single *Drosophila melanogaster* RPD3 protein, and a pair of proteins in *Caenorhabditis elegans*. HDAC1-related proteins have also been identified in several other organisms, including chicken *(10)*, *Xenopus laevis* *(11)*, *Danio rerio* *(12)*, *Arabidopsis thaliana* *(9)*, maize *(13,14)*, and bacteria *(4)*.

The existence of an HDAC1/HDAC2 subclass within class I highlights the high degree of similarity that exists between these two enzymes: in mammals, HDAC1 and HDAC2 exhibit approx 82% identity, and their genomic organization is almost identical *(15,16)*. This indicates that HDAC1 and HDAC2 arose from a relatively recent gene duplication and suggests that they have probably undergone little functional divergence either from their common ancestor or from each other *(9)*. Indeed, both HDAC1 and HDAC2 are widely expressed nuclear proteins, they are found in similar protein complexes (*see* the section entitled HDAC1-Associated Protein Complexes, below), and they have been shown to heterodimerize *(16–18)*. Furthermore, HDAC1 appears to influence the expression of HDAC2, and vice versa (*see* the section entitled HDAC1 and the Regulation of Cell Cycle Progression, Proliferation, and Differentiation). However, the observation that HDAC1 deletion leads to embryonic lethality in the mouse *(19)* indicates that, despite some functional overlap, HDAC1 and HDAC2 also have distinct and nonredundant biological functions.

STRUCTURAL AND FUNCTIONAL
CHARACTERISTICS OF HDAC1

Structural Organization and Transcriptional Regulation of the HDAC1 Gene

Sequence analysis and chromosomal fluorescent *in situ* hybridization have shown that HDAC1 maps to mouse chromosome 4 and human chromosome 1p34.1; in both cases, linkage to the genes encoding the myristoylated alanine-rich protein C kinase substrate (MARCKS)-related protein (MRP) and lymphocyte-specific protein tyrosine kinase (LCK) is conserved *(5,15)*. In mammals, the HDAC1 gene is about 30 kb in length and comprises 14 exons interrupted by 13 introns *(15)*. The HDAC1 open reading frame is 1446 bp long and encodes a 482-amino acid protein with a molecular mass of approx 55 kDa *(3–5)*.

The HDAC1 promoter is rich in GC, lacks a TATA box consensus sequence, and contains two transcription factor binding sites that are crucial for its full activity: a CCAAT box that is recognized by the transcriptional regulator NF-Y and a distal GC box to which members of the SP family can bind *(20)*. NF-Y and SP1/SP3 have been found to regulate the transcriptional activation or repression of HDAC1 synergistically by recruiting either histone acetyltransferases (HATs) or HDACs, respectively, to the HDAC1 promoter. This indicates that the HDAC1 gene itself is regulated by the balanced action of acetylating and deacetylating enzymes. In particular, HDAC1 has been found to be recruited to its own promotor by NF-Y and SP1/SP3, thereby mediating its own repression via a negative feedback loop *(20)*. HDAC1 transcription has also been shown to be induced by a two-step mechanism involving stabilization of histone H3 phosphoacetylation by growth factor-mediated activation of the mitogen-activated protein (MAP) kinase pathway and removal of HDACs and/or recruitment of HATs at the HDAC1 promoter *(21)*.

Structural and Functional Organization of the HDAC1 Protein

HDAC1 is a metalloenzyme containing three important functional domains: (1) an N-terminal HDAC association domain (HAD; residues 1–53), which is essential for HDAC1 homodimerization, association with HDAC2 as well as other proteins, and catalytic activity *(18)*; (2) a central zinc-binding catalytic domain termed HDAC consensus motif (residues 25–303), which contains several conserved histidine and aspartate residues and forms the active site pocket of the enzyme *(18,22)*; and (3) a C-terminal lysine-rich domain (residues 438–482) containing the core nuclear localization signal (NLS) KKAKRVKT *(18)* and the IACEE motif involved in the interaction with the pocket proteins pRB, p107, and p130 *(23–25)*. Interestingly, a truncated HDAC1 protein lacking the NLS can still translocate into the nucleus through association with an intact HDAC1 protein *(18)*, and Taplick and colleagues *(18)* have therefore proposed that homodimerization plays a pivotal role in the activity of the enzyme. The HDAC1 protein is also a target for various posttranslational modifications *(26–28)*. Phosphorylation of serine residues in the C-terminal portion of the protein appears to promote HDAC1 enzymatic activity *(27)*, whereas sumoylation of lysine residues in the same domain seems to be required for transcriptional repression by HDAC1 *(28)*. Acetylation of the protein also appears to enhance its enzymatic activity (J. Taplick and C. Seiser, unpublished data).

TRANSCRIPTIONAL REPRESSION MEDIATED BY HDAC1

HDAC1 Substrate Specificity

HDACs are believed to repress transcription mainly through deacetylation of the histone tails that protrude from the nucleosomes, resulting in local modification of chromatin structure *(7)*. HDAC1 has been shown to deacetylate all four core histones in vitro and appears to preferentially deacetylate specific lysine residues on histone H4 *(29)*. The enzyme has also been found to deacetylate a subset of histones H3 and H4 in vivo *(19)*. In addition to histones, HDAC1 can also deacetylate nonhistone proteins, such as the tumor suppressor p53 *(30,31)*, the transcription factors E2F1 *(32,33)* and YY1 *(34)*, and proliferating cell nuclear antigen (PCNA) *(35)*.

HDAC1-Associated Protein Complexes

HDAC1, together with the closely related enzyme HDAC2, is generally found in multiprotein complexes that are recruited to DNA by various transcription factors. To date, three complexes containing HDAC1 and HDAC2 have been characterized in mammals: the corepressor complex SIN3, the nucleosome remodeling and deacetylase complex (NuRD), and the CoREST complex *(8)*. The SIN3 and NuRD complexes both contain HDAC1, HDAC2, retinoblastoma-associated protein (RbAp)46, and RbAp48, a protein originally copurified with human HDAC1 *(3)*. In addition, mSin3A, SAP18, and SAP30 are associated with the SIN3 complex, whereas Mi-2α/Mi-2β (also called CHD3/CHD4) and MTA2 are found in the NuRD complex. The CoREST complex also contains both HDAC1 and HDAC2, as well as CoREST and LSD1, a recently identified lysine-specific histone demethylase *(8,35a)*.

A large number of transcription factors have been identified that recruit HDAC1-associated complexes to specific promoters in order to mediate transcriptional repression. These include regulators of cell cycle progression, proliferation, differentiation, and development *(7,8,16,36,37)*. In addition to transcriptional repression through protein complexes, HDAC1 can also fulfil its repressive function through direct interaction with DNA binding proteins such as SP1/SP3, YY1, PCNA, the pocket proteins pRB, p107, and p130, and the tumor suppressors p53 and BRCA1 *(7,30,38)*.

HDAC1 AND THE REGULATION OF CELL CYCLE PROGRESSION, PROLIFERATION, AND DIFFERENTIATION

HDAC1 was originally identified in the mouse as a growth factor-inducible protein *(4)* and its expression has been found to correlate with proliferation in various tissues, embryonic stem (ES) cells, and several transformed cell lines *(4,19)*, thereby suggesting a link between HDAC1 and regulation of cellular proliferation. Indeed, both overexpression of HDAC1 in mouse fibroblasts and disruption of the gene in mouse embryos and ES cells have been shown to severely perturb proliferation and cell cycle progression *(4,19)*, indicating that maintenance of cell type-specific deacetylase levels is crucial for unrestricted proliferation. In line with this idea, HDAC2 and HDAC3 protein levels have been found to be upregulated in the absence of HDAC1 *(19)*, and loss of HDAC2 appears to cause overexpression of HDAC1 (S. Chiocca, personal communication). It is, however, important to note that the effects of HDAC1-mediated transcriptional repression on the regulation of cell cycle progression, proliferation, and differentiation are diverse and seem to be dependent on HDAC1 molecular partners, as will be discussed in the following sections.

HDAC1 and the Pocket Proteins

The involvement of HDAC1 in the control of cell cycle progression is underscored by its interaction with the three members of the retinoblastoma family of transcriptional repressors, the pocket proteins pRB, p107, and p130, via the IACEE motif *(23–25,39,40)*. Hypophosphorylated pocket proteins recruit HDAC1 early in G1 and repress cell cycle progression by binding to and inhibiting members of the E2F family of transcription factors. Upon phosphorylation of pocket proteins by cyclin-dependent kinase (CDK)/cyclin complexes, the HDAC1/pocket protein/E2F complex is abrogated, allowing E2F factors to activate a series of genes required for G1/S phase transition and DNA synthesis, including cyclin A and cyclin E *(41)*. CDK4/6/cyclin D2 complexes have been shown to be particularly effective at phosphorylating pRB and consequently inhibiting the pRB-HDAC1 interaction at the G1/S phase transition, thus promoting cyclin E expression *(42)*. Although recruitment of HDAC1 by pRB is clearly crucial for repression of E2F-responsive genes, a recent report has shown that HDAC1 does not cooperate with pRB to repress E2F1-mediated cell death. In contrast, in this particular case, HDAC1 inhibits the effects of pRB on E2F1 by a mechanism that does not involve deacetylase activity but requires the IACEE motif *(43)*.

HDAC1 and the MAD/MAX Heterodimer

A further indication of the role of HDAC1 in the control of cell growth and proliferation is its association with the MAD/MAX heterodimer. In proliferating cells, MYC/MAX heterodimer activates transcription of genes required for cellular growth. Upon differentiation, however, MYC is replaced by MAD, and the MAD/MAX heterodimer represses transcription of the growth-stimulatory genes through recruitment of the SIN3/HDAC1/2 corepressor complex *(44–47)*.

Promotion of Cellular Proliferation by HDAC1

The recruitment of HDAC1 by the pocket proteins and the MAD/MAX complex clearly demonstrates the involvement of the protein in repression of cellular proliferation. However, targeted disruption of HDAC1 in the mouse has revealed that the enzyme is also essential for unrestricted proliferation *(19)*. HDAC1 homozygous mutant (–/–) embryos are severely growth retarded and exhibit a proliferation defect that is associated with elevated levels of the CDK inhibitors p21 and p27 and with a decrease in cyclin-associated activity. Similar phenotypes were also observed in HDAC1–/– ES cells. Consistent with these findings, the p21 promoter has been found to be associated with hyperacetylated histones in the absence of HDAC1 *(19)*, and HDAC1 has been shown to be recruited to the p21 promoter by direct interaction with the transcription factor SP1 *(48)*. The tumor suppressor p53 is known to activate p21 in response to DNA damages, thereby inducing cell cycle arrest and apoptosis *(49)*. Interestingly, p53 is also recruited to the p21 promoter through direct interaction with SP1 *(48,50)* and has been shown to compete with HDAC1 for the regulation of p21 expression following DNA damage *(48)*. Taken together, these findings indicate that HDAC1 is a crucial negative regulator of p21 transcriptional activity, although the possibility cannot be excluded that other HDACs may also be involved in the repression of p21 *(51)*.

In addition to inhibition of p21, HDAC1 has also been shown to repress p53 function by direct deacetylation of the protein *(30,31)*. Acetylation of p53 stabilizes and activates the protein in response to genotoxic stress, while deacetylation appears to provide a rapid mechanism to inhibit p53-mediated cell cycle arrest and apoptosis and to restore normal cell growth once DNA repair is completed *(52)*. This probably occurs through recruitment of HDAC1 by MDM2—a key negative regulator of p53—thereby inducing p53 deacetylation and allowing MDM2 to ubiquitinate the protein, which is then targeted for degradation *(53)*. Although acetylation clearly activates p53 function, it appears not to be essential for the transactivation of p21 following DNA damage; however, p53 acetylation strongly enhances its binding to the p21 promoter in vivo *(52,54)*.

HDAC1 and Nuclear Receptors

Nuclear receptors are a large family of ligand-induced transcription factors that regulate a variety of physiological processes, including development and differentiation. Furthermore, nuclear receptors are well-characterized examples of HDAC-recruiting proteins *(55)*. Thyroid hormone receptors and retinoic acid receptors have been shown to repress transcription through recruitment of the SIN3/HDAC1/2 complex in the absence of ligand *(7)*. HDAC1 has also been found to associate with a variety of transcriptional cofactors that bind to and block nuclear receptors in the presence of agonists, such as MTA1 *(56)*, receptor-interacting protein 140 (RIP140; *57*), and the repressor of estrogen receptor activity (REA; *58*). Furthermore, a recent report has shown that HDAC1 can directly interact with and suppress the transcriptional activity of estrogen receptor-α (ER-α) in breast cancer cells *(59)*.

HDAC1 and Differentiation Processes

The involvement of HDAC1 in differentiation processes is highlighted by its interaction with the myogenic activator MyoD. In undifferentiated myoblasts, HDAC1 associates with MyoD, leading to repression of genes involved in skeletal muscle differentiation. Upon induction of myoblast differentiation, the interaction between HDAC1 and MyoD is abrogated, allowing MyoD to activate the myogenic program *(60,61)*. It has been shown that hypophosphorylated pRB can displace HDAC1 from MyoD upon differentiation, thereby reducing the repressive effect of HDAC1 on MyoD; subsequently, HDAC1/pRB complexes are found in differentiated myotubes, where they appear to maintain irreversible cell cycle arrest *(61)*. In particular, Mal and Harter *(62)* have shown that HDAC1 and MyoD are present at the myogenin promoter in undifferentiated myoblasts and that replacement of HDAC1 by the HAT P/CAF leads to MyoD-mediated differentiation, thereby suggesting that acetylation is an important step in skeletal muscle differentiation. Recently, a role for HDAC1 and HDAC2 in the regulation of intestinal epithelium differentiation has also been demonstrated in vivo: expression of both proteins was found to decrease upon differentiation of the intestinal epithelium, whereas their overexpression blocked the expression of certain differentiation markers *(63)*.

OTHER BIOLOGICAL FUNCTIONS OF HDAC1

Transcriptional repression mediated by HDAC1 clearly plays a crucial role in regulation of cell cycle progression, proliferation, and differentiation. However, increasing evidence indicates that HDAC1 can also influence various other biological processes by mechanisms that do not necessarily involve transcriptional repression, as will be discussed in the following sections.

HDAC1 and DNA Replication

PCNA is a crucial component of the DNA replication machinery *(64)*. Physical interaction between HDAC1 and PCNA has been found to cause deacetylation of the protein and appears to be linked to dissociation of PCNA from the DNA and completion of replication *(35,38)*. This suggests that HDAC activity is essential for the formation of proper chromatin structure following DNA synthesis. Whether deacetylation is the cause, or the consequence, of PCNA dissociation from the DNA polymerase remains, however, to be elucidated. HDAC1 has also been shown to interact directly with the enzyme DNA topoisomerase II in the context of the NuRD complex *(65,66)*. Topoisomerase II is involved in DNA unwinding during replication and transcription and also participates in genetic recombination, chromosome condensation, and apoptosis *(67)*. The association between the two enzymes appears to be essential for apoptosis induced by the DNA topoisomerase II poison eposide, and it has been proposed that chromatin remodeling by the NuRD/HDAC1 complex is necessary for topoisomerase II-mediated DNA rearrangements *(66)*.

HDAC1 and the G2/M Checkpoint

A link between HDAC1 and the G2/M checkpoint has been suggested by the finding that the enzyme forms a complex with Hus1 and Rad9, two Rad proteins that are involved in the mitotic checkpoint induced by DNA damage or DNA replication block *(68)*. It has been proposed that the Rad proteins/HDAC1 complex could associate with PCNA to form a ring-like structure around the DNA at the G2/M checkpoint. This complex could then recruit the nucleosome remodeling NuRD complex to facilitate DNA repair and/or restore the native chromatin conformation once DNA has been repaired *(68)*.

Additional evidence for the involvement of HDAC1 in mitotic processes comes from the observation that the protein associates with human and mouse metaphase centromeres, as well as with all other major regions of pericentric and nonpericentric heterochromatin *(69)*. In particular, HDAC1 and MBD3, a component of the NuRD complex, have been found to colocalize with Aurora A, a kinase that is crucial for centrosome separation and bipolar spindle assembly (70), at the centrosomes in the early M phase (71). Furthermore, the SIN3/HDAC1/2 complex-associated protein Sds3 has recently been shown to be essential for deacetylation of pericentric heterochromatin histones and proper chromosome segregation (72), suggesting that HDAC1 and/or HDAC2 play an important role in mitotic processes.

HDAC1 and Chromatin Modifications

Increasing evidence indicates that HDAC1 is an intrinsic part of the epigenetic circuit regulating chromatin modification and remodeling. Consistent with this idea, various reports have shown that HDAC1 interacts with several other chromatin and DNA-modifying enzymes. For instance, it has recently been reported that HDAC1 is recruited by the HAT p300 and interferes with the p300-dependent transcriptional activation of p53 and MyoD, thereby suggesting that HATs and HDACs could associate to control gene expression (73). A link between histone methylation and deacetylation has been demonstrated by the finding that HDAC1, HDAC2, and HDAC3 interact with the histone methyltransferase Suv39H1 (74). Association of HDACs and Suv39H1 could play a role in heterochromatin silencing and/or transcriptional repression by pRB. In addition, the Polycomb group (PcG) complex EED/EZH2 has been found to interact with HDAC1 and HDAC2 (75). The EED-EZH2 complex mediates transcriptional repression in part via its intrinsic histone methyltransferase activity (76), and its silencing function appears to require HDAC activity (75). Recently, work by Shi and colleagues (76a) has also raised the possibility that, within the CoREST complex, the HDAC activity of HDAC1 and HDAC2 may collaborate with the histone demethylase activity of LSD1 to create a repressive chromatin environment. Conflicting results have however been reported (76b) and discrepancies between the two studies still need to be resolved.

In addition to histone methylation, DNA methylation has also been found to cooperate with histone deacetylation to modulate chromatin remodeling and transcriptional silencing (77). Methyl-CpG binding proteins such as MeCP2 and MBD2 have been shown to interact with HDAC1 and to repress transcription in an HDAC-dependent manner (77). Furthermore, HDAC1 has been found to mediate transcriptional repression through association with the DNA methyltransferases DNMT1 (78,79), DNMT3A (80), DNMT3B (81), and DNMT3L (82). In particular, HDAC1 has been shown to form a complex with DNMT1, pRB, and E2F1 to repress transcription from promoters containing E2F1 binding sites (79).

Defense Mechanisms Against Viral Infection

In recent years, evidence has emerged that HDAC1 is involved in cellular defense against viral infection. For example, viral transcription mediated by open reading frame 50 (ORF50), an activator of early and late genes in the lytic cycle of the Kaposi's sarcoma-associated herpesvirus, is repressed upon association with HDAC1 *(83,84)*. Furthermore, inhibition of HDAC activity appears to be important for viral infection. For example, Gam1, an early gene product essential for the replication of the avian adenovirus CELO, can interact with HDAC1 and inhibit its enzymatic activity *(85)*. The bovine herpesvirus 1 immediate-early protein (bICP0) has also been shown to associate with HDAC1 and activate transcription by interfering with MAD/MAX-dependent transcriptional repression, thereby promoting viral infection in differentiated cells *(86)*. Viral transforming proteins such as the human papillomavirus oncoprotein E7 are also known to interfere with the binding of HDAC1 to pRB, thereby promoting cell cycle progression *(23–25)*. Although blocking of HDAC activity appears to be important for viral activity, it may also have negative consequences for the virus, as HDAC inhibition has been reported to activate cellular mechanisms to fight against the viral infection *(87)*. In line with this idea, a recent clinical study by Lerhman and colleagues *(87a)* has suggested that inhibition of HDAC1 in resting CD4+ T cells could contribute to elimination of human immunodeficiency virus (HIV) infection in human patients.

HDAC1 Is Essential for Mouse Embryonic Development

Various studies have demonstrated the role of the HDAC1-containing complexes SIN3 and NuRD in specific developmental processes *(36)*. Direct evidence for the crucial role of HDAC1 itself during embryonic development comes from the analysis of an HDAC1 knockout mouse model *(19)*. Whereas the absence of one HDAC1 allele does not impair mouse viability, targeted disruption of both HDAC1 alleles severely perturbs embryonic development and leads to lethality before E10.5. In addition to reduced cellular proliferation (*see* section entitled Promotion of Cellular Proliferation by HDAC1), HDAC1–/– embryos display various developmental defects such as abnormal head and allantois formation. Although increased levels of HDAC2 and HDAC3 proteins have been found in HDAC1–/– embryos and ES cells, these two class I enzymes could not complement the loss of HDAC1. Accordingly, the deacetylase activity of the SIN3 and NuRD complexes was significantly reduced in HDAC1–/– ES cells *(19)*. Taken together, these findings indicate that HDAC1 plays a crucial and unique role during mouse embryonic development and that the integrity of HDAC1-containing complexes is essential for proper development.

Additional evidence for the crucial role of HDAC1 during development comes from the analysis of HDAC1 mutation in other organisms. Mutation of the HDAC1 ortholog RPD3 in *Drosophila melanogaster* perturbs segmentation and results in embryonic lethality *(88)*. In *Caenorhabditis elegans*, inhibition of maternal and zygotic HDA-1 expression also leads to embryonic lethality *(89)*, whereas mutation of zygotic HDA-1 only causes defects in postembryonic gonadogenesis *(90)*. Embryonic lethality is also associated with deletion of HDAC1 in *Danio rerio (91)*, and a detailed analysis of the mutant phenotype has revealed that HDAC1 is specifically required to maintain neurogenesis in the zebrafish central nervous system during embryogenesis *(12)*.

HDAC1 and Cancer

Extensive studies have shown that HDAC inhibitors induce cell cycle arrest, differentiation, and/or apoptosis in a variety of transformed cell lines, as well as in tumor-bearing animals. Consequently, these inhibitory compounds are currently in phase I and II clinical trials for antitumor therapy *(92,93)*. Several mechanisms can be proposed to explain the antitumor effects of HDAC inhibitors. The general view is that accumulation of acetylated histones and nonhistone proteins leads to activation or repression of a specific subset of genes and molecular pathways crucial for repression of tumor cell growth. This mechanism is consistent with the finding that the expression of only a limited number of genes is affected by HDAC inhibitors *(94)*. With increasing evidence for HDACs involvement in molecular and cellular processes other than transcriptional regulation, it is also reasonable to hypothesize that HDAC inhibitors exert their effects by directly interfering with DNA replication or mitotic division. Finally, based on the observation that tumor cells (which by definition exhibit alterations in various molecular pathways involved in cell growth and differentiation) are much more sensitive to the effects of HDAC inhibitors than normal cells *(92)*, we propose that activation or repression of specific genes and pathways by HDAC inhibitors may generate conflicting signals in tumor cells, leading to cell death or apoptosis.

The antitumor effects of HDAC inhibitors clearly suggest that HDACs play a major role in cancer development. However, as most HDAC inhibitors affect the activity of several enzymes, it is difficult to identify the particular HDACs involved in tumor formation. One way to evaluate the importance of specific HDACs in cancer is through analysis of their expression levels in tumors. Recent reports have indicated that HDAC1 is upregulated in gastric and prostate cancers *(95–98)*, and in both cases, its overexpression has been shown to correlate with downregulation of gelsolin *(97,98)*, a known target of HDAC inhibitors *(94)*. Furthermore, HDAC1 knockdown in human cervical carcinoma cells has been found to induce changes in cellular morphology and to inhibit proliferation, thereby suggesting that HDAC1 is essential for tumor cell survival *(99)*. Interestingly, downregulation of HDAC1 expression has been shown to be associated with cellular differentiation in a variety of human breast tumor cell lines *(100)*.

One mechanism by which HDAC inhibitors appear to repress tumor cell growth is through the activation of the tumor suppressor p21, which is required for inhibition of cell cycle progression *(92)*. As noted above *(see* section entitled Promotion of Cellular Proliferation by HDAC1), HDAC1 is a crucial negative regulator of p21. A recent report has shown that transcriptional activation of p21 by the HDAC inhibitor suberoylanilide hydroxamic acid (SAHA) is accompanied by a marked reduction in HDAC1 bound at the p21 promoter *(51)*. Furthermore, displacement of HDAC1 from the p21 promoter by the pRB binding protein Che-1 *(101,102)* has been shown to activate p21 and consequently inhibit proliferation in human colon carcinoma cell lines *(103)*. Taken together, these findings strongly suggest that HDAC1 could promote tumor formation through selective repression of p21. Another mechanism by which HDAC1 could promote tumorigenesis is via suppression of ER-α *(see* the section entitled HDAC1 and Nuclear Receptors), whose loss is known to be critical for breast cancer progression *(59)*. Finally, it has been reported that HDAC1 expression can be induced by hypoxia in a lung carcinoma cell line, leading to downregulation of the tumor suppressors p53 and von Hippel-Lindau factor and stimulation of hypoxia-induced angiogenesis *(104)*. These findings suggest that HDAC1 could influence tumor progression by promoting angiogenesis.

CONCLUDING REMARKS AND FUTURE DIRECTIONS

The crucial role of HDAC1 in the regulation of cell cycle progression, proliferation, and differentiation via transcriptional repression of specific target genes has clearly been demonstrated since the identification of the protein in 1996. In addition, evidence has recently emerged showing that HDAC1 can influence various cellular processes, such as DNA replication and chromosome segregation, independently of transcriptional repression. Moreover, HDAC1-mediated transcriptional activation of interferon-stimulated genes (ISGs) has recently been reported *(105,106)* and HDAC1 with its associated enzymatic activity has been found to be necessary for the proper induction of the ISGs interferon regulatory factor 1 (IRF1) and guanylate binding protein 2 (GBP2) (G. Zupkovitz and C. Seiser, unpublished data). Importantly, cumulative observations indicate that HDAC1 is involved in tumor formation and/or progression and is a crucial target for HDAC inhibitors in cancer therapy. The development of selective inhibitors is critical to better understand the exact role played by HDAC1 in normal and neoplastic cells. In this respect, it is interesting to note that the HDAC inhibitors MS-27-275 and SB-429201 have recently been shown to preferentially inhibit HDAC1 *(107)* and so may prove extremely useful for future analyses of the biological functions of HDAC1.

ACKNOWLEDGMENTS

We thank B. Schuettengruber and S. Winter for critical comments on the manuscript and S. Chiocca for sharing unpublished data. We apologize to all authors whose work could not be referenced owing to space limitations. This work was supported by the Austrian Science Fund (FWF grant P14909-B12) and the GEN-AU program of the Austrian Government.

REFERENCES

1. Kijima M, Yoshida M, Sugita K, Horinouchi S, Beppu T. Trapoxin, an antitumor cyclic tetrapeptide, is an irreversible inhibitor of mammalian histone deacetylase. J Biol Chem 1993;268:22,429–22,435.
2. Yoshida M, Horinouchi S, Beppu T. Trichostatin A and trapoxin: novel chemical probes for the role of histone acetylation in chromatin structure and function. Bioessays 1995;17:423–430.
3. Taunton J, Hassig CA, Schreiber SL. A mammalian histone deacetylase related to the yeast transcriptional regulator Rpd3p. Science 1996;272:408–411.
4. Bartl S, Taplick J, Lagger G, Khier H, Kuchler K, Seiser C. Identification of mouse histone deacetylase 1 as a growth factor-inducible gene. Mol Cell Biol 1997;17:5033–5043.
5. Furukawa Y, Kawakami T, Sudo K, et al. Isolation and mapping of a human gene (RPD3L1) that is homologous to RPD3, a transcription factor in *Saccharomyces cerevisiae*. Cytogenet Cell Genet 1996;73:130–133.
6. Vidal M, Gaber RF. RPD3 encodes a second factor required to achieve maximum positive and negative transcriptional states in *Saccharomyces cerevisiae*. Mol Cell Biol 1991;11:6317–6327.
7. Cress WD, Seto E. Histone deacetylases, transcriptional control, and cancer. J Cell Physiol 2000;184:1–16.
8. Grozinger CM, Schreiber SL. Deacetylase enzymes: biological functions and the use of small-molecule inhibitors. Chem Biol 2002;9:3–16.
9. Gregoretti IV, Lee YM, Goodson HV. Molecular evolution of the histone deacetylase family: functional implications of phylogenetic analysis. J Mol Biol 2004;338:17–31.
10. Sun JM, Chen HY, Moniwa M, Samuel S, Davie JR. Purification and characterization of chicken erythrocyte histone deacetylase 1. Biochemistry 1999;38:5939–5947.
11. Ladomery M, Lyons S, Sommerville J. *Xenopus* HDm, a maternally expressed histone deacetylase, belongs to an ancient family of acetyl-metabolizing enzymes. Gene 1997;198:275–280.
12. Cunliffe VT. Histone deacetylase 1 is required to repress Notch target gene expression during zebrafish neurogenesis and to maintain the production of motoneurones in response to hedgehog signalling. Development 2004;131:2983–2995.

13. Rossi V, Hartings M, Motto M. Identification and characterization of an RPD3 homologue from maize (*Zea mays* L.) that is able to complement an rpd3 null mutant of *Saccharomyces cerevisiae*. Mol Gen Genet 1998;258:288–296.
14. Lechner T, Lusser A, Pipal A, et al. RPD3-type histone deacetylases in maize embryos. Biochemistry 2000;39:1683–1692.
15. Khier H, Bartl S, Schuettengruber B, Seiser C. Molecular cloning and characterization of the mouse histone deacetylase 1 gene: integration of a retrovirus in 129SV mice. Biochim Biophys Acta 1999;1489:365–373.
16. de Ruijter AJM, van Gennip AH, Caron HN, Kemp S, van Kuilenburg ABP. Histone deacetylases (HDACs): characterization of the classical HDAC family. Biochem J 2003;370:737–749.
17. Hassig CA, Tong JK, Fleischer TC, et al. A role for histone deacetylase activity in HDAC1-mediated transcriptional repression. Proc Natl Acad Sci U S A 1998;95:3519–3524.
18. Taplick J, Kurtev V, Kroboth K, Posch M, Lechner T, Seiser C. Homo-oligomerisation and nuclear localisation of mouse histone deacetylase 1. J Mol Biol 2001;308:27–38.
19. Lagger G, O'Carroll D, Rembold M, et al. Essential function of histone deacetylase 1 in proliferation control and CDK inhibitor repression. EMBO J 2002;21: 2672–2681.
20. Schuettengruber B, Simboeck E, Khier H, Seiser C. Autoregulation of mouse histone deacetylase 1 expression. Mol Cell Biol 2003;23:6993–7004.
21. Hauser C, Schuettengruber B, Bartl S, Lagger G, Seiser C. Activation of the HDAC1 gene by cooperative histone phosphorylation and acetylation. Mol Cell Biol 2002;22:7820–7830.
22. Marmorstein R. Structure of histone deacetylases: insights into substrate recognition and catalysis. Structure (Camb) 2001;9:1127–1133.
23. Brehm A, Miska EA, McCance DJ, Reid JL, Bannister AJ, Kouzarides T. Retinoblastoma protein recruits histone deacetylase to repress transcription. Nature 1998;391:597–601.
24. Ferreira R, Magnaghi-Jaulin L, Robin P, Harel-Bellan A, Trouche D. The three members of the pocket proteins family share the ability to repress E2F activity through recruitment of a histone deacetylase. Proc Natl Acad Sci U S A 1998;95: 10,493–10,498.
25. Magnaghi-Jaulin L, Groisman R, Naguibneva I, et al. Retinoblastoma protein represses transcription by recruiting a histone deacetylase. Nature 1998;391: 601–605.
26. Cai R, Kwon P, Yan-Neale Y, Sambuccetti L, Fischer D, Cohen D. Mammalian histone deacetylase 1 protein is posttranslationally modified by phosphorylation. Biochem Biophys Res Commun 2001;283:445–453.
27. Pflum MK, Tong JK, Lane WS, Schreiber SL. Histone deacetylase 1 phosphorylation promotes enzymatic activity and complex formation. J Biol Chem 2001;276:47,733–47,741.
28. David G, Neptune MA, DePinho RA. SUMO-1 modification of histone deacetylase 1 (HDAC1) modulates its biological activities. J Biol Chem 2002;277: 23,658–23,663.
29. Johnson CA, Turner BM. Histone deacetylases: complex transducers of nuclear signals. Semin Cell Dev Biol 1999;10:179–188.
30. Juan LJ, Shia WJ, Chen MH, et al. Histone deacetylases specifically down-regulate p53-dependent gene activation. J Biol Chem 2000;275: 20,436–20,443.

31. Luo J, Su F, Chen D, Shiloh A, Gu W. Deacetylation of p53 modulates its effect on cell growth and apoptosis. Nature 2000;408:377–381.

32. Martinez-Balbas MA, Bauer UM, Nielsen SJ, Brehm A, Kouzarides T. Regulation of E2F1 activity by acetylation. EMBO J 2000;19:662–671.

33. Marzio G, Wagener C, Gutierrez MI, Cartwright P, Helin K, Giacca M. E2F family members are differentially regulated by reversible acetylation. J Biol Chem 2000;275:10,887–10,892.

34. Yao YL, Yang WM, Seto E. Regulation of transcription factor YY1 by acetylation and deacetylation. Mol Cell Biol 2001;21:5979–5991.

35. Naryzhny SN, Lee H. The post-translational modifications of proliferating cell nuclear antigen: acetylation, not phosphorylation, plays an important role in the regulation of its function. J Biol Chem 2004;279:20,194–20,199.

35a. Shi Y, Lan F, Matson C, et al. Histone demethylation mediated by the nuclear amine oxidase homolog LSD1. Cell 2004;119:941–953.

36. Ahringer J. NuRD and SIN3 histone deacetylase complexes in development. Trends Genet 2000;16:351–356.

37. Ng HH, Bird A. Histone deacetylases: silencers for hire. Trends Biochem Sci 2000;25:121–126.

38. Milutinovic S, Zhuang Q, Szyf M. Proliferating cell nuclear antigen associates with histone deacetylase activity, integrating DNA replication and chromatin modification. J Biol Chem 2002;277:20,974–20,978.

39. Luo RX, Postigo AA, Dean DC. Rb interacts with histone deacetylases to repress transcription. Cell 1998;92:463–473.

40. Stiegler P, De Luca A, Bagella L, Giordano A. The COOH-terminal region of pRb2/p130 binds to histone deacetylase 1 (HDAC1), enhancing transcriptional repression of the E2F-dependent cyclin A promoter. Cancer Res 1998;58:5049–5052.

41. Wade PA. Transcriptional control at regulatory checkpoints by histone deacetylases: molecular connections between cancer and chromatin. Hum Mol Genet 2001;10:693–698.

42. Takaki T, Fukasawa K, Suzuki-Takahashi I, Hirai H. Cdk-mediated phosphorylation of pRB regulates HDAC binding in vitro. Biochem Biophys Res Commun 2004;316:252–255.

43. Pennaneach V, Barbier V, Regazzoni K, Fotedar R, Fotedar A. Rb inhibits E2F-1-induced cell death in a LXCXE-dependent manner by active repression. J Biol Chem 2004;279:23,376–23,383.

44. Hassig CA, Fleischer TC, Billin AN, Schreiber SL, Ayer DE. Histone deacetylase activity is required for full transcriptional repression by mSin3A. Cell 1997;89:341–347.

45. Laherty CD, Yang WM, Sun JM, Davie JR, Seto E, Eisenman RN. Histone deacetylases associated with the mSin3 corepressor mediate mad transcriptional repression. Cell 1997;89:349–356.

46. Sommer A, Hilfenhaus S, Menkel A, et al. Cell growth inhibition by the Mad/Max complex through recruitment of histone deacetylase activity. Curr Biol 1997;7:357–365.

47. Li J, Lin Q, Wang W, Wade P, Wong J. Specific targeting and constitutive association of histone deacetylase complexes during transcriptional repression. Genes Dev 2002;16:687–692.

48. Lagger G, Doetzlhofer A, Schuettengruber B, et al. The tumor suppressor p53 and histone deacetylase 1 are antagonistic regulators of the cyclin-dependent kinase inhibitor p21/WAF1/CIP1 gene. Mol Cell Biol 2003;23:2669–2679.

49. Levine AJ. p53, the cellular gatekeeper for growth and division. Cell 1997;88:323–331.
50. Koutsodontis G, Tentes I, Papakosta P, Moustakas A, Kardassis D. Sp1 plays a critical role in the transcriptional activation of the human cyclin-dependent kinase inhibitor p21(WAF1/Cip1) gene by the p53 tumor suppressor protein. J Biol Chem 2001;276:29,116–29,125.
51. Gui CY, Ngo L, Xu WS, Richon VM, Marks PA. Histone deacetylase (HDAC) inhibitor activation of p21WAF1 involves changes in promoter-associated proteins, including HDAC1. Proc Natl Acad Sci U S A 2004;101:1241–1246.
52. Brooks CL, Gu W. Ubiquitination, phosphorylation and acetylation: the molecular basis for p53 regulation. Curr Opin Cell Biol 2003;15:164–171.
53. Ito A, Kawaguchi Y, Lai CH, et al. MDM2-HDAC1-mediated deacetylation of p53 is required for its degradation. EMBO J 2002;21:6236–6245.
54. Luo J, Li M, Tang Y, Laszkowska M, Roeder RG, Gu W. Acetylation of p53 augments its site-specific DNA binding both in vitro and in vivo. Proc Natl Acad Sci U S A 2004;101:2259–2264.
55. Privalsky ML. The role of corepressors in transcriptional regulation by nuclear hormone receptors. Annu Rev Physiol 2004;66:315–360.
56. Mazumdar A, Wang RA, Mishra SK, et al. Transcriptional repression of oestrogen receptor by metastasis-associated protein 1 corepressor. Nat Cell Biol 2001;3:30–37.
57. Wei LN, Hu X, Chandra D, Seto E, Farooqui M. Receptor-interacting protein 140 directly recruits histone deacetylases for gene silencing. J Biol Chem 2000;275:40,782–40,787.
58. Kurtev V, Margueron R, Kroboth K, Ogris E, Cavailles V, Seiser C. Transcriptional regulation by the repressor of estrogen receptor activity via recruitment of histone deacetylases. J Biol Chem 2004;279:24,834–24,843.
59. Kawai H, Li H, Avraham S, Jiang S, Avraham HK. Overexpression of histone deacetylase HDAC1 modulates breast cancer progression by negative regulation of estrogen receptor alpha. Int J Cancer 2003;107:353–358.
60. Mal A, Sturniolo M, Schiltz RL, Ghosh MK, Harter ML. A role for histone deacetylase HDAC1 in modulating the transcriptional activity of MyoD: inhibition of the myogenic program. EMBO J 2001;20:1739–1753.
61. Puri PL, Iezzi S, Stiegler P, et al. Class I histone deacetylases sequentially interact with MyoD and pRb during skeletal myogenesis. Mol Cell 2001;8: 885–897.
62. Mal A, Harter ML. MyoD is functionally linked to the silencing of a muscle-specific regulatory gene prior to skeletal myogenesis. Proc Natl Acad Sci U S A 2003;100:1735–1739.
63. Tou L, Liu Q, Shivdasani RA. Regulation of mammalian epithelial differentiation and intestine development by class I histone deacetylases. Mol Cell Biol 2004;24:3132–3139.
64. Maga G, Hubscher U. Proliferating cell nuclear antigen (PCNA): a dancer with many partners. J Cell Sci 2003;116:3051–3060.
65. Tsai SC, Valkov N, Yang WM, Gump J, Sullivan D, Seto E. Histone deacetylase interacts directly with DNA topoisomerase II. Nat Genet 2000;26:349–353.
66. Johnson CA, Padget K, Austin CA, Turner BM. Deacetylase activity associates with topoisomerase II and is necessary for etoposide-induced apoptosis. J Biol Chem 2001;276:4539–4542.
67. Austin CA, Marsh KL. Eukaryotic DNA topoisomerase II beta. Bioessays 1998;20:215–226.

68. Cai RL, Yan-Neale Y, Cueto MA, Xu H, Cohen D. HDAC1, a histone deacety-lase, forms a complex with Hus1 and Rad9, two G2/M checkpoint Rad proteins. J Biol Chem 2000;275:27,909–27,916.

69. Craig JM, Earle E, Canham P, Wong LH, Anderson M, Choo KH. Analysis of mammalian proteins involved in chromatin modification reveals new metaphase centromeric proteins and distinct chromosomal distribution patterns. Hum Mol Genet 2003;12:3109–3121.

70. Dutertre S, Descamps S, Prigent C. On the role of aurora-A in centrosome function. Oncogene 2002;21:6175–6183.

71. Sakai H, Urano T, Ookata K, et al. MBD3 and HDAC1, two components of the NuRD complex, are localized at Aurora-A-positive centrosomes in M phase. J Biol Chem 2002;277:48,714–48,723.

72. David G, Turner GM, Yao Y, Protopopov A, DePinho RA. mSin3-associated protein, mSds3, is essential for pericentric heterochromatin formation and chromosome segregation in mammalian cells. Genes Dev 2003;17:2396–2405.

73. Simone C, Stiegler P, Forcales SV, et al. Deacetylase recruitment by the C/H3 domain of the acetyltransferase p300. Oncogene 2004;23:2177–2187.

74. Vaute O, Nicolas E, Vandel L, Trouche D. Functional and physical interaction between the histone methyl transferase Suv39H1 and histone deacetylases. Nucleic Acids Res 2002;30:475–481.

75. Otte AP, Kwaks TH. Gene repression by Polycomb group protein complexes: a distinct complex for every occasion? Curr Opin Genet Dev 2003;13:448–454.

76. Cao R, Zhang Y. The functions of E(Z)/EZH2-mediated methylation of lysine 27 in histone H3. Curr Opin Genet Dev 2004;14:155–164.

76a. Shi YJ, Matson C, Lan F, Iwase S, Baba T, Shi Y. Regulation of LSD1 histone demethylase activity by its associated factors. Mol Cell 2005;19:857–864.

76b. Lee MG, Wynder C, Cooch N, Shiekhattar R. An essential role for CoREST in nucleosomal histone 3 lysine 4 demethylation. Nature 2005;437:432–435.

77. Dobosy JR, Selker EU. Emerging connections between DNA methylation and histone acetylation. Cell Mol Life Sci 2001;58:721–727.

78. Fuks F, Burgers WA, Brehm A, Hughes-Davies L, Kouzarides T. DNA methyltransferase Dnmt1 associates with histone deacetylase activity. Nat Genet 2000;24:88–91.

79. Robertson KD, Ait-Si-Ali S, Yokochi T, Wade PA, Jones PL, Wolffe AP. DNMT1 forms a complex with Rb, E2F1 and HDAC1 and represses transcription from E2F-responsive promoters. Nat Genet 2000;25:338–342.

80. Fuks F, Burgers WA, Godin N, Kasai M, Kouzarides T. Dnmt3a binds deacety-lases and is recruited by a sequence-specific repressor to silence transcription. EMBO J 2001;20:2536–2544.

81. Geiman TM, Sankpal UT, Robertson AK, Zhao Y, Zhao Y, Robertson KD. DNMT3B interacts with hSNF2H chromatin remodeling enzyme, HDACs 1 and 2, and components of the histone methylation system. Biochem Biophys Res Commun 2004;318:544–555.

82. Deplus R, Brenner C, Burgers WA, et al. Dnmt3L is a transcriptional repressor that recruits histone deacetylase. Nucleic Acids Res 2002;30:3831–3838.

83. Gwack Y, Byun H, Hwang S, Lim C, Choe J. CREB-binding protein and histone deacetylase regulate the transcriptional activity of Kaposi's sarcoma-associated herpesvirus open reading frame 50. J Virol 2001;75:1909–1917.

84. Lu F, Zhou J, Wiedmer A, Madden K, Yuan Y, Lieberman PM. Chromatin remodeling of the Kaposi's sarcoma-associated herpesvirus ORF50 promoter correlates with reactivation from latency. J Virol 2003;77:11,425–11,435.

85. Chiocca S, Kurtev V, Colombo R, et al. Histone deacetylase 1 inactivation by an adenovirus early gene product. Curr Biol 2002;12:594–598.

86. Zhang Y, Jones C. The bovine herpesvirus 1 immediate-early protein (bICP0) associates with histone deacetylase 1 to activate transcription. J Virol 2001;75: 9571–9578.

87. Shestakova E, Bandu MT, Doly J, Bonnefoy E. Inhibition of histone deacetylation induces constitutive derepression of the beta interferon promoter and confers antiviral activity. J Virol 2001;75:3444–3452.

87a. Lehrman G, Hogue IB, Palmer S, et al. Depletion of latent HIV-1 infection in vivo: a proof-of-concept study. Lancet 2005;366:549–555.

88. Mannervik M, Levine M. The Rpd3 histone deacetylase is required for segmentation of the *Drosophila* embryo. Proc Natl Acad Sci U S A 1999;96:6797–6801.

89. Shi Y, Mello C. A CBP/p300 homolog specifies multiple differentiation pathways in *Caenorhabditis elegans*. Genes Dev 1998;12:943–955.

90. Dufourcq P, Victor M, Gay F, Calvo D, Hodgkin J, Shi Y. Functional requirement for histone deacetylase 1 in *Caenorhabditis elegans* gonadogenesis. Mol Cell Biol 2002;22:3024–3034.

91. Golling G, Amsterdam A, Sun Z, et al. Insertional mutagenesis in zebrafish rapidly identifies genes essential for early vertebrate development. Nat Genet 2002; 31:135–140.

92. Marks P, Rifkind RA, Richon VM, Breslow R, Miller T, Kelly WK. Histone deacetylases and cancer: causes and therapies. Nat Rev Cancer 2001;1: 194–202.

93. Kelly WK, O'Connor OA, Marks PA. Histone deacetylase inhibitors: from target to clinical trials. Expert Opin Investig Drugs 2002;11:1696–1713.

94. Marks PA, Miller T, Richon VM. Histone deacetylases. Curr Opin Pharmacol 2003;3:344–351.

95. Choi JH, Kwon HJ, Yoon BI, et al. Expression profile of histone deacetylase 1 in gastric cancer tissues. Jpn J Cancer Res 2001;92:1300–1304.

96. Patra SK, Patra A, Dahiya R. Histone deacetylase and DNA methyltransferase in human prostate cancer. Biochem Biophys Res Commun 2001;287: 705–713.

97. Halkidou K, Gaughan L, Cook S, Leung HY, Neal DE, Robson CN. Upregulation and nuclear recruitment of HDAC1 in hormone refractory prostate cancer. Prostate 2004;59:177–189.

98. Kim JH, Choi YK, Kwon HJ, Yang HK, Choi JH, Kim DY. Downregulation of gelsolin and retinoic acid receptor beta expression in gastric cancer tissues through histone deacetylase 1. J Gastroenterol Hepatol 2004;19:218–224.

99. Glaser KB, Li J, Staver MJ, Wei RQ, Albert DH, Davidsen SK. Role of class I and class II histone deacetylases in carcinoma cells using siRNA. Biochem Biophys Res Commun 2003;310:529–536.

100. Zhou Q, Melkoumian ZK, Lucktong A, Moniwa M, Davie JR, Strobl JS. Rapid induction of histone hyperacetylation and cellular differentiation in human breast tumor cell lines following degradation of histone deacetylase-1. J Biol Chem 2000;275:35,256–35,263.

101. Fanciulli M, Bruno T, Di Padova M, et al. Identification of a novel partner of RNA polymerase II subunit 11, Che-1, which interacts with and affects the growth suppression function of Rb. FASEB J 2000;14:904–912.

102. Bruno T, De Angelis R, De Nicola F, et al. Che-1 affects cell growth by interfering with the recruitment of HDAC1 by Rb. Cancer Cell 2002;2:387–399.

103. Di Padova M, Bruno T, De Nicola F, et al. Che-1 arrests human colon carcinoma cell proliferation by displacing HDAC1 from the p21WAF1/CIP1 promoter. J Biol Chem 2003;278:36,496–36,504.
104. Kim MS, Kwon HJ, Lee YM, et al. Histone deacetylases induce angiogenesis by negative regulation of tumor suppressor genes. Nat Med 2001;7:437–443.
105. Nusinzon I, Horvath CM. Interferon-stimulated transcription and innate antiviral immunity require deacetylase activity and histone deacetylase 1. Proc Natl Acad Sci U S A 2003;100:14,742–14,747.
106. Klampfer L, Huang J, Swaby LA, Augenlicht L. Requirement of histone deacty-lase activity for signaling by STAT1. J Biol Chem 2004;279:30,358–30,368.
107. Hu E, Dul E, Sung CM, et al. Identification of novel isoform-selective inhibitors within class I histone deacetylases. J Pharmacol Exp Ther 2003;307:720–728.

2 Biochemistry of Multiprotein HDAC Complexes

Alejandro Vaquero, PhD,
Michael Scher, PhD,
and Danny Reinberg, PhD

CONTENTS

SUMMARY

Histone deacetylases perform an important role in the regulation of transcription by modifying the histone components of chromatin. This imparts specific restrictions to transcription and contributes to the proper coordination of gene expression. In order to perform these functions and to achieve proper modulation of their activity, HDACs associate with other proteins, and in some cases, even with themselves. The purification and analyses of these complexes during the last few years has changed our view of the functions of these enzymes, as well as how they are regulated and interconnect with other chromatin-related activities. We are starting to understand how a limited number of HDACs can perform such a variety of functions. Here we review all the known HDAC-containing complexes including classes I, II, and III and we

From: *Cancer Drug Discovery and Development*
Histone Deacetylases: *Transcriptional Regulation and Other Cellular Functions*
Edited by: E. Verdin © Humana Press Inc., Totowa, NJ

Acronyms and Abbreviations

Abf-1	Activated B-cell factor-1
ACF1	ATP-utilizing chromatin assembly and remodeling factor 1
ADA3	Transcriptional adapter 3
ALL-1, (same as MLL, HRX, HTRX)	Acute lymphoblastic leukemia 1
AP-1	Activator protein 1
APPL-1,-2	Adaptor protein containing PH domain, PTB domain, and leucine zipper motif 1,2
ASAP	Apoptosis- and splicing-associated protein
BAF57,-60a,-170	BRG1-associated factor 57, 60a, 170
BCH110	BRAF-HDAC component 110
Bcl6	B-cell lymphoma 6
BRG1	Brm/SWI2-related gene 1
BTB/POZ	BR-C, ttk, and bab/poxvirus and zinc finger
CaMK	Ca^{2+}/calmodulin-dependent kinase cells
CoREST	Corepressor of REST
Cpr1p	Cyclophilin A peptidyl-prolyl isomerase
C-Ski	Sloan-Kettering virus isolates
CtBP	Carboxyl-terminal binding protein
CTCF	CCCTC-binding factor
CTIP2	Chicken ovalbumin upstream promoter transcription factor-interacting protein 2
DNMT1	DNA (cytosine-5)-methyltransferases
Ebi	Epidermal growth factor receptor regulator
Eto	Eight twenty-one transcription factor
EuHMT	Euchromatic histone-lysine N-methyltransferase
FAD^+	Flavin adenine dinucleotide
FLO10	Flocculation factor 10
FOXO	Forkhead box
G9a	Euchromatic histone-lysine N-methyltransferase
GSP2	G protein pathway suppressor
HES	Homeobox gene in ES
HML	Silent mating type loci L
HMR	Silent mating type loci R

(Continued on p. 26)

summarize the implications of their composition to the function for HDACs in vivo.

Key Words: *BCH110,* chromatin, CoRest, HDAC1-11, deacetylation, histone tails, *MBD2, MeCP1, Mi2, MTA1, MTA2, MTA3,* NCoR/SMRT, NURD, RENT complex, repression, *Sin3, Sirt1-7,* TEL complex.

INTRODUCTION

The year 1996 was a momentous one for members of the chromatin community. Two reports provided the long-awaited connection between chromatin and the regulation of gene expression. In one report, Allis and coworkers *(1)* described a histone acetyltransferase and discovered that it was *GCN5,* whose gene had been previously identified in yeast using a genetic screen that scored for transcriptional regulators. In a second report, Schreiber and coworkers *(2),* revealed that a histone deacetylase (HDAC) resides in a mammalian homolog of yeast *RPD3,* a gene isolated in genetic screens scoring for transcriptional repressors. These two seminal findings, together with subsequent observations demonstrating that the enzymatic activities of *Gcn5* and *Rpd3* are regulated through their association with other proteins opened the door for chromatin research in the context of transcriptional regulation. We now know that many transcription regulators contain activities that covalently modify the histone tails. In this chapter we describe the different HDACs and their regulation.

HDACs perform an important role in the proper regulation of cellular functions through their connection with chromatin and transcriptional regulation. To perform these functions and to achieve proper modulation of their activity, HDACs associate with other proteins and in some cases even with themselves. The purification and analyses of these complexes during the last nine years has changed our view of the functions of these enzymes, as well as how they are regulated and interconnect with other chromatin-related activities. These endeavors have begun to reveal how a limited number of HDACs can perform such a variety of functions *(3,4).*

CLASS I HDACs

Class I HDAC members, which are defined by their homology to the yeast HDAC *Rpd3,* are *HDAC1, -2, -3, -8,* and *-11 (5).* Complexes have been described for HDAC-1, -2, and -3, whereas little is known about the proteins interacting with *HDAC8* and *-11.* Class I deacetylases access specific regions of DNA, yet they lack DNA binding activity. Access to DNA is facilitated through the large number of transcription and chromatin-related factors that interact with and recruit class I HDACs to specific chromosomal regions. These include the sequence-specific DNA binding

Acronyms and Abbreviations *(Continued)*

Hos2p	High osmolarity sensitivity two
HOXA9	Homeobox protein A9
Hst1	Homolog of Sir2p, 1
HTLV-1	Type I human T-cell leukemia virus
Ini1	Integrase interactor protein 1
IR10	WD-repeat protein
ISWI	Imitation-switch
KAP-1	KRAB-interacting protein 1
KRAB	Krüppel associated box
Ku70	Lupus Ku autoantigen protein p70
Mad/Max	MAX dimerization protein 1/MYC associated factor X
MAPK	Mitogen activated protein kinases
MARK	Microtubule affinity regulating kinase
MBD	Methyl-CpG binding domain
MeCP2	Methyl-CpG binding protein 2 gene
MEF2	Myocyte enhancer factor 2
Mi2	Dermatomyositis-specific autoantigen
MITR	MEF2-interacting transcription repressor
MLL-1	Myeloid/lymphoid leukemia 1
Mnt	MYC antagonist
MTA2	Metastasis-associated protein 2
Mxi1	Max interactor 1
Myb	Avian myeloblatosis virus oncogene
Nan1p	Net1-associated nuclear protein
NCoR	Nuclear receptor corepressor
Net1p	Nucleolar silencing establishing factor and telophase regulator 1
NF-κB	Nuclear factor κ-B
NLS	Nuclear localization signal
Nop1	Nuclear protein one
NoRC	Nucleolar chromatin remodeling complex
NuRD	Nucleosome remodeling and histone deacetylase
ORC1	Origin replication complex 1
PCAF	p300/CBP associated factor

(Continued on p. 28)

factors *YY1 (6)*, *Mad-Max (7)*, *Runx2 (8)*, *RBP-1 (9)*, and *Sp1 (10)*, the insulator factor *CTCF (11)*, the corepressors *Sin3 (12,13)*, *SMRT*, and *NCoR (14,15)*, the DNA methyltransferase *DNMT1 (16)*, and the H3 histone methyltransferase *Suv39H1 (17)*, among others. The retinoblastoma protein *Rb*, a regulator of cell growth, also binds *HDAC1 (18)*. Additionally, promyelocytic leukemia is caused by an oncoprotein, produced by fusion of the *PML* and *RAR*-α genes, which recruits class I HDACs to repress transcription of specific genes *(19)*. Class I members exhibit very weak activity in isolation and their multiple functions require interactions with specific factors that modulate the response to different stimuli. Thus, class I HDACs are found in vivo as part of protein complexes that provide the appropriate structural, functional, and regulatory environment to elicit their activity.

HDAC1 and HDAC2 Complexes

The Sin3 HDAC Complex: From Yeast to Humans

Sin3 was discovered to be a global repressor of transcription in yeast *(20)*. *Sin3* functions as a suppressor of the transcriptional activator *Swi5*, which is required for expression of the HO gene. Null mutations in Sin3 consistently relieve the requirement for *Swi5* in *HO* expression *(21,22)*, implicating *Sin3* as a repressor of transcription. *Sin3* is a 175-kDa protein that contains four putative, paired amphipatic helix (PAH) domains *(23)* but is devoid of known DNA binding domains. *Sin3* is directed to target sites through association with other proteins. The Sin3-PAH domains have been found to be involved in protein–protein interactions and to mediate interactions with the DNA binding and transcriptional repressors *Mad*, *Mxi1*, and *Mnt*, which are discussed later *(12,13,24,25)*.

Yeast *Rpd3* and *Sin3*

The histone deacetylase that defines class I HDACs is the budding yeast enzyme *Rpd3*. It was shown to be the enzymatic component of a multiprotein complex *(2,26)*. *Rpd3* was originally isolated as a repressor of the same set of genes repressed by *Sin3 (27)*. This suggested a genetic link between *Sin3* and *Rpd3*, and, as expected, they were shown to exist together in a large multiprotein complex *(28)*. As with *Sin3*, *Rpd3* did not exhibit DNA binding activity, indicating the need for its interaction with DNA binding proteins to facilitate its access to chromatin for transcriptional repression.

HDAC1 and HDAC2

Whether it be a single cell of budding yeast or multicellular organisms, the regulation of gene expression requires the same basic components, such as HDACs.

Acronyms and Abbreviations *(Continued)*

PHD	Plant homeodomain
PML	Promyelocytic leukemia
PPAR-γ	Peroxisome proliferator activated receptor, gamma
Pyr	Pyrimidin-rich binding, SW1/SNF related complex
Rab5	
RAD21	Radiation-sensitive mutant 21
Rap1	Repressor/activator protein 1
RAR-α	Retinoic acid receptor α
RAS	Harvey sarcoma virus transforming gene
RbAp	Retinoblastoma-associated protein
RBP-1	Retinoblastoma binding protein 1
RENT	Regulator of nucleolar silencing and telophase
REST/NRSF	RE1-silencing transcription factor/Neuronal restricted silencing factor
RORγ	Retinoid-related orphan receptor γ
Rpd3	Reduced potassium dependency three
RunX2	Runt-related transcription factor 2
SA1/SA2	Stromal antigen 1/2
SANT	SWI3, ADA2, NCoR, and TFIIIB B
Sap	Sin3 associated protein
SBE	Smad-binding element
SET	SU(VAR)3-9, enhancer of Zeste, Trithorax
SFL1p	Suppressor gene for flocculation 1
SID	Sin3 interacting domain
Sif2p	SIR4 interacting factor 2
Sin3	Switch-independent three
Sir2p	Silent information regulator 2
siRNA	Small interfering RNA
SirT1	Sir2-like (Sirtuin)1
SMC	Structural maintenance of chromosomes factors
SMRT	Silencing mediator for retionoid and thyroid hormone receptors
SNF2h	Sucrose nonfermenting 2 homolog
Sntp	Two SANT domains

(Continued on p. 30)

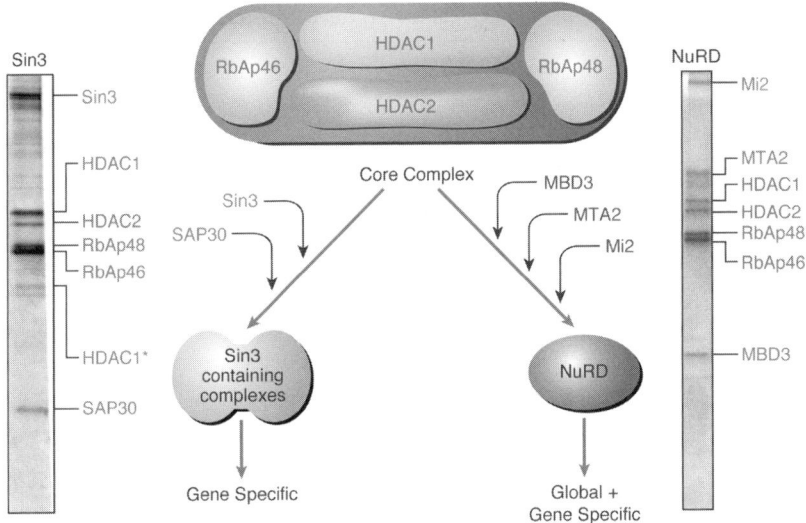

Fig. 1. Polypeptides composing the Sin3 and NuRD corepressor complexes. The scheme in the middle of the figure illustrates the core complex of the Sin3 and NuRD repressor complexes, composed of histone deacetylases 1 and 2 *(HDAC1/HDAC2)* and the histone binding proteins *RbAp 46* and *48*. This core complex can interact with *SAP30* and *Sin3* or with *MBD3*, *MTA2*, and *Mi2*, forming the Sin3 and NuRD corepressor complexes, respectively. The Sin3 complex interacts directly or indirectly with sequence-specific DNA binding proteins repressing expression of specific genes. The NuRD complex represses transcription more globally but also interacts with gene-specific transcription factors *(see* Fig. 2). For abbreviations, *see* Acronyms and Abbreviations table. *See* Color Plate 1 following p. 180.

Affinity pull-down experiments using the HDAC inhibitor trapoxin resulted in the isolation of human *HDAC1* and *RbAp48* and the novel finding that *HDAC1* contains the enzymatic activity *(2)*. A multiprotein complex was demonstrated to exist in human cells upon the isolation of a human Sin3-HDAC complex *(25,29,30)*. The complex contained the class *I HDAC1* and *HDAC2*, *hSin3*, and the histone chaperones retinoblastoma-associated proteins *(RbAp) 48* and *46*, as well as two novel proteins termed *Sap18* and *Sap30* (Sin3-associated proteins of 18 and 30 kDa, respectively; Fig. 1; *see* Color Plate 1 following p. 180). These components function together to impart specificity to the complex with respect to its localization to certain regions of the genome as well as to regulate its transient activity. Although initial studies described *Sap18* as part of the Sin3 complex *(25)*, the majority of *Sap18* isolated from HeLa cells was actually found in a complex that did not contain *Sin3* or *HDAC1/2*; it appears to function during apoptosis and in the regulation of splicing (ASAP) *(31)*.

Acronyms and Abbreviations *(Continued)*

Sp1	Specificity protein-1
Srg3	SWI3-related gene product 3
Sum1p	Suppressor of uncontrolled mitosis
Suv39H1	Suppressior of position-effect variegation 3-9 homolog 1
Swi/Snf	Switch/sucrose nonfermenting
SWI3	Matting-type switching defective mutant 3
TAFI68	TBP-associated factors Pol I 68
Tax	HTLV-1 trans-acting transcriptional activator
TBL1	Transducin β-like protein 1
TBLR1	Transducin β-like related protein 1
TEL complex	Telomere complex
TFIIIB	RNA polymerase III transcription factor B
TGF-β	Transforming growth factor β
TSA	Trichostatin A
Tup1	Deoxythymidine monophosphate uptake factor 1
UbcH5	E2 ubiquitin conjugating enzyme H5
Ume6p	UAS_{PHR1} multi copy enhancer six
WCRF180 (same as ACF1)	Williams syndrome transcription factor-related chromatin remodeling factor 180
XFIM	X-linked mental retardation, zinc finger protein 261
YIL112w	Ankyrin repeats-containing protein
YY1	Yin-yang 1

Sap30 was also shown to be present and genetically linked to a Sin3 complex in budding yeast, suggesting that the Sin3 complex performs conserved functions in all eukaryotes in terms of gene repression *(32)*. Analyses of *Sap30* resulted in the isolation of two Sin3-containing complexes from human cells, the Sin3 complex described above and a complex containing the p53 binding candidate tumor suppressor *p33^INGI^ (33)*. The interaction of *p33^INGI^* with *Sin3* is mediated through *Sap30*. Interestingly, our studies *(33)* as well as those of others *(34)* revealed that the Sin3-HDAC complex can also interact with the Swi/Snf chromatin remodeling complex. Again, *Sap30* was found to link the Sin3-HDAC complex to Swi/Snf *(33)*. *Sap18* was not isolated in these complexes, providing further evidence that it is probably not a member of the Sin3 complex.

It is clear that the class I HDACs present in the complex provide the enzymatic activity, whereas Sin3 appears to function as a switchboard that coordinates the interaction between HDACs and sequence-specific DNA binding proteins (*see* Fig. 1 and the NurD section). The RbAp proteins appear to have a role in stabilizing the interaction of this complex with the core histones present in nucleosomes. The Sin3-HDAC complex may also impart substrate specificity once it is recruited to chromatin. Its role in vivo was confirmed with chromatin immunoprecipitation (ChIP) experiments performed in a yeast strain in which *Rpd3* was deleted. This strain exhibited increased acetylation of all histone residues, except for H4 lysine-16 *(35)*. In vitro, the human Sin3-HDAC complex was able to deacetylate all of the core histones when in isolation, but not when composing nucleosomes, suggesting that chromatin remodeling precedes deacetylation in vivo *(32)*.

Sin3 protein from human or yeast is large and capable of multiple interactions. In yeast, the DNA binding and transcriptional repressor of meiotic genes *Ume6p* interacts with the Sin3-HDAC complex and specifically interacts with *Sin3* in a yeast two-hybrid screen *(36)*. Repression by *Ume6p* depends on the enzymatic activity of *Rpd3*.

In higher organisms, a number of transcriptional regulators were shown to bind the Sin3 complex and direct it to specific genes. These are the zinc finger DNA binding proteins *Ikaros* and *Aiolos* *(37)*, the helix-loop-helix heterodimers of the Mad family *Mad/Max* and *Mxi1/Max*, and the Sin3-interacting domain (SID) containing the protein Mnt, which interacts with *Max* *(38)*. *C-Ski* was also found to interact with *Sin3*. *C-Ski* is part of a complex containing *Smad3/4* that binds to the Smad DNA binding element (SBE) and is involved in transforming growth factor (TGF)-β signaling *(39)*. NoRC, an *SNF2h*-containing nucleolar chromatin remodeling complex that represses ribosomal gene transcription, has also been shown to recruit *Sin3* *(40)*. *MeCP2*, a methyl binding domain (MBD)-containing protein that binds to and represses promoters containing methylated CpG, also appears to recruit the Sin3 complex specifically *(41)*. The corepressors NCoR/SMRT bind to unliganded nuclear hormone receptors and recruit the Sin3 complexes to repress transcription at the receptor-targeted genes *(14,15,20)*. The interaction with *NCoR* is mediated through both *Sin3* and *Sap30*, as *Sap30* appears to stabilize the interaction with NCoR/SMRT *(42)*.

Interaction between the class I HDACs and the corepressor COOH-terminal binding protein *(CtBP)* has been reported. *CtBP* was originally discovered based on its interaction with the C terminus of the adenovirus *E1A* protein and was later found to bind the *Drosophila* DNA binding proteins *Hairy, Snail, Krüppel*, and mammalian *Krüppel-like factor 3 (BKLF/KLF3)*. Interestingly, CtBP-mediated repression of transcription has been reported to be sensitive to the HDAC inhibitor TSA at some promoters and insensitive at others *(43)*. *CtBP* was found to retain transcriptional repression in *Drosophila* embryos deficient in *Rpd3*, suggesting that *CtBP* can repress transcription through alternate means *(43)*.

Class I HDACs are thus highly regulated by virtue of their association with Sin3. This is evident by Sin3-mediated interaction with disparate sequence-specific DNA binding proteins and also through *Sin3* interaction with other corepressors such as *CtBP* and NCor/SMRT that interact with other sequence-specific DNA binding proteins. HDACs are thus directed to target genes and participate in their regulation during differentiation and development and in response to specific environmental stimuli.

NuRD

In higher eukaryotes, there is another group of complexes comparable in abundance and diversity of function to Sin3-containing complexes. The term nucleosome remodeling and deacetylase complex (NuRD; also NURD or NRD) encompasses a group of complexes from *Caenorhabditis elegans* to mammals that are involved in gene silencing, cell cycle progression, and development *(44–48)*. NuRD contains the core components of the Sin3 complex (Fig. 1), but associates with a different set of polypeptides *(Mi2, MTA2, and MBD3)*, which target the complex to different sites in the genome. Additionally, NuRD can associate with different polypeptides, resulting in the formation of "supra"-NuRD complexes exhibiting diverse NuRD-dependent functions. NuRD imparts a new strategy to the functioning of HDAC complexes as it contains two different types of chromatin-modifying activities: histone deacetylation (regulation through covalent modification of histones) and ATP-dependent chromatin remodeling activities (nucleosome mobilization/alteration). Thus, in the NuRD context, optimal deacetylation involves the ATP-remodeling machinery such that the histone tails are presented in the proper configuration *(49)*. The presence of an activity that mobilizes/alters nucleosome structure in NuRD is compatible with its having a more general function in the maintenance of global chromatin structure.

As in the case of the Sin3-HDAC complexes, NuRD complexes must be brought to the chromatin vicinity to perform their function. This is accomplished in different ways (Fig. 2; *see* Color Plate 2 following p. 180). First, specific DNA binding transcription factors can recruit NuRD to specific genes, as in the case of the HOX genes *(50,51)*. Second, certain factors with broader DNA binding capacity, such as the CpG-methyl binding protein *MBD2*, recruit NuRD to certain genomic regions containing methylated-DNA (Fig. 2), such that the target may outreach a single gene *(52)*. Third, some studies have shown that NuRD complexes can perform housekeeping roles in the general regulation of chromatin, through a constitutive association that is independent of recruiters *(53)*. This may contribute to the more general dynamics of chromatin structure through the processes

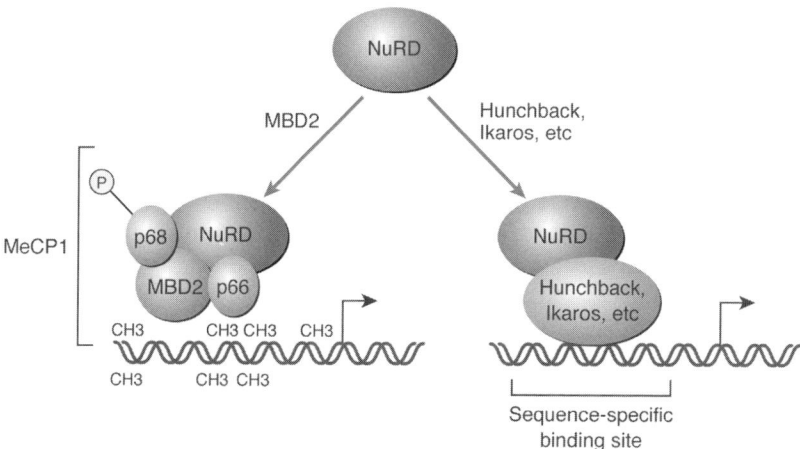

Fig. 2. The NuRD complex. This complex can interact with sequence-specific DNA binding proteins and thus be directed to specific genes, as illustrated on the right side. NuRD can also interact with *MBD2* and a polypeptide that exist in phosphorylated (p68) and unphosphorylated (p66) forms. This arrangement of polypeptides composes the MeCP1 complex. The *MBD2* subunit tethers the complex to CpG-methylated DNA. For abbreviations, *see* Acronyms and Abbreviations table. *See* Color Plate 2 following p. 180.

of acetylation and deacetylation. This function is probably related to the capacity of NuRD to bind to the histone H3 tails *(54,55)*.

That NuRD can be recruited to sites independent of sequence-specific DNA binding proteins may be related to its association with an activity that alters/mobilizes nucleosomes. This is in contrast to the Sin3 complex that is recruited to specific promoters through interactions with sequence-specific DNA binding proteins, although, in general, these proteins can also recruit factors that alter the structure of nucleosomes. Although the NuRD complex can target specific genes through interaction with sequence-specific DNA binding proteins, this appears to be much more restricted relative to the case of Sin3. NuRD appears to function in a more global manner, based on its recruitment to the histone H3 tail and CpG-methylated DNA.

Components of the NuRD Complexes

All NuRD complexes share a similar organization that includes a core complex identical to that of Sin3, containing *HDAC1* and *HDAC2* in mammals (or *Rpd3* in lower organisms) and *RbAp46/48*. In the case of NuRD, however, the complex also contains *MBD3* and *MTA1/2* and the ATP-dependent chromatin-remodeling protein Mi2 (Fig. 1). In fact, many

NuRD complexes with different properties and specificities have been isolated *(56)*.

This heterogeneity is one of the defining traits of NuRD complexes. It is evidenced not only by the presence or absence of certain factors but also by the variability among family members of the components that are integral. The most logical explanation of this phenomenon is an evolutionary one: the proteins that were unique in lower organisms diversified to perform new specific functions in a progressively more complex environment within the context of these complexes *(48)*.

With regard to the NuRD-specific proteins, *Mi2* (the dermatomyositis-specific autoantigen) exhibits the least variability. *Mi2* exists in two forms, *Mi2α* (or *CHD3*) and *Mi2β* (or *CHD4*) *(57)*. Although the predominant form in the NuRD complexes is *Mi2β*, reports indicate the presence of *Mi2α* in some of the complexes *(46,56)*. *Mi2* is important for NuRD enzymatic activity and for recruiting NuRD to multiple targets. Thus, *Mi2* can interact with multiple factors like the corepressor *KAP-1* through its KRAB domain *(58)*, the retinoid-related orphan receptor *(RORg)* *(59)*, the zinc finger transcription factor *Ikaros* in lymphocytes *(51)*, and the *Drosophila* transcriptional repressors *Tramtrack69 (60)* and *Hunchback (50)*.

Probably the most important paradigm of variability in proteins composing NuRD is the MTA family of metastasis-associated proteins (or MTAs). These have three members in vertebrates, *MTA1–3,* that have been implicated in cancer progression, metastasis, cell differentiation, and cell type-specific transcription *(56, 61)*. *MTA1* and *MTA3* are present in different isoforms, bringing the total number of proteins to six (*MTA1, MTA1s, MTA1-ZG29p, MTA2, MTA3*, and *MTA3L*) *(62)*. All three MTAs have been found in NuRD complexes and, based on their distinctive patterns of expression and performance, they may be responsible for one level of specificity in the functioning of the NuRD complexes. For instance, *MTA1* and *MTA3* expression is cell type specific, in contrast to the ubiquitous *MTA2* *(56,61,63)*. This suggests that *MTA2* may be involved in the housekeeping functions of NuRD, whereas the other two components may participate in specialized repression. *MTA2*, for example, interacts with the multifunctional transcription factor *YY1*, whereas *MTA1* does not *(61)*.

MTA1 is detected in multiple cancer cells and its presence is associated with the uncontrolled growth and invasive properties of multiple types of tumors *(56,61,64)*. Although its main function is not completely known, it is commonly believed that it may involve the recruitment of the NuRD complex to specific genes.

MTA3 seems to be highly expressed in breast cancer, and its expression and function seem to be dependent on the activation of the estrogen receptor. In particular, *MTA3* inhibits the expression of the transcription factor *Snail* by bringing NuRD to its promoter *(65)*. *Snail* is a key factor for the expression of the E-cadherin glycoproteins involved in cell adhesion; thus defects in *Snail* expression would impact on tumor suppression, development, and cell polarity *(56,65)*.

Similar to *Mi2*, in addition to their recruitment function, MTA proteins are also important for NuRD activity. Reconstitution studies showed that the core NuRD complex has a remarkably weak HDAC activity and that its optimal activity in vitro requires the presence of the MTA2 SANT domain *(52)*. SANT domains (from S̲WI3, A̲DA3, N̲CoR, and T̲FII-IB) *(66)* resemble the DNA binding domains of Myb-related DNA binding proteins and are also present in transcription factors and in proteins associated with HDAC class I complexes like CoREST and SMRT (*see* sections entitled CoREST Complex and HDAC3 Complexes below).

Finally, another important component of the NuRD complex is a member of the MBD family of methyl-DNA (mCpG) binding proteins found in higher eukaryotes and involved in transcription repression and DNA repair *(67)*. Of the four different MBD proteins *(MBD1–4)* found in mammals, only *MBD3* seems unable to bind to CpG methyl-DNA directly *(52)*. This is in spite of its extensive homology to the well-studied CpG methyl-DNA binding protein *MBD2* and the fact that the *MBD3* orthologs in lower organisms can bind to CpG-methylated DNA *(68)*. *MBD3* is the only member of the family that is present constitutively in the NuRD complexes.

Although MBD2 is not a component of the NuRD complexes, it can recruit NuRD to CpG-methylated DNA regions (Fig. 2). *MBD2* copurifies with NuRD in the large supercomplex termed MeCP1 *(52,69, see* that section just below). Notably, the link between DNA methylation and NuRD activity suggests a functional link between histone deacetylation and methylated DNA regions.

Interestingly, the composition of the NuRD complexes found in lower organisms provides a clue to the common origin of *MBD2* and *MBD3*. For instance, the *Drosophila* NuRD complex contains MBD2/3, an ortholog to *MBD2* and *MBD3* that possesses characteristics of both proteins *(4,48,56,70)*.

Supra-NuRD Complexes

In some cases, NuRD has been found as part of larger complexes, or supercomplexes, that incorporate a considerable number of factors and that, in general, seem to be involved in highly specific functions.

MECP1 COMPLEX. The MeCP1 complex is able to bind to CpG-methylated DNA containing more than 10 methyl-cytosines and participates in gene repression *(71)*. MeCP1 is formed by an MBD3-containing NuRD complex in conjunction with *MBD2* and the two associated proteins *p66* and *p68* (Fig. 2). The p68 protein is a posttranslationally modified version of *p66*, and both seem to be implicated in the recruitment of MeCP1 to specific loci

(72). MeCP1 can also interact with *APPL1* and *APPL2*, two effectors of the GTPase *Rab5* that are involved in signal transduction and endocytosis *(73)*. Although the functional relevance of these interactions is currently unknown, they may signify a new level of regulation by MeCP1 upon cellular exposure to external stimuli.

COHESIN COMPLEX. Recent studies suggest that NuRD might be involved in functions other than transcriptional silencing, as a cohesin complex was isolated in association with NuRD *(74)*. The isolated complex contains the ISWI-type of ATP-dependent remodeling factor *SNF2h*, the *MBD3*-containing NuRD complex, *MBD2*, and the core-cohesin complex. The core cohesin complex is formed by *SMC1, SMC3, SA1/SA2, RAD21* *(75,76)*, and WCRF180, also known as Acf1, which is the partner of *SNF2h* in the human and *Drosophila ACF/WCRF* complex *(77)*.

ChIP studies identified regions of Alu repeats within the X chromosome that are in association with the isolated NuRD-cohesin complex *(74)*. The role of NuRD in this context has yet to be characterized.

ALL-1 COMPLEX. The largest complex described thus far as containing NuRD is ALL-1. This complex is apparently composed of approx 30 polypeptides and is probably greater than 3 Mda in size *(78)*. The trithorax protein *ALL-1* (also known as *MLL, HRX,* or *HTRX*) contains a histone lysine methyltransferase activity with specificity for lysine-4 of the histone H3 tail *(79)*. ALL-1 is essential for the development of hematopoietic stem cells *(80)*. Leukemias involving translocation phenomena generate chimeric proteins containing ALL-1 fused to other partners *(80)*.

The putative ALL-1 complex also included subunits of the RNA polymerase II-associated TFIID complex, as well as subunits of the chromatin remodeling complexes *SNF2h, Swi/Snf, NuRD,* and *Sin3*. Apparently, all these components were found to coexist at the promoter of the *HoxA9* gene in vivo *(78)*. However, it is our belief that ALL-1 may not represent a unique complex. From the data reported thus far, we cannot exclude the possibility that this group of distinct, but functionally related, complexes associate transiently, rather than as a biochemically stable entity in the cell.

The ALL-1/MLL-1 proteins function in transcriptional activation as ALL-1 to methylate lysine-4 of histone H3, which is known to be involved in transcription activity *(78)*. The presence of HDACs is consistent with the need to deacetylate specific residues in histone H3 for their subsequent methylation. However, the exact role of NuRD is unclear given that NuRD is displaced from the histone H3 tail upon methylation of histone H3 lysine-4 *(55)*. Moreover, duplication in activities in this supracomplex is perplexing. For example, the Sin3 complex is also present, and, in addition to *Mi2*, the complex also has two additional ATP remodeling activities, Swi/Snf and *SNF2h*. The existence of this supracomplex in vivo would appear to require additional validation.

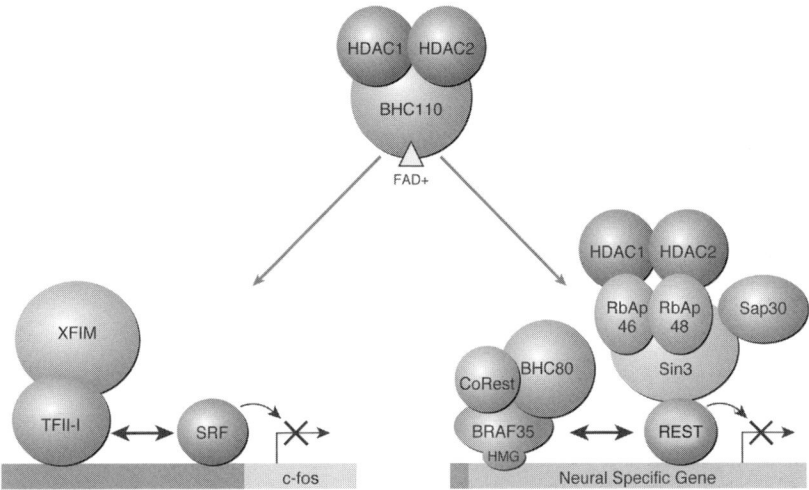

Fig. 3. BCH10-containing complexes. This lesser known group of *HDAC1/2*-containing proteins is formed by the complexes CoREST and XFIM. Both contain a core of *HDAC1/2* and *BCH110*, a FAD$^+$ binding protein with unknown function. CoREST participates together with the Sin3-containing complex in repression mediated by the factor *REST*, which is responsible for silencing of the neuronal-specific genes (right). The CoREST complex can bind to DNA through the HMG domain of *BRAF35*. The XFIM complex is involved in the control of basal c-fos gene repression (left) and is probably recruited to the c-Fos promoter by serum response factor *(SRF)* which interacts with the DNA-binding factor *TFII-I*. For abbreviations, *see* Acronyms and Abbreviations table. *See* Color Plate 3 following p. 180.

PYR. PYR is a SWI/SNF-related complex that binds to DNA containing pyrimidine-rich sequences located between the human fetal and adult β-globin-like genes *(81)*. Interestingly, this DNA binding activity is specific to adult hematopoietic cells. The complex contains the lymphocyte-specific transcription factor *Ikaros*, the NuRD core complex except for *HDAC1*, and at least five SWI/SNF complex-related proteins—*Brg1, Baf57, Baf60a, Srg3, Ini1*, and *Baf170 (82)*. The function of PYR is not known, but it might be involved in the switch between fetal and adult β-globin expression.

BHC110-CONTAINING COMPLEXES

In recent years, a new group of *HDAC1/2*-containing-complexes has been described *(83–86)*. They all contain a core complex formed by HDAC1/2 and the FAD$^+$ binding protein *BHC110* (Fig. 3; *see* Color Plate 3 following p. 180). The complexes also contain other proteins that confer specificity of function. Two complexes have been described thus far, but preliminary data are suggestive of more to come *(86)*. These complexes are involved in transcriptional repression, although, in contrast to NuRD- and

Sin3-containing complexes, the subset of genes affected is more restricted, with repression seemingly more specialized *(85,87,88)*.

CoREST Complex

The CoREST/BHC mammalian complex was identified by different investigators as a group of proteins that cofractionated with CoREST, a corepressor of the transcription factor REST/NRSF *(83–85)*. *REST* is responsible for the maintenance of long-term repression of neuronal-specific genes in nonneuronal cells *(89)*. *REST* exerts its function by binding to the Sin3-containing complex through its N-terminal domain *(90)* and also the CoREST complex through its C-terminal region *(91)*. The CoREST complex is formed by six subunits: the core complex, *CoREST*, BRCA2-associated factor 35 *(BRAF35)*, and *BHC80* (Fig. 3) *(85)*.

CoREST contains two SANT domains, only the first of which (SANT1) is involved in the interaction with HDACs, being essential for *HDAC1* activation *(83)*. The other component of the CoREST complex, *BRAF35*, was originally discovered as a component of the breast cancer-related factor *BRCA2* complex, in which it plays a structural role *(92)*. Its main feature is the presence of an HMG domain that confers an ability to bind DNA, which is critical for the repressive activity of the CoREST complex in vivo *(85)*.

There is not much known about *BHC80*, except that it contains one PHD and two leucine zipper domains *(85,93)*, all of which are involved in protein–protein interactions. However, in contrast to the ubiquitous *BRAF35*, the presence of *BHC80* is highly tissue specific, perhaps reflective of a specialized role *(85,93)*.

Interestingly, a supracomplex that contains the CoREST complex was isolated through affinity purification of the corepressor *CtBP* *(94,95)*. Among the factors comprising this complex are two histone methyltransferases responsible for dimethylation of lysine-9 in the histone H3 tail, i.e., *G9A* and *EuHMT* *(96,97)*. However, as in the case of the ALL-1 complex, there are outstanding issues regarding the existence of such a native complex. These include the fact that the complex seems to contain all of CoREST and that *CtBP* is capable of engaging in interaction with multiple factors; therefore, whether the studies uncovered a supracomplex or a mixed population of *CtBP* complexes remains an open question. Once again, this species may actually be a composite isolated in vitro rather than an entity that exists in vivo. This remains to be clarified.

XFIM Complex

The XFIM complex contains, in addition to the same core complex as CoREST, the factor *XFIM*, a candidate for X-linked mental retardation, and the DNA binding protein *TFII-I* (Fig. 3) *(86)*. Interestingly, this complex of about 1 MDa contains four molecules of XFIM and is specifically

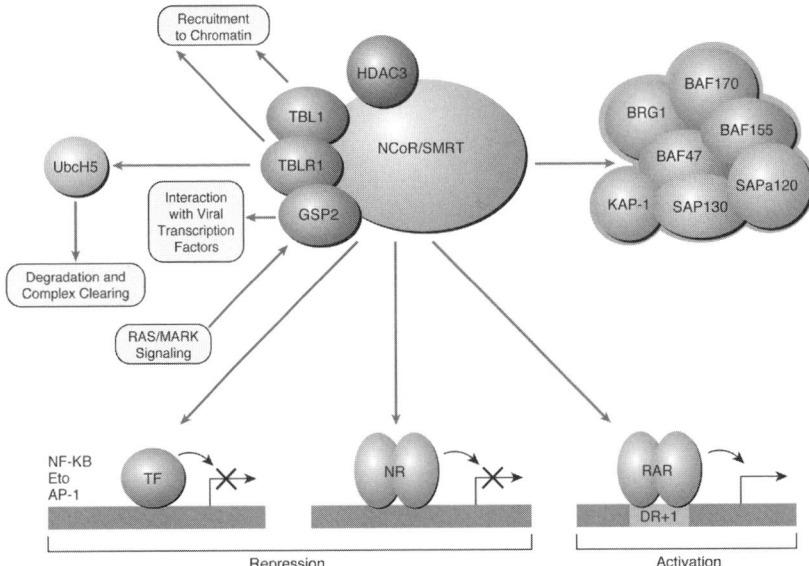

Fig. 4. *HDAC3* complex. On the one hand, the core HDAC3 complex consisting of NCoR/SMRT and *HDAC3* can form a complex together with *TBL1*, *TBLR1*, and *GSP2* (left part of the figure), although they have not been found in all cases. On the other hand, interaction with SWI/SNF proteins together with KAP1, *SAP130*, and *SAP3a120*, has been described. The role of the first complex is repression of specific genes recruited by transcription factors and by nuclear receptors (NRs). However, reports have also described the involvement of the complex in activation, in the case of retinoic acid receptor *(RAR)* binding to the DR-1 elements. For abbreviations, *see* Acronyms and Abbreviations table. *See* Color Plate 4 following p. 180.

recruited to the *c-Fos* promoter by *TFII-I (98,99)*. The XFIM complex seems to be involved in the tight control of *c-Fos* gene expression *(86)*. Whereas *c-Fos* levels are tightly repressed, growth factors and other stimuli induce an immediate activation of *c-Fos* gene expression, which then returns to the repressed state soon after the stimulus is gone. ChIP studies have shown that, in vivo, components of the XFIM complex are present at the promoter before and after the stimuli, but not during activation, suggesting an important role for the complex in maintaining a repressed state *(86)*.

HDAC3 Complexes

Like *HDAC1* and *HDAC2, HDAC3* is involved in transcriptional repression, but *HDAC3* function seems to be less global. In fact, *HDAC3* is involved in repression of a specific group of genes, in particular those connected with nuclear receptor signaling (Fig. 4; *see* Color Plate 4 following p. 180) *(100–102)*. Interestingly, some reports have also found

a role for *HDAC3* in the transcriptional activation of specific genes responsive to the retinoic acid hormone receptor *(103;* Fig. 4). In accordance
with this, *hos2*, the *HDAC3* homolog in yeast, has been reported to be
involved in both repression and activation of specific genes *(104)*.

This more restricted function is also reflected by the nature of the
HDAC3-containing complexes. So far, different groups have described the
purification of several *HDAC3*-containing complexes *(102,105–108)*, and
although it is still not clear whether all the subunits reported actually com-
pose the same or disparate complexes, the common constituents are
HDAC3 and the nuclear hormone corepressors NCoR/SMRT *(109)*.

Most of the *HDAC3*-containing complexes described are rather large
(1–2 MDa), most of them contain many common subunits, and the combined sizes of the subunits described do not match the complex size
observed by gel filtration chromatography *(105,108)*. These observations
suggest that there might actually be only a few disparate *HDAC3* complexes, in contrast to the case with NuRD. The most convincingly studied
complex *(105–108)* appeared to contain *HDAC3*, NCoR/SMRT, transducin
β-like protein *(TBL1)*, transducin β-like related protein *(TBLR1)*, and the
G-protein pathway suppressor 2 *(GSP2)*. Other associated proteins were
present in substochiometric amounts, for example, the coronin-like actin
binding protein *IR10* (Fig. 4). Although most reports found *TBL1* as part
of the complex *(105–108)*, others did not *(102)*. Discrepancies also
involved *GSP2* and *TBLR1*, which were reported by only one *(107)* and
two *(107,108)* groups, respectively. Additional work is needed to clarify
the nature of these complexes.

NCoR and *SMRT* have been extensively studied because of their wide-
ranging role in transcriptional repression from general to cell-type specific, mediated through their interaction with a variety of transcription
factors, such as nuclear factor-κB (*NF-κB*) *(110)*, *Eto (111)*, *AP-1 (112)*,
homodomain-containing factors *(113)*, and others. However, they also
have a particularly important function in hormone receptor signaling
(109,114,115). Interestingly, NCoR/SMRT binds to class II HDACs (see
below). The enormous implications of the multiple functions associated
with NCoR/SMRT fit well with the embryonic lethality observed in *NCoR*
knockout mice, with defects in development and cell differentiation *(103)*.
In the context of the *HDAC3*-containing complexes, NCoR/SMRT are not
only important for the function of the complexes and for interaction with
the hormone receptor machinery and other regulators (see above), but are
also required for proper *HDAC3* activity. As in the case of the MTA proteins in NuRD and of REST in the CoREST complex, the presence of
SANT domains in SMRT is required for full *HDAC3* enzymatic activity
(116). However, of the two SANT domains contained in each of these
proteins, only the first seems to be involved in this function, in both
cases *(117)*.

TBL1 has intrinsic transcriptional repressive activity and is highly related to *Ebi*, a regulator of epidermal growth receptor signaling in *Drosophila (118)*. *TBL1* contains six WD40 repeats that apparently confer chromatin binding ability *(105,108)*. WD40 repeats are also found in eukaryotic corepressors such as *Streptomyces cerevisiae Tup1 (119)* and *Drosophila Groucho (120)*, and they can recruit HDACs *(Rpd3) (121)*. *Tup1* and *Groucho* also exhibit an intrinsic repressive activity, independent of HDACs, which may be related to their interactions with the basal transcription machinery *(122,123)*. The role of *TBL1*, together with *TBLR1*, may be analogous to the histone chaperones *RbAp46/48* in *HDAC1*-containing complexes.

TBLR1 is highly related to *TBL1* in that it also contains six WD40 repeats and possesses chromatin binding ability *(105,108)*. Using specific siRNA methodology, *TBL1* and *TBLR1* were found to be necessary, but functionally redundant, when tested for repression by unliganded thyroid hormone receptor *(108)*. However, other studies on natural promoters in vivo suggested that *TBLR1* is actually required for clearance of the complex. This entails the recruitment of an ubiquitination complex consisting of the conjugating enzyme *UbcH5* that brings along components of the 19S proteasome degradation system *(110,112)*.

GSP2, or *AMF-1*, is involved in the regulation of the RAS/MAPK pathway *(124)*, interacts with the viral transcription factor *Tax* encoded by T-cell lymphotrophic virus type I (HTLV-I) *(107)*, and can also repress *JNK1*-activating activity *(107,124)*.

IR10 contains three WD40 repeats, although it is not highly related to *TBL1* or *TBLR1 (125)*. IR10 interacts with *NcoR*, but not *SMRT (107)*. It is found in substochiometric amounts in association with the *HDAC3* core complex formed by *HDAC1/2* and *BCH110* (Fig. 3); its function remains unknown. Interestingly, a related complex has been found in yeast, SET3C *(126)*. SET3C contains: the SET and PHD domain containing protein *Set3p*, *Hos2p*, the homolog of *HDAC3*, *Sif2p*, a WD40-repeat protein homolog of *TBL1*, *Sntp*, which, like NCoR/SMRT, is a SANT domain-containing protein, and *YIL112w*, which contains ankyrin repeats involved in protein-protein interactions. It also contains *Cpr1p* and the class III HDAC *Hst1* (*see* Class III HDACs section).

One group also reported the purification of another HDAC3-NCor/SMRT-containing complex that included the core of the ATP-dependent chromatin-remodeling SWI/SNF complex, the corepressor *KAP-1*, the splicing-related factor *SAP130*, and the splicing factor *3a120* *(127)*. The SWI/SNF core complex is formed by the SWI/SNF enzyme *BRG1* and associated proteins *Baf170*, *Baf155*, and *Baf47* (Fig. 4) *(128)*. Although functional data are lacking, the presence of the SWI/SNF core complex may facilitate access of the deacetylase to the chromatin substrate, as in the case of *Mi2* in NuRD.

CLASS II HDACs

The budding yeast *Hda1* is the enzyme that defines this family *(24)*. In humans, class II HDACs are subdivided into classes IIa and IIb *(129)*. As with the class I HDACs, the enzymes of this family perform a wide variety of highly regulated functions. These enzymes also do not contain DNA binding activity, suggesting interactions with other proteins in order to repress transcription *(1,3,129)*. This aspect of class II HDACs will be discussed.

HDAC Class IIa

Class IIa HDACs consist of *HDAC4, -5, -7, -9*, and a splice variant of HDAC9 that contains only the N-terminus region of the protein, designated myocyte enhancer factor 2 *(MEF2)* interacting transcription repressor *(MITR) (130)*. Many interactions regulate the ability of class IIa HDACs to repress transcription (*see* next section). A striking feature of class IIa HDACs, however, is their ability to shuttle between the nucleus and cytoplasm *(1,3,129)*. The cytoplasmic chaperon protein *14-3-3 (131)* is responsible for cytoplasmic sequestration of class IIa enzymes. *14-3-3* binds to the HDAC that is phosphorylated on one or two of the three N-terminal serines by calcium calmodulin-dependent protein kinase *(CaMK)*, which is activated after Ca^{2+} release *(132*; Fig. 5; *see* Color Plate 5 following p. 180). Once the HDAC reaches the cytoplasm and is thus phosphorylated, complex formation with 14-3-3 sequesters the enzyme in the cytoplasm, thwarting its ability to repress transcription.

CLASS IIA INTERACTING PROTEINS

Many of the interactions that allow the different class IIa HDACs to repress transcription have been discovered (Fig. 5) *(1,3,129,130)*. Class IIa enzymes bind to the corepressor SMRT/NCoR complex described earlier (which includes *HDAC3*) *(116,133)*. SMRT/NCoR can also be recruited by the human protooncogene *Bcl6 (134)*. *Bcl6* is a BTB/POZ-zinc finger transcriptional repressor that, upon overexpression, protects B-cell lines from apoptosis induced by DNA damage. In keeping with this activity, recent studies have shown that overexpression of *Bcl6* suppresses *p53* expression *(135)*. However, it has also been reported that *Bcl6* binds to the N-terminus of class IIa HDACs *(136)*. This suggests that *Bcl6* can recruit either the SMRT/NCoR complex, which can then recruit a class IIa HDAC, or the class IIa HDAC directly. Class IIa HDACs do not exhibit enzymatic activity in isolation *(129,130)* but only in complex with the SMRT/NCoR corepressor complex *(137)*. However, given that this corepressor complex contains the class I *HDAC3*, and that it is enzymatically active without class IIa enzymes, the class IIa HDACs may be redundant.

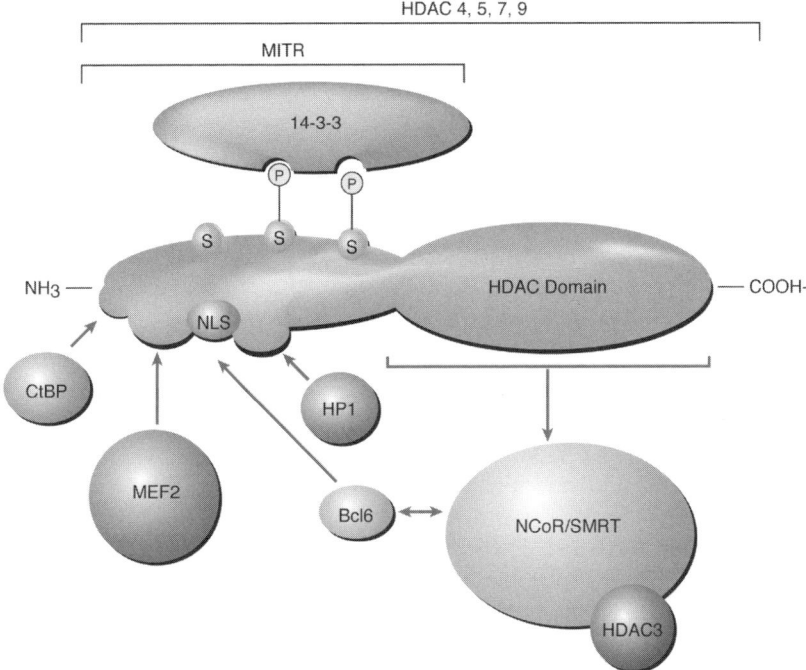

Fig. 5. HDAC IIa interactions. The domain structure of class IIa HDACs is shown. The MITR domain is illustrated. Serines that can be phosphorylated by *CaMK* are represented by S. The phosphorylated proteins *(MITR, HDACs 4/5/7/9)* interact with *14-3-3*. Other interaction partners of the class Iia HDACs are illustrated. For abbreviations, *see* Acronyms and Abbreviations table. *See* Color Plate 5 following p. 180.

More likely, the enzymatic activity of the full complex (containing both HDACs) may target histone polypeptides as well as nonhistone substrates. This remains to be elucidated.

MEF2 is an important DNA binding transcriptional regulator *(138)*. It is involved in the regulation of myogenesis, in negative selection of developing thymocytes, and in transcriptional regulation of the Epstein-Barr virus (EBV) *(139)*. Class IIa HDACs bind to *MEF2* through a highly conserved 17-amino acid N-terminal motif (Fig. 5) *(129,130,140)*. When a class IIa HDAC is present in the nucleus bound to *MEF2* at a promoter, the gene is repressed *(140,141)*. However, when the HDAC becomes phosphorylated, the interaction is lost and the HDAC becomes sequestered in the cytoplasm, inducing activation of myogenesis in muscle cells, for example *(139,141,142)*. Another protein that was found to interact with *HDAC4*, *-5*, and *MITR*, through specific regions of their N-termini, is the transcriptional repressor *CtBP (143)*, which was discussed earlier toward the end of the section entitled HDAC1 and HDAC2, as it also interacts with class I HDACs. Heterochromatin protein 1 *(HP1)* has been reported to interact with *HDAC4, -5,* and *MITR* through a distinct region in their N-termini (Fig. 5) *(144)*. *HP1* binds methylated histone H3 lysine-9 and interacts with histone lysine methyltransferase *SUV39H1 (145,146)*. The interaction between *HP1* and *HDAC4, -5,* and *MITR* is lost following phosphorylation of the class IIa HDACs by *CaMK*. Because silent *MEF2* genes are methylated at lysine-9 of histone H3 *(144)* and this methylation has been shown to be a chromatin repressive mark, these findings suggest a possible mechanism whereby deacetylation by a class IIa HDAC precedes methylation to allow for repression *(144)*.

A recent finding illustrates a tissue-specific role for class II HDACs. *HDAC4* gain of function and loss of function mutants display similar phenotypes as the corresponding mutants of *RUNX2*, the DNA binding transcription factor that is involved in bone development; *HDAC4* and *RUNX2* were also shown to interact physically *(147)*.

HDAC Class IIb

Class IIb consists of *HDAC6* and *-10*. As an *HDAC10* complex has not been described, this section focuses on *HDAC6*. *HDAC6* was found to be a α-*tubulin* deacetylase *(149,150)*; it also binds polyubiquitin chains on misfolded proteins. Recently, a link with Parkinson's disease was revealed when *HDAC6* was found to interact with cytoplasmic *dynein*, a microtubule minus end-directed motor protein *(148)* necessary for the transport of misfolded proteins *(148)*. This evidence suggests that *HDAC6* is an adapter protein that allows aggregated, misfolded, and polyubiquitinated proteins *(151)* to come together with dynein *(152)*, with subsequent transport to aggresomes. Tubulin hyperacetylation is correlated with more stable microtubules *(130)*. Thus acetylation and deacetylation of tubulin may be important for the movement of such misfolded proteins along the microtubules, highlighting the role of *HDAC6* in this transport. Moreover, *HDAC6* colocalizes with ubiquitin conjugates and α-*synuclein* in structures resembling neuronal inclusion bodies, i.e., Lewy bodies, a defining feature of Parkinson's disease *(153)*.

CLASS III HDACs

Class III HDACs are related to the yeast NAD⁺-dependent HDAC silent information regulator 2 *(Sir2p)*, which is involved in gene silencing through the generation of heterochromatin-like compacted chromatin that is hypoacetylated in histone H3 and H4 tails. Yeast has four SIR silent information regulator (SIR) proteins, all involved in the formation of specialized repressed chromatin, but only *Sir2p* possesses enzymatic activity on its own *(154–156)*.

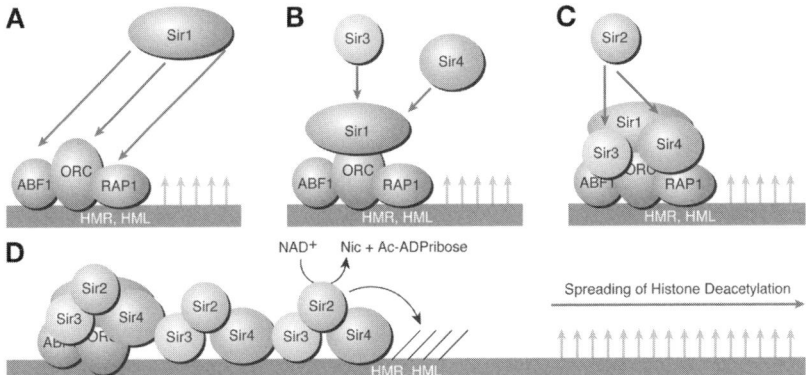

Fig. 6. Sequential model of *Sir2p* action at the mating-type Loci. **(A)** *Sir1p* is responsible for establishment of silencing of the loci, by binding to the factors *Rap1p*, *Abf1p*, and the origin replication complex (ORC). **(B)** *Sir3p* and *Sir4p* are then recruited and bind directly to histone tails. **(C)** *Sir3p* and *Sir4p* recruit, in turn, *Sir2p*. **(D)** Deacetylation and compaction of chromatin occurs in the presence of NAD⁺. The initial assembly of the triplex Sir2p-Sir3p-Sir4p induces the recruitment of more molecules whose spread extends over a few kilobases. For abbreviations, *see* Acronyms and Abbreviations table. (Adapted from ref. *160*.) *See* Color Plate 6 following p. 180.

Class III HDACs include homologs of *Sir2p* in all higher organisms, including 7 homologs in humans *(SirT1–7) (157,158)*. In addition, proteins with some similarity to *Sir2p* have been found in bacteria *(157)*. In yeast, a family of four proteins with similarity to *Sir2p* called homologs of Sir2p *(Hst)1–4p* has also been defined, although not much is known about their function *(158)*. Interestingly, Hstps are probably the true orthologs of the class III members of higher organisms because the SIR machinery is absent in higher eukaryotes. Other evidence supporting this idea is the cellular localization and specificity of these proteins. For instance, *Hst1p* might be the ortholog of *SirT1* and *Hst2p* the ortholog of *SirT2* and *SirT3 (158,159)*.

Yeast Sir2p

Together with the other Sir proteins, *Sir2p* is involved in the formation of specialized compacted chromatin regions in three specific loci in yeast: telomeres, mating-type (HML and HMR) and rDNA repeats in the nucleolus *(160)*. However, only *Sir2p* is required in all three loci. *Sir3p* and *Sir4p* are involved in mating-type loci regulation and telomeres, whereas *Sir1p* is only involved in mating-type loci *(161)*.

Genetic and biochemical studies suggest a model of sequential recruitment in *Sir2p*-mediated silencing (Fig. 6; *see* Color Plate 6 following p. 180) *(154,155,162)*. For instance, in the mating-type loci,

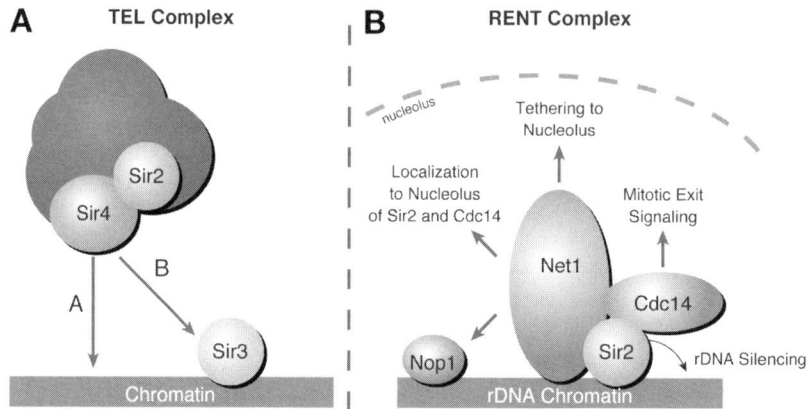

Fig. 7. *Sir2p*-containing complexes. (**A**) TEL complex components are not fully identified but contain *Sir2p* and *Sir4p* and perhaps partially challenge the sequential model. However, these two models need not be exclusive and together may explain the arrival of the TEL complex at the chromatin. The "A" arrow indicates that TEL could bind independently to chromatin through *Sir4p*, and the "B" arrow shows that Sir3p would be responsible for recruitment of the complex to chromatin. (**B**) The RENT complex and its subunits bound to rDNA genes. The functions of the RENT subunits are indicated. For abbreviations, *see* Acronyms and Abbreviations table. *See* Color Plate 7 following p. 180.

Sir1p is involved in the establishment of silencing by binding to the origin replication complex subunit 1 *(ORC1)*, *Rap1*, and *Abf-1*. After *Sir1p* binding, *Sir3p* and *Sir4p* bind to chromatin through interactions with histones H3 and H4 and bring in *Sir2p (154,155,162)*.

However, the situation seems to be more complex than this model would suggest. Some studies found that *Sir2p* is essentially present in two large complexes in the cell *(163–165)*. The first one is called the TEL complex *(163)*, a large species of about 800 kDa that contains *Sir2p*, *Sir4p*, and other uncharacterized proteins, but not *Sir1p* or *Sir3p* (Fig. 7; *see* Color Plate 7 following p. 180). The presence of *Sir2p* and *Sir4p* in the TEL complex suggests that the arrival of *Sir2p* at the chromatin is dependent on the capacity of *Sir4p* to bind chromatin. However, because *Sir3p* binds to *Sir4p (166,167)*, it is also possible that *Sir3p* mediates the recruitment of the TEL complex. Additional studies are required to reconcile these observations.

The second complex is called regulator of nucleolar silencing and telophase exit (RENT) *(164,165)*, which is only present in the nucleolus and contains *Sir2p*, *Cdc14p*, *Net1p*, and *Net1*-associated nucleolar protein *(Nan1p)* (Fig. 7). RENT is involved in mitotic exit control, rDNA silencing, and nucleolar localization of *Nop1*, a factor involved in nucleolar pre-rRNA processing *(168)*. *Cdc14p* is a protein phosphatase that belongs to the mitotic exit network (MEN) *(169)*. *Net1p* is a key factor in the RENT complex, as it is responsible for tethering the complex to the nucleolus *(165)*. Because of the presence of *Net1p*, *Sir2p* and *Cdc14p* localize to the nucleolus, where they can exert their function. It is possible that *Net1p* is also the factor responsible for bringing *Sir2p* to the rDNA repeats. *Net1p* can also stimulate RNA polymerase I activity by binding directly to the enzyme *(170)*.

Hst1 and SirT1

Hst1p is probably the best known of the Hst proteins. *Hst1p* is the closest member of the class III HDACs to *Sir2p*, and its main function seems to be related to the repression of middle sporulation genes *(171,172)*.

Hst1p forms two different complexes in yeast cells (Fig. 8; *see* Color Plate 8 following p. 180). One such complex *(171,172)*, together with the DNA binding transcriptional repressor *Sum1p*, participates in middle sporulation gene repression and accounts for almost all the cellular *Hst1p* *(173)*. The second complex that has been described is SET3C *(126)*, the yeast counterpart of HDAC3-containing NCoR/SMRT in higher organisms that also participates in meiotic repression and sporulation. However, *Hst1p* does not seem to be responsible for the activity of the complex, leaving open the possibility that this complex participates in other functions *(126)*. Interestingly, *Hos2p* and *Set3p* have also been found to be involved in the transcriptional activation of certain genes *(104)*. It is unknown whether this function is mediated by SET3C or by an alternative complex that contains both subunits.

SIRT1

SirT1 is the member of the human Sir2 family that is closest to *Sir2p*, and it has been reported to deacetylate histones and nonhistone substrates *(174)*. All core histones are substrates in vitro, but *SirT1* exhibits a preference for acetylated lysine-16 of histone H4 and acetylated lysine-9 of histone H3 as well as acetylated lysine-26 of histone H1b (or H1.4) in vitro and in vivo *(175)*. The nonhistone targets are *p53 (176,177)*, *TAFI68 (178)*, *BCL6 (179)*, FOXO transcription factors *(180,181)*, *Ku70 (182)*, and NF-κB *(RelA/p65) (183)*.

SirT1 functions in transcriptional repression and heterochromatin formation, muscle differentiation *(184)*, inhibition of senescence and apoptosis induced by *p53 (176,177)*, life span extension *(182)*, stress response *(180,181)*, and inhibition of axonal degeneration *(185)*. *SirT1* interacts with multiple factors, most of them transcription factors, which seem to recruit *SirT1* to chromatin specific regions. Among these are *p53 (176,177)*, *CTIP2 (186)*, *HES1* and *HES2 (187)*, *FOXO (180,181)*,

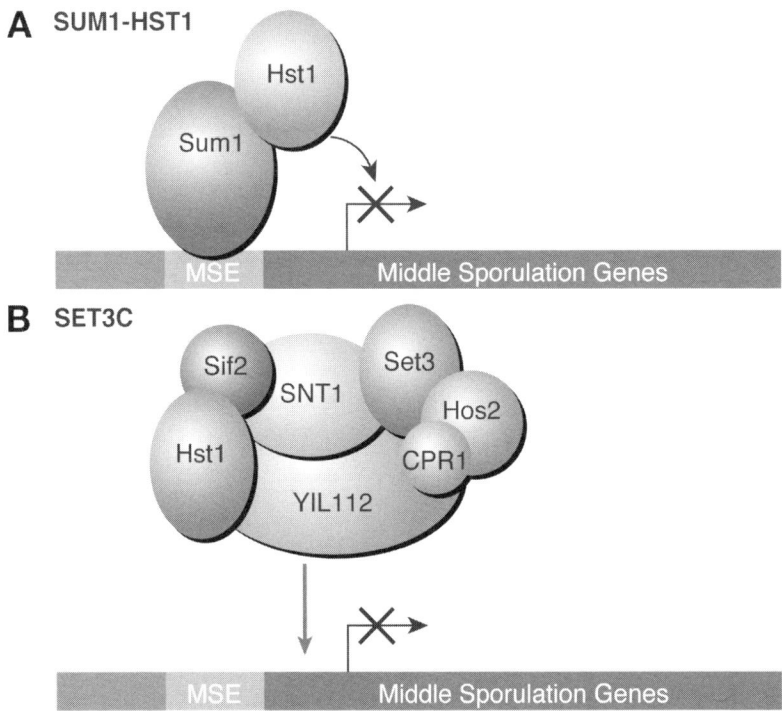

Fig. 8. *Hst1p* complexes. Two complexes have been described that contain *Hst1p*.
(A) *Hst1p* sum1p participates in the repression of middle sporulation genes by the
binding of Sum1p to the middle sporulation elements (MSEs). **(B)** *Hst1p* was
found to be part of SET3C, a complex containing *Hos2p* that also participates in
middle sporulation gene repression. However, *Hst1p* is not required for the activity of the complex. For abbreviations, *see* Acronyms and Abbreviations table. *See*
Color Plate 8 following p. 180.

NF-κB *(183)*, *NCoR* and *SMRT (188)*, *PPAR-γ (188)* and the histone
acetyltransferase PCAF *(184)*. Importantly, SirT1 also interacts with histone *H1b (175)*, and recent studies have demonstrated that recruitment of
SirT1 to specific genes results in the formation of repressed chromatin
(175). This includes the recruitment of histone *H1b* and the modification
of the histone H3 and H4 tails with "marks" that are the signature of
repressed chromatin.

The native form of *SirT1* is a homomultimer of about 350–400 kDa
that most likely corresponds to a trimer *(175)*, although minor amounts of
the enzyme may be present in other complexes. This fits well with predic-
tions of trimer formation based on structural studies of other members of
the class III family *(189)*.

Hst2p, SirT2, and SirT3

Hst2p is a homolog of *Sir2p* in yeast and is part of the class III NAD$^+$-dependent HDACs *(157)*. It has been shown to be one of the most enzymatically active of the class III enzymes *(190)*. It is completely sequestered in the cytoplasm, suggesting a substrate other than histones *(191)*. The function of *Hst2p* remains largely unknown, as a multiprotein complex has not been isolated. Some evidence suggests that *Hst2p* is involved in the cell cycle as well as in epigenetic regulation of a select group of genes *(174,192)*. However, given its cytoplasmic localization, it is unclear how and when Hst2p could travel to the nuclei to participate in these functions.

SIRT2

In humans, *SirT2* and *SirT3* appear to have the closest homology to *Hst2p (157,158)*. *SirT2* may be most homologous, given its almost exclusive localization to the cytoplasm *(190,193)*. *SirT2* was shown to colocalize with tubulin as well as to be able to deacetylate acetylated α-*tubulin (193)*. Immunoprecipitation experiments with *SirT2* brought down the other known tubulin deactylase *HDAC6*, suggesting a functional complex between these proteins *(193)*. This is an interesting function that must have been acquired during evolution considering that acetylated tubulin has not been found in budding yeast. This also suggests that human *SirT2* and *Hst2p* may share an even more basic function. Multiprotein complexes containing *SirT2* have not yet been characterized. *SirT2* has been shown to be upregulated during mitosis and can affect the cell cycle when overexpressed *(194)*. Both *Hst2p* and *SirT2* have been shown to inhibit starfish oocyte maturation in microinjection experiments, and *Hst2p* was also shown to delay starfish embryonic cell division in similar experiments using daughter blastomeres *(195)*.

It is also a possibility that *SirT2* and *Hst2p* silence genes. Both *Hst1p* and *Hst2p* are recruited specifically by *Sfl1p* to a specific region of the *FLO10* promoter located near the telomere and are required for silencing of the gene *(191)*. Deletion of *Sir2p* had no effect on this silencing. Both of these findings suggest that *Hst1p* and *Hst2p* (and probably *SirT2*) participate in complex protein interactions yet to be discovered.

SIRT3

SirT3 is an equally interesting protein. Although it is closely related to *Hst2p* and *SirT2*, it has been reported to be a mitochondrial protein *(196,197)*. *SirT3* has not been found in a multiprotein complex, leaving its role unclarified for the present. *SirT3* has been shown to be cleaved at the N terminus by an interaction with matrix-processing peptidase *(MPP)* once it has reached the mitochondria, resulting in a truncated form of *SirT3 (196,197)*.

S<small>IR</small>T4–7

SirT4–7 have the least homology to *Sir2p* and remain virtually unstudied.

REFERENCES

1. Brownell JE, Zhou J, Ranalli T, et al. Tetrahymena histone acetyltransferase A: a homolog to yeast Gcn5p linking histone acetylation to gene activation. Cell 1996;84:843–851.
2. Taunton J, Hassig CA, Schreiber SL. A mammalian histone deacetylase related to the yeast transcriptional regulator Rpd3p. Science 1996;272:408–411.
3. de Ruijter AJ, van Gennip AH, Caron HN, Kemp S, van Kuilenburg AB. Histone deacetylases (HDACs): characterization of the classical HDAC family. Biochem J 2003;370:737–749.
4. Kuzmichev A, Reinberg D. Role of histone deacetylase complexes in the regulation of chromatin metabolism. Curr Top Microbiol Immunol 2001;254:35–58.
5. Cress WD, Seto E. Histone deacetylases, transcriptional control, and cancer. J Cell Physiol 2000;184:1–16.
6. Yang WM, Inouye C, Zeng Y, Bearss D, Seto E. Transcriptional repression by YY1 is mediated by interaction with a mammalian homolog of the yeast global regulator RPD3. Proc Natl Acad Sci U S A 1996;93:12,845–12,850.
7. Grandori C, Cowley SM, James LP, Eisenman RN. The Myc/Max/Mad network and the transcriptional control of cell behavior. Annu Rev Cell Dev Biol 2000;16:653–699.
8. Javed A, Guo B, Hiebert S, et al. Groucho/TLE/R-esp proteins associate with the nuclear matrix and repress RUNX (CBF(alpha)/AML/PEBP2(alpha)) dependent activation of tissue-specific gene transcription. J Cell Sci 2000;113:2221–2231.
9. Lai A, Kennedy BK, Barbie DA, et al. RBP1 recruits the mSIN3-histone deacetylase complex to the pocket of retinoblastoma tumor suppressor family proteins found in limited discrete regions of the nucleus at growth arrest. Mol Cell Biol 2001;21:2918–2932.
10. Sowa Y, Orita T, Minamikawa S, et al. Histone deacetylase inhibitor activates the WAF1/Cip1 gene promoter through the Sp1 sites. Biochem Biophys Res Commun 1997;241:142–150.
11. Lutz M, Burke LJ, Barreto G, et al. Transcriptional repression by the insulator protein CTCF involves histone deacetylases. Nucleic Acids Res 2000;28: 1707–1713.
12. Ayer DE, Lawrence QA, Eisenman RN. Mad-Max transcriptional repression is mediated by ternary complex formation with mammalian homologs of yeast repressor Sin3. Cell 1995;80:767–776.
13. Schreiber-Agus N, Chin L, Chen K, et al. An amino-terminal domain of Mxi1 mediates anti-Myc oncogenic activity and interacts with a homolog of the yeast transcriptional repressor SIN3. Cell 1995;80:777–786.
14. Nagy L, Kao HY, Chakravarti D, et al. Nuclear receptor repression mediated by a complex containing SMRT, mSin3A, and histone deacetylase. Cell 1997;89: 373–380.
15. Heinzel T, Lavinsky RM, Mullen TM, et al. A complex containing N-CoR, mSin3 and histone deacetylase mediates transcriptional repression. Nature 1997;387:43–48.

16. Fuks F, Burgers WA, Brehm A, et al. DNA methyltransferase Dnmt1 associates with histone deacetylase activity. Nat Genet 2000;24:88–91.

17. Czermin B, Schotta G, Hulsmann BB, et al. Physical and functional association of SU(VAR)3-9 and HDAC1 in *Drosophila*. EMBO Rep 2001;2:915–919.

18. Luo RX, Postigo AA, Dean DC. Rb interacts with histone deacetylase to repress transcription. Cell 1998;92:463–473.

19. Khan MM, Nomura T, Kim H, et al. Role of PML and PML-RARalpha in Mad-mediated transcriptional repression. Mol Cell 2001;7:1233–1243.

20. Ayer DE. Histone deacetylases: transcriptional repression with SINers and NuRDs. Trends Cell Biol 1999;9:193–198.

21. Nasmyth K, Stillman D, Kipling D. Both positive and negative regulators of HO transcription are required for mother-cell-specific mating-type switching in yeast. Cell 1987;48:579–587.

22. Sternberg PW, Stern MJ, Clark I, Herskowitz I. Activation of the yeast HO gene by release from multiple negative controls. Cell 1987;48:567–577.

23. Wang H, Clark I, Nicholson PR, Herskowitz I, Stillman DJ. The *Saccharomyces cerevisiae* SIN3 gene, a negative regulator of HO, contains four paired amphipathic helix motifs. Mol Cell Biol 1990;10:5927–5936.

24. Koskinen PJ, Ayer DE, Eisenman RN. Repression of Myc-Ras cotransformation by Mad is mediated by multiple protein–protein interactions. Cell Growth Differ 1995;6:623–629.

25. Zhang Y, Iratni R, Erdjument-Bromage H, Tempst P, Reinberg D. Histone deacetylases and SAP18, a novel polypeptide, are components of a human Sin3 complex. Cell 1997;89:357–364.

26. Rundlett SE, Carmen AA, Kobayashi R, Bavykin S, Turner BM, Grunstein M. HDA1 and RPD3 are members of distinct yeast histone deacetylase complexes that regulate silencing and transcription. Proc Natl Acad Sci U S A 1996;93: 14,503–14,508.

27. Vidal M, Gaber RF. RPD3 encodes a second factor required to achieve maximum positive and negative transcriptional states in *Saccharomyces cerevisiae*. Mol Cell Biol 1991;11:6317–6327.

28. Kasten MM, Dorland S, Stillman DJ. A large protein complex containing the yeast Sin3p and Rpd3p transcriptional regulators. Mol Cell Biol 1997;17: 4852–4858.

29. Hassig CA, Fleischer TC, Billin AN, Schreiber SL, Ayer DE. Histone deacetylase activity is required for full transcriptional repression by mSin3A. Cell 1997;89:341–347.

30. Laherty CD, Yang WM, Sun JM, Davie JR, Seto E, Eisenman RN. Histone deacetylases associated with the mSin3 corepressor mediate mad transcriptional repression. Cell 1997;89:349–356.

31. Schwerk C, Prasad J, Degenhardt K, et al. ASAP, a novel protein complex involved in RNA processing and apoptosis. Mol Cell Biol 2003;23: 2981–2990.

32. Zhang Y, Sun ZW, Iratni R, et al. SAP30, a novel protein conserved between human and yeast, is a component of a histone deacetylase complex. Mol Cell 1998;1021–1031.

33. Kuzmichev A, Zhang Y, Erdjument-Bromage H, Tempst P, Reinberg D. Role of the Sin3-histone deacetylase complex in growth regulation by the candidate tumor suppressor p33(ING1). Mol Cell Biol 2002;22:835–848.

34. Sif S, Saurin AJ, Imbalzano AN, Kingston RE. Purification and characterization of mSin3A-containing Brg1 and hBrm chromatin remodeling complexes. Genes Dev 2001;15:603–618.
35. Suka N, Suka Y, Carmen AA, Wu J, Grunstein M. Highly specific antibodies determine histone acetylation site usage in yeast heterochromatin and euchromatin. Mol Cell 2001;8:473–479.
36. Kadosh D, Struhl K. Repression by Ume6 involves recruitment of a complex containing Sin3 corepressor and Rpd3 histone deacetylase to target promoters. Cell 1997;89:365–371.
37. Koipally J, Renold A, Kim J, Georgopoulos K. Repression by Ikaros and Aiolos is mediated through histone deacetylase complexes. EMBO J 1999;18: 3090–3100.
38. Hurlin PJ, Queva C, Eisenman RN. Mnt, a novel Max-interacting protein is coexpressed with Myc in proliferating cells and mediates repression at Myc binding sites. Genes Dev 1997;11:44–58.
39. Ng HH, Bird A. Histone deacetylases: silencers for hire. Trends Biochem Sci 2000;25:121–126.
40. Zhou Y, Santoro R, Grummt I. The chromatin remodeling complex NoRC targets HDAC1 to the ribosomal gene promoter and represses RNA polymerase I transcription. EMBO J 2002;21:4632–4640.
41. Jones PL, Veenstra GJ, Wade PA, et al. Methylated DNA and MeCP2 recruit histone deacetylase to repress transcription. Nat Genet 1998;19:187–191.
42. Laherty CD, Billin AN, Lavinsky RM, et al. SAP30, a component of the mSin3 corepressor complex involved in N-CoR-mediated repression by specific transcription factors. Mol Cell 1998;2:33–42.
43. Chinnadurai G. CtBP, an unconventional transcriptional corepressor in development and oncogenesis. Mol Cell 2002;9:213–224.
44. Zhang Y, LeRoy G, Seelig HP, Lane WS Reinberg D. The dermatomyositis-specific autoantigen Mi2 is a component of a complex containing histone deacetylase and nucleosome remodeling activities. Cell 1998;95:279–289.
45. Wade PA, Jones PL, Vermaak D, Wolffe AP. A multiple subunit Mi-2 histone deacetylase from *Xenopus laevis* cofractionates with an associated Snf2 superfamily ATPase. Curr Biol 1998;8:843–846.
46. Xue Y, Wong J, Moreno GT, Young MK, Cote J, Wang W. NURD, a novel with both ATP-dependent chromatin-remodeling and histone deacetylase activities. Mol Cell 1998;2:851–861.
47. Tong JK, Hassig CA, Schnitzler GR, Kingston RE, Schreiber SL. Chromatin deacetylation by an ATP-dependent nucleosome remodeling complex. Nature 1998;395:917–921.
48. Ahringer J. NuRD and SIN3 histone deacetylase complexes in development. Trends Genet 2000;16:351–356.
49. Becker PB, Hörz W. ATP-dependent nucleosome remodeling. Annu Rev Biochem 2002;71:247–273.
50. Kehle J, Beuchle D, Treuheit S, et al. dMi-2, a hunchback-interacting protein that functions in polycomb repression. Science 1998;282:1897–1900.
51. Kim J, Sif S, Jones B, et al. Ikaros DNA-binding proteins direct formation of chromatin remodeling complexes in lymphocytes. Immunity 1999;10:345–355.
52. Zhang Y, Ng HH, Erdjument-Bromage H, Tempst P, Bird A, Reinberg D. Analysis of the NuRD subunits reveals a histone deacetylase core complex and a connection with DNA methylation. Genes Dev 1999;13:1924–1935.

53. Li J, Lin Q, Wang W, Wade P, Wong J. Specific targeting and constitutive association of histone deacetylase complexes during transcriptional repression. Genes Dev 2002;16:687–692.

54. Nishioka K, Chuikov S, Sarma K, et al. Set9, a novel histone H3 methyltransferase that facilitates transcription by precluding histone tail modifications required for heterochromatin formation. Genes Dev 2002;16:479–489.

55. Zegerman P, Canas B, Pappin D, Kouzarides T. Histone H3 lysine 4 methylation disrupts binding of nucleosome remodeling and deacetylase (NuRD) repressor complex. J Biol Chem 2002;277:11,621–11,624.

56. Bowen NJ, Fujita N, Kajita M, Wade PA. Mi-2/NurD: multiple complexes for many purposes. Biochim Biophys Acta 2004;1677:52–57.

57. Woodage T, Basrai MA, Baxevanis AD, Hieter P, Collins FS. Characterization of the CHD family of proteins. Proc Natl Acad Sci U S A 1997;94:11,472–11,477.

58. Schultz DC, Friedman JR, Rauscher FJ 3rd. Targeting histone deacetylase complexes via KRAB-zinc finger proteins: the PHD and bromodomains of KAP-1 form a cooperative unit that recruits a novel isoform of the Mi-2alpha subunit of NuRD. Genes Dev 2001;15:428–443.

59. Johnson DR, Lovett JM, Hirsch M, Xia F, Chen JD. NuRD complex component Mi-2b binds to and represses RORg-mediated transcriptional activation. Biochem Biophys Res 2004;714–718.

60. Murawsky CM, Brehm A, Badenhorst P, Lowe P, Becker PB, Travers AA. Tramtrack69 interacts with the dMi-2 subunit of the *Drosophila* NuRD chromatin remodeling complex. EMBO Rep 2001;21:1089–1094.

61. Yao YL, Yang WM. The metastasis-associated proteins 1 and 2 form distinct protein complexes with histone deacetylase activity. J Biol Chem 2003;278: 42,560–42,568.

62. Kumar R, Wang RA, Bagheri-Yarmand R. Emerging roles of MTA family members in human cancers. Semin Oncol 2003;30:30–37.

63. Fujita N, Jaye DL, Geigerman C, et al. MTA3 and the Mi-2/NuRD complex regulate cell fate during B lymphocyte differentiation. Cell 2004;119:75–86.

64. Toh Y, Pencil SD, Nicolson GL. A novel candidate metastasis-associated gene, mta1, differentially expressed in highly metastatic mammary adenocarcinoma cell lines. cDNA cloning, expression, and protein analyses. J Biol Chem 1994;269:22,958–22,963.

65. Fujita N, Jaye DL, Kajita M, Geigerman C, Moreno CS, Wade PA. MTA3, a Mi-2/NuRD complex subunit, regulates an invasive growth pathway in breast cancer. Cell 2003;113:207–219.

66. Aasland R, Stewart AF, Gibson T. The SANT domain: a putative DNA-binding domain in the SWI-SNF and ADA complexes, the transcriptional co-repressor N-CoR and TFIIIB. Trends Biochem Sci 1996;21:87, 88.

67. Hendrich B, Bird A. Identification and characterization of a family of mammalian methyl-CpG binding proteins. Mol Cell Biol 1998;18:6538–6547.

68. Wade PA, Gegonne A, Jones PL, Ballestar E, Aubry F, Wolffe AP. Mi-2 complex couples DNA methylation to chromatin remodelling and histone deacetylation. Nat Genet 1999;23:62–66.

69. Feng Q, Zhang Y. The MeCP1 complex represses transcription through preferential binding, remodeling, and deacetylating methylated nucleosomes. Genes Dev 2001;15:827–832.

70. Roder K, Hung MS, Lee TL, et al. Transcriptional repression by *Drosophila* methyl-CpG-binding proteins. Mol Cell Biol 2000;20:7401–7409.

71. Meehan RR, Lewis JD, McKay S, Kleiner EL, Bird AP. Identification of a mammalian protein that binds specifically to DNA containing methylated CpGs. Cell 1989;58:499–507.
72. Feng Q, Cao R, Xia L, Erdjument-Bromage H, Tempst P, Zhang Y. Identification and functional characterization of the p66/p68 components of the MeCP1 complex. Mol Cell Biol 2002;22:536–546.
73. Miaczynska M, Christoforidis S, Giner A, et al. APPL proteins link Rab5 to nuclear signal transduction via an endosomal compartment. Cell 2004;116:445–456.
74. Hakimi MA, Bochar DA, Schmiesing JA, et al. A chromatin remodelling complex that loads cohesin onto human chromosomes. Nature 2002;418: 994–998.
75. Michaelis C, Ciosk R, Nasmyth K. Cohesins: chromosomal proteins that prevent premature separation of sister chromatids. Cell 1997;91:35–45.
76. Tomonaga T, Nagao K, Kawasaki Y, et al. Characterization of fission yeast cohesin: essential anaphase proteolysis of Rad21 phosphorylated in the S phase. Genes Dev 2000;14:2757–2770.
77. Dmitry V, Kadonaga J. The many faces of chromatin remodeling: SWItching beyond transcription. Cell 2001;106:523–525.
78. Nakamura T, Mori T, Tada S, et al. ALL-1 is a histone methyltransferase that assembles a supercomplex of proteins involved in transcriptional regulation. Mol Cell 2002;10:1119–1128.
79. Milne TA, Briggs SD, Brock HW, et al. MLL targets SET domain methyltransferase activity to Hox gene promoters. Mol Cell 2000;10:1107–1117.
80. Ernst P, Wang J, Korsmeyer SJ. The role of MLL in hematopoiesis and leukemia. Curr Opin Hematol 2002;9:282–287.
81. O'Neill D, Yang J, Erdjument-Bromage H, Bornschlegel K, Tempst P, Bank A. Tissue-specific and developmental stage-specific DNA binding by a mammalian SWI/SNF complex associated with human fetal-to-adult globin gene switching. Proc Natl Acad Sci U S A 1999;96:349–354.
82. O'Neill DW, Schoetz SS, Lopez RA, et al. An ikaros-containing chromatin-remodeling complex in adult-type erythroid cells. Mol Cell Biol 2000;20:7572–7582.
83. You A, Tong JK, Grozinger CM, Schreiber SL. CoREST is an integral component of the CoREST-human histone deacetylase complex. Proc Natl Acad Sci U S A 2001:98:1454–1458.
84. Humphrey GW, Wang Y, Russanova VR, et al. Stable histone deacetylase complexes distinguished by the presence of SANT domain proteins CoREST/kiaa0071 and Mta-L1. J Biol Chem 2001;276:6817–6824.
85. Hakimi MA, Bochar DA, Chenoweth J, Lane WS, Mandel G, Shiekhattar R. A core-BRAF35 complex containing histone deacetylase mediates repression of neuronalspecific genes. Proc Natl Acad Sci U S A 2002;99:7420–7425.
86. Hakimi MA, Dong Y, Lane WS, Speicher DW, Shiekhattar R. A candidate X-linked mental retardation gene is a component of a new family of histone deacetylase containing complexes. J Biol Chem 2003;278:7234–7239.
87. Andres ME, Burger C, Peral-Rubio MJ, et al. CoREST: a functional corepressor required for regulation of neural-specific gene expression. Proc Natl Acad Sci U S A 1999;96:9873–9878.
88. Kim DW, Cheriyath V, Roy AL, Cochran BH. TFII-I enhances activation of the c-fos promoter through interactions with upstream elements. Mol Cell Biol 1998;18:3310–3320.

89. Jones FS, Meech R. Knockout of REST/NRSF shows that the protein is a potent repressor of neuronally expressed genes in non-neural tissues. Bioessays 1999;21:372–376.

90. Grimes JA, Nielsen SJ, Battaglioli E, et al. The co-repressor mSin3A is a functional component of the REST-CoREST repressor complex. J Biol Chem 2000;275:9461–9467.

91. Ballas N, Battaglioli E, Atouf F, et al. Regulation of neuronal traits by a novel transcriptional complex. Neuron 2001;31:353–365.

92. Marmorstein LY, Kinev AV, Chan GK, et al. A human BRCA2 complex containing a structural DNA binding component influences cell cycle progression. Cell 2001;104:247–257.

93. Iwase S, Januma A, Miyamoto K, et al. Characterization of BHC80 in BRAF-HDAC complex, involved in neuron-specific gene repression. Biochem Biophys Res Commun 2004;322:601–608.

94. Shi Y, Sawada J, Sui G, et al. Coordinated histone modifications mediated by a CtBP corepressor complex. Nature 2003;422:735–738.

95. Chinnadurai G. CtBP family proteins: more than transcriptional corepressors. Bioessays 2003;25:9–12.

96. Tachibana M, Sugimoto K, Nozaki M, et al. G9a histone methyltransferase plays a dominant role in euchromatic histone H3 lysine 9 methylation and is essential for early embryogenesis. Genes Dev 2002;16:1779–1791.

97. Ogawa H, Ishiguro K, Gaubatz S, Livingston DM, Nakatani Y. A complex with chromatin modifiers that occupies E2F- and Myc-responsive genes in G0 cells. Science 2002;296:1132–1136.

98. Roy AL. Biochemistry and biology of the inducible multifunctional transcription factor TFII-I. Gene 2001;274:1–13.

99. Grueneberg DA, Henry RW, Brauer A, et al. A multifunctional DNA-binding protein that promotes the formation of serum response factor/homeodomain complexes: identity to TFII-I. Genes Dev 1997;11:2482–2493.

100. Bertos NR, Wang AH, Yang XJ. Class II histone deacetylases: structure, function, and regulation. Biochem Cell Biol 2001;79:243–252.

101. Ishizuka T, Lazar MA. The N-CoR/histone deacetylase 3 complex is required for repression by thyroid hormone receptor. Mol Cell Biol 2003;23:5122–5131.

102. Wen YD, Perissi V, Staszewski LM, et al. The histone deacetylase-3 complex contains nuclear receptor corepressors. Proc Natl Acad Sci U S A 2000;97:7202–7207.

103. Jepsen K, Hermanson O, Onami TM, et al. Combinatorial roles of the nuclear receptor corepressor in transcription and development. Cell 2000;102:753–763.

104. Wang A, Kurdistani SK, Grunstein M. Requirement of Hos2 histone deacetylase for gene activity in yeast. Science 2002;298:1412–1414.

105. Guenther MG, Lane WS, Fischle W, Verdin E, Lazar MA, Shiekhattar R. A core SMRT corepressor complex containing HDAC3 and TBL1, a WD40-repeat protein linked to deafness. Genes Dev 2000;14:1048–1057.

106. Li J, Wang J, Nawaz Z, Liu JM, Qin J, Wong J. Both corepressors proteins SMRT and NCor exist in large protein complexes containing HDAC3. EMBO J 2000;19:4342–4350.

107. Zhang J, Kalkum M, Chait BT, Roeder RG. The N-CoR-HDAC3 nuclear receptor corepressor complex inhibits the JNK pathway through the integral subunit GPS2. Mol Cell 2002;9:611–623.

108. Yoon HG, Chan DW, Huang ZQ, et al. Purification and functional characterization of the human N-CoR complex: the roles of HDAC3, TBL1 and TBLR1. EMBO J 2003;22:1336–1346.
109. Glass CK, Rosenfeld MG. The coregulator exchange in transcriptional functions of nuclear receptors. Genes Dev 2000;14:121–141.
110. Perissi V, Aggarwal A, Glass CK, Rose DW, Rosenfeld MG. A corepressor/coactivator exchange complex required for transcriptional activation by nuclear receptors and other regulated transcription factors. Cell 2004;116:511–526.
111. Lutterbach B, Westendorf JJ, Linggi B, et al. ETO, a target of t(8;21) in acute leukemia, interacts with the N-CoR and mSin3 corepressors. Mol Cell Biol 1998;18:7176–7184.
112. Ogawa S, Lozach J, Jepsen K, et al. A nuclear receptor corepressor transcriptional checkpoint controlling activator protein 1-dependent gene networks required for macrophage activation. Proc Natl Acad Sci U S A 2004;101:14,461–14,466.
113. Asahara H, Dutta S, Kao HY, Evans RM, Montminy M. Pbx-Hox heterodimers recruit coactivator-corepressor complexes in an isoform-specific manner. Mol Cell Biol 1999;19:8219–8225.
114. Ordentlich P, Downes M, Evans RM. Corepressors and nuclear hormone receptor function. Curr Top Microbiol Immunol 2001;254:101–116.
115. Rosenfeld MG, Glass CK. Coregulator codes of transcriptional regulation by nuclear receptors. J Biol Chem 2001;276:36,865–36,868.
116. Guenther MG, Barak O, Lazar MA. The SMRT and N-CoR corepressors are activating cofactors for histone deacetylase 3. Mol Cell Biol 2001;21:6091–6101.
117. Yu J, Li Y, Ishizuka T, Guenther MG, Lazar MA. A SANT motif in the SMRT corepressor interprets the histone code and promotes histone deacetylation. EMBO J 2003;22:3403–3410.
118. Dong X, Tsuda L, Zavitz KH, et al. ebi regulates epidermal growth factor receptor signaling pathways in *Drosophila*. Genes Dev 1999;13:954–965.
119. Edmondson DG, Smith MM, Roth SY. Repression domain of the yeast global repressor Tup1 interacts directly with histones H3 and H4. Genes Dev 1996;10:1247–1259.
120. Chen G, Nguyen PH, Courey AJ. A role for Groucho tetramerization in transcription repression. Mol Cell Biol 1998;18:7259–7268.
121. Chen G, Fernandez J, Mische S, Courey AJ. A functional interaction between the histone deacetylase Rpd3 and the corepressor groucho in *Drosophila* development. Genes Dev 1999;13:2218–2230.
122. Carlson M. Genetics of transcriptional regulation in yeast: connections to the RNA polymerase II CTD. Annu Rev Cell Dev Biol 1997;13:1–23.
123. Redd MJ, Arnaud MB, Johnson AD. A complex composed of tup1 and ssn6 represses transcription in vitro. J Biol Chem 1997;11,193–11,197.
124. Jin DY, Teramoto H, Giam CZ, Chun RF, Gutkind JS, Jeang KT. A human suppressor of c-Jun N-terminal kinase 1 activation by tumor necrosis factor alpha. J Biol Chem 1997;272:25,816–25,823.
125. Zaphiropoulos PG, Toftgard R. cDNA cloning of a novel WD repeat protein mapping to the 9q22.3 chromosomal region. DNA Cell Biol 1996;15:1049–1056.
126. Pijnappel WWMP, Schaft D, Roguev A, et al. The *S. cerevisiae* SET3 complex includes two histone deacetylases, Hos2 and Hst1, and is a meiotic-specific repressor of the sporulation gene program. Genes Dev 2001;15: 2991–3004.

127. Underhill C, Qutob MS, Yee SP, Torchia J. A novel nuclear receptor corepressor complex, N-CoR, contains components of the mammalian SWI/SNF complex and the corepressors KAP-1. J Biol Chem 2000;51:40,463–40,470.

128. Wang W, Xue Y, Zhou S, Kuo A, Cairns BR, Crabtree GR. Diversity and specialization of mammalian SWI/SNF complexes. Genes Dev 1996;10:2117–2130.

129. Fischle W, Kiermer V, Dequiedt F, Verdin E. The emerging role of class II histone deacetylases. Biochem Cell Biol 2001;79:337–348.

130. Verdin E, Dequiedt F, Kasler HG. Class II histone deacetylases: versatile regulators. Trends Genet 2003;19:286–293.

131. Mackintosh C. Dynamic interactions between 14-3-3 proteins and phosphoproteins regulate diverse cellular processes. Biochem J 2004;381:329–342.

132. McKinsey TA, Zhang CL, Olson EN. Activation of the myocyte enhancer factor-2 transcription factor by calcium/calmodulin-dependent protein kinase-stimulated binding of 14-3-3 to histone deacetylase 5. Proc Natl Acad Sci U S A 2000;97:14,400–14,405.

133. Huang EY, Zhang J, Miska EA, Guenther MG, Kouzarides T, Lazar MA. Nuclear receptor corepressors partner with class II histone deacetylases in a Sin3-independent repression pathway. Genes Dev 2000;14:45–54.

134. Dhordain P, Albagli O, Lin RJ, et al. Corepressor SMRT binds the BTB/POZ repressing domain of the LAZ3/BCL6 oncoprotein. Proc Natl Acad Sci U S A 1997;94:10,762–10,767.

135. Phan RT, Dalla-Favera R. The BCL6 proto-oncogene suppresses p53 expression in germinal-centre B cells. Nature 2004;432:635–639.

136. Huynh KD, Fischle W, Verdin E, Bardwell VJ. BCoR, a novel corepressor involved in BCL-6 repression. Genes Dev 2000;14:1810–1823.

137. Fischle W, Dequiedt F, Hendzel MJ, et al. Enzymatic activity associated with class II HDACs is dependent on a multiprotein complex containing HDAC3 and SMRT/N-CoR. Mol Cell 2002;9:45–57.

138. Naya FJ, Olson E. MEF2: a transcriptional target for signaling pathways controlling skeletal muscle growth and differentiation. Curr Opin Cell Biol 1999;11:683–688.

139. McKinsey TA, Zhang CL, Olson EN. Control of muscle development by dueling HATs and HDACs. Curr Opin Genet Dev 2001;11:497–504.

140. Lu J, McKinsey TA, Zhang CL, Olson EN. Regulation of skeletal myogenesis by association of the MEF2 transcription factor with class II histone deacetylases. Mol Cell 2000;6:233–244.

141. Dressel U, Bailey PJ, Wang SC, Downes M, Evans RM, Muscat GE. A dynamic role for HDAC7 in MEF2-mediated muscle differentiation. J Biol Chem 2001;276:17,007–17,013.

142. Li X, Song S, Liu Y, Ko SH, Kao HY. Phosphorylation of the histone deacetylase 7 modulates its stability and association with 14-3-3 proteins. J Biol Chem 2004;279:34,201–34,208.

143. Zhang CL, McKinsey TA, Lu JR, Olson EN. Association of COOH-terminal-binding protein (CtBP) and MEF2-interacting transcription repressor (MITR) contributes to transcriptional repression of the MEF2 transcription factor. J Biol Chem 2001;276:35–39.

144. Zhang CL, McKinsey TA, Olson EN. Association of class II histone deacetylases with heterochromatin protein 1: potential role for histone methylation in control of muscle differentiation. Mol Cell Biol 2002;22:7302–7312.

145. Bannister AJ, Zegerman P, Partridge JF, et al. Selective recognition of methylated lysine 9 on histone H3 by the HP1 chromo domain. Nature 2001;410:120–124.
146. Lachner M, O'Carroll D, Rea S, Mechtler K, Jenuwein T. Methylation of histone H3 lysine 9 creates a binding site for HP1 proteins. Nature 2001;410:116.
147. Vega RB, Matsuda K, Oh J, et al. Histone deacetylase 4 controls chondrocyte hypertrophy during skeletogenesis. Cell 2004;119:555–566.
148. Kawaguchi Y, Kovacs JJ, McLaurin A, Vance JM, Ito A, Yao TP. The deacetylase HDAC6 regulates aggresome formation and cell viability in response to misfolded protein stress. Cell 2003;115:727–738.
149. Zhang Y, Li N, Caron C, et al. HDAC-6 interacts with and deacetylates tubulin and microtubules in vivo. EMBO J 2003;22:1168–1179.
150. Matsuyama A, Shimazu T, Sumida Y, et al. In vivo destabilization of dynamic microtubules by HDAC6-mediated deacetylation. EMBO J 2002;21:6820–6831.
151. Hook SS, Orian A, Cowley SM, Eisenman RN. Histone deacetylase 6 binds polyubiquitin through its zinc finger (PAZ domain) and copurifies with deubiquitinating enzymes. Proc Natl Acad Sci U S A 2002;99:13,425–13,430.
152. Hubbert C, Guardiola A, Shao R, et al. HDAC6 is a microtubule-associated deacetylase. Nature 2002;417:455–458.
153. Tran PB, Miller RJ. Aggregates in neurodegenerative disease: crowds and power? Trends Neurosci 1999;22:194–197.
154. Gartenberg MR. The Sir proteins of *Saccharomyces cerevisiae*: mediators of transcriptional silencing and much more. Curr Opin Microbiol 2000;3:132–137.
155. Guarente L. Sir2 links chromatin silencing, metabolism, and aging. Genes Dev 2000;14:1021–1026.
156. Imai S, Armstrong CM, Kaeberlein M, Guarente L. Transcriptional silencing and longevity protein Sir2 is an NAD-dependent histone deacetylase. Nature 2000;403:795–800.
157. Frye RA. Characterization of five human cDNAs with homology to the yeast SIR2 gene: Sir2-like proteins (sirtuins) metabolize NAD and may have protein ADP-ribosyltransferase activity. Biochem Biophys Res Commun 1999;260:273–279.
158. Frye RA. Phylogenetic classification of prokaryotic and eukaryotic Sir2-like proteins. Biochem Biophys Res Commun 2000;273:793–798.
159. Guarente L. Diverse and dynamic functions of the Sir silencing complex. Nat Genet 1999;23:281–285.
160. Cockell MM, Gasser SM. The nucleolus: nucleolar space for RENT. Curr Biol 1999;9:R575, R576.
161. Gottschling DE. Gene silencing: two faces of SIR2. Curr Biol 2000;10:R708–R711.
162. Moazed D. Enzymatic activities of Sir2 and chromatin silencing. Curr Opin Cell Biol 2001;13:232–238.
163. Ghidelli S, Donze D, Dhillon N, Kamakaka RT. Sir2p exists in two nucleosome-binding complexes with distinct deacetylase activities. EMBO J 2001;20:4522–4535.
164. Straight AF, Shou W, Dowd GJ, et al. Net1, a Sir2-associated nucleolar protein required for rDNA silencing and nucleolar integrity. Cell 1999;97:245–256.
165. Shou W, Seol JH, Shevchenko A, et al. Exit from mitosis is triggered by Tem1-dependent release of the protein phosphatase Cdc14 from nucleolar RENT complex. Cell 1999;97:233–244.
166. Hecht A, Strahl-Bolsinger S, Grunstein M. Spreading of transcriptional repressor SIR3 from telomeric heterochromatin. Nature 1996;383:92–96.

167. Moazed D, Johnson D. A deubiquitinating enzyme interacts with SIR4 and regulates silencing in *S. cerevisiae*. Cell 1996;86:667–677.
168. Tollervey D, Hurt EC. The role of small nucleolar ribonucleoproteins in ribosome synthesis.
169. Taylor GS, Liu Y, Baskerville C, Charbonneau H. The activity of Cdc14p, an oligomeric dual specificity protein phosphatase from *Saccharomyces cerevisiae*, is required for cell cycle progression. J Biol Chem 1997;272:24,054–24,063.
170. Shou W, Sakamoto KM, Keener J, et al. Net1 stimulates RNA polymerase I transcription and regulates nucleolar structure independently of controlling mitotic exit. Mol Cell 2001;8:45–55.
171. Xie J, Pierce M, Gailus-Durner V, Wagner M, Winter E, Vershon AK. Sum1 and Hst1 repress middle sporulation-specific gene expression during mitosis in *Saccharomyces cerevisiae*. EMBO J 1999;18:6448–6454.
172. Sutton A, Heller RC, Landry J, Choy JS, Sirko A, Sternglanz R. A novel form of transcriptional silencing by Sum1-1 requires Hst1 and the origin recognition complex. Mol Cell Biol 2001;21:3514–3522.
173. Robert F, Pokholok DK, Hannett NM, et al. Global position and recruitment of HATs and HDACs in the yeast genome. Mol Cell 2004;16:199–209.
174. Blander G, Guarente L. The Sir2 family of protein deacetylases. Annu Rev Biochem 2004;73:417–435.
175. Vaquero A, Scher M, Lee D, Erdjument-Bromage H, Tempst P, Reinberg D. Human SirT1 interacts with histone H1 and promotes formation of facultative heterochromatin. Mol Cell 2004;16:93–105.
176. Vaziri H, Dessain SK, Ng Eaton E, et al. hSIR2(SIRT1) functions as an NAD-dependent p53 deacetylase. Cell 2001;107:149–159.
177. Luo J, Nikolaev AY, Imai S, et al. Negative control of p53 by Sir2alpha promotes cell survival under stress. Cell 2001;107:137–148.
178. Muth V, Nadaud S, Grummt I, Voit R. Acetylation of TAF(I)68, a subunit of TIF-IB/SL1, activates RNA polymerase I transcription. EMBO J 2001;20:1353–1362.
179. Bereshchenko OR, Gu W, Dalla-Favera R. Acetylation inactivates the transcriptional repressor BCL6. Nat Genet 2002;32:606–613.
180. Brunet A, Sweeney LB, Sturgill JF, et al. Stress-dependent regulation of FOXO transcription factors by the SIRT1 deacetylase. Science 2004;303:2011–2015.
181. Motta MC, Divecha N, Lemieux M, et al. Mammalian SIRT1 represses forkhead transcription factors. Cell 2004;116:551–563.
182. Cohen HY, Miller C, Bitterman KJ, et al. Calorie restriction promotes mammalian cell survival by inducing the SIRT1 deacetylase. Science 2004;305:390–392.
183. Yeung F, Hoberg JE, Ramsey CS, et al. Modulation of NF-kappaB-dependent transcription and cell survival by the SIRT1 deacetylase. EMBO J 2004;23:2369–2380.
184. Fulco M, Schiltz RL, Iezzi S, et al. Sir2 regulates skeletal muscle differentiation as a potential sensor of the redox state. Mol Cell 2003;12:51–62.
185. Araki T, Sasaki Y, Milbrandt J. Increased nuclear NAD biosynthesis and SIRT1 activation prevent axonal degeneration. Science 2004;305:1010–1013.
186. Senawong T, Peterson VJ, Avram D, et al. Involvement of the histone deacetylase SIRT1 in chicken ovalbumin upstream promoter transcription factor (COUP-TF)-interacting protein 2-mediated transcriptional repression. J Biol Chem 2003;278:43,041–43,050.
187. Takata T, Ishikawa F. Human Sir2-related protein SIRT1 associates with the bHLH repressors HES1 and HEY2 and is involved in HES1- and HEY2-mediated transcriptional repression. Biochem Biophys Res Commun 2003;301:250–257.

188. Picard F, Kurtev M, Chung N, et al. Sirt1 promotes fat mobilization in white adipocytes by repressing PPAR-gamma. Nature 2004;429:771–776.
189. Zhao K, Chai X, Clements A, Marmorstein R. Structure and autoregulation of the yeast Hst2 homolog of Sir2. Nat Struct Biol 2003;10:864–871.
190. Landry J, Sutton A, Tafrov ST, et al. The silencing protein SIR2 and its homologs are NAD-dependent protein deacetylases. Proc Natl Acad Sci U S A 2000;97: 5807–5811.
191. Perrod S, Cockell MM, Laroche T, et al. A cytosolic NAD-dependent deacetylase, Hst2p, can modulate nucleolar and telomeric silencing in yeast. EMBO J 2001;20:197–209.
192. Halme A, Bumgarner S, Styles C, Fink GR. Genetic and epigenetic regulation of the FLO gene family generates cell-surface variation in yeast. Cell 2004;116: 405–415.
193. North BJ, Marshall BL, Borra MT, Denu JM, Verdin E. The human Sir2 ortholog, SIRT2, is an NAD$^+$-dependent tubulin deacetylase. Mol Cell 2003;11:437–444.
194. Dryden SC, Nahhas FA, Nowak JE, Goustin AS, Tainsky MA. Role for human SIRT2 NAD-dependent deacetylase activity in control of mitotic exit in the cell cycle. Mol Cell Biol 2003;23:3173–3185.
195. Borra MT, O'Neill FJ, Jackson MD, et al. Conserved enzymatic production and biological effect of O-acetyl-ADP-ribose by silent information regulator 2-like NAD$^+$-dependent deacetylases. J Biol Chem 2002;277:12,632–12,641.
196. Onyango P, Celic I, McCaffery JM, Boeke JD, Feinberg AP. SIRT3, a human SIR2 homologue, is an NAD-dependent deacetylase localized to mitochondria. Proc Natl Acad Sci U S A 2002;99:13,653–13,658.
197. Schwer B, North BJ, Frye RA, Ott M, Verdin E. The human silent information regulator (Sir)2 homologue hSIRT3 is a mitochondrial nicotinamide adenine dinucleotide-dependent deacetylase. J Cell Biol 2002;158:647–657.

3 The Biology of HDAC3

Edward Seto, PhD

Contents

SUMMARY

Histone deacetylase 3 (HDAC3) is one of four members of the human class I histone deacetylases that repress transcription by deacetylation of histones. This review describes our current knowledge regarding its structure, function, mechanisms of action, and regulation.

Key Words: HDAC3, transcription regulation, histone modification, NCoR/SMRT.

INTRODUCTION

In 1996, a major breakthrough in the study of histone deacetylase (HDAC) came with the purification and cloning of the first human HDAC

From: *Cancer Drug Discovery and Development*
Histone Deacetylases: *Transcriptional Regulation and Other Cellular Functions*
Edited by: E. Verdin © Humana Press Inc., Totowa, NJ

Acronyms and Abbreviations

AML-MTG16	Acute myelogenous leukemia-myeloid translocation gene 16
Arg	Arginine
Bmal1	Brain and muscle Arnt-like protein 1
cDNA	Complementary DNA
ChIP	Chromatin immunoprecipitation
COUP-TF	Chicken ovalbumin upstream promoter transcription factor
CRM1	Chromosome region maintenance 1
DAD	Deacetylase-activating domain
DAX1	Dosage sensitive sex reversal (adrenal hypoplasia congenita gene on the X chromosome)
DFNA1	Deafness, autosomal dominant nonsyndromic sensorineural 1
Dlk1	Delta-like 1
EGF	Epidermal growth factor
ER-α	Estrogen receptor-α
FISH	Fluorescence *in situ* hybridization
GATA-1	GATA-binding transcription factor 1
GDF11	Growth/differentiation factor 11
GM-CSF	Granulocyte/macrophage colony-stimulating factor
GPS2	G protein pathway suppressor 2
GRIA1	Glutamate receptor, ionotropic, AMPA 1
HDA	Histone deacetylase A
HDAC	Histone deacetylase
HOS	HDA one similar
HSP70	Heat shock protein 70
HSPC	Hematopoietic stem progentior cell
IITLV1	Human T-cell leukemia virus type 1
ICSBP	Interferon consensus sequence-binding protein
IE1	Immediate-early 1
IFN-γ	Interferon-γ
IL-1β	Interleukin-1β
IκBα	Inhibitor of κ Bα
JDP2	Jun dimerization protein 2
JNK	c-Jun amino-terminal kinase
KLF6	Krüppel-like factor-6

(Continued on p. 64)

enzyme, HDAC1 (originally called HD1) *(1)*. The predicted amino acid sequence derived from the complete cDNA sequence of HDAC1 revealed a high degree of similarity to the yeast transcriptional regulator RPD3 *(2)*. That same year, a transcriptional corepressor protein (later called HDAC2), also with high homology to yeast RPD3, was identified from a yeast two-hybrid experiment with the human YY1 transcription factor *(3)*. Similar to previous experiments used to characterize HDAC1, immuno-precipitation of HDAC2 from human cells followed by enzymatic assays showed that HDAC2 contained HDAC activity *(4)*. HDAC1 and HDAC2 exist together in multiprotein complexes, and many transcription factors target HDAC1 and HDAC2 to specific promoters to repress transcription (reviewed in refs. *5* and *6*).

The excitement in the HDAC field did not end with the discoveries of HDAC1 and HDAC2. Shortly afterward, three papers independently reported the findings of an additional human HDAC, HDAC3. By screening the NCBI database of expressed sequence tags, two groups found several cDNAs that encode a protein, HDAC3, with similarity to the yeast RPD3 yet distinct from HDAC1 and HDAC2 *(4,7)*. Using mRNA differential display, a third group independently identified HDAC3 in phyto-hemaggtutinin (PHA)-activated T cells *(8)*. The discovery of HDAC3 immediately introduced another layer of complexity to the studies of HDAC and opened up new opportunities to explore additional mechanisms by which HDACs might regulate gene expression. Many unexpected and exceedingly interesting findings resulted from attempts to understand the functions and mechanisms of action of HDAC3. In the following sections, I will review the work from many different laboratories that contributed to our current understanding of this fascinating protein.

GENE AND PROTEIN STRUCTURE OF HDAC3

The predicted amino acid sequence of HDAC3 has an open reading frame of 428 residues with a theoretical molecular mass of 49 kDa and a calculated isoelectric point of 4.9 *(4,7,8)*. A protein motif search (http://hits.isb-sib.ch) revealed that HDAC3 has a conserved HDAC domain (residues 4–316) and one repeat unit of the Pumilio RNA-binding domain (residues 182–200). The RNA binding domain of the *Drosophila* Pumilio protein regulates mRNA translation and stability by binding to a specific sequence in the 3′ untranslated region of mRNA *(9–13)*. It consists of eight imperfect repeats of about 35 amino acids and has been found in a number of eukaryotic proteins. The significance of the presence of a single repeat in HDAC3 is not known at this time.

In humans, close to 20 HDACs have been identified to date, and they can be divided into at least three classes *(14–18)*. Within class I HDACs

Acronyms and Abbreviations *(Continued)*

MAPKK	Mitogen-activated protein kinase kinase
MusTRD1/BEN	Muscle transcription factor II-I repeat domain-containing protein 1/binding factor for early enhancer
MYC	Myelocytomatosis oncogene
NCBI	National Center for Biotechnology Information
NCoR	Nuclear receptor corepressor
NF-κB	Nuclear factor κB
PBMC	Peripheral blood mononuclear cell
PHA	Phytohemagglutinin
PIAS	Protein inhibitor of activated STAT
Pit-1	Pituitary-specific transcription factor
PMA	Phorbol-12-myristate-13-acetate
PP4	Protein serine/threonine phosphatase 4
PPAR-γ	Peroxisome proliferator-activated receptor-γ
Rb	Retinoblastoma tumor suppressor protein
RbAp48	Rb-associated protein 48
RBP1	Retinoblastoma-binding protein 1
RelA	v-rel reticuloendotheliosis viral oncogene homolog A
RIP140	Receptor-interacting protein 140
RPD3	Reduced potassium dependency 3
SANT	SWI-SNF, ADA, NCoR, TFIIB
SET	Suppressor of position effect variegation 3-9, enhancer-of-zeste, trithorax
siRNA	Small-interfering RNA (also known as short-interfering RNA)
SIRT	Sirtuin
SMRT	Silencing mediator of retinoid and thyroid hormone receptors
SNP	Single-nucleotide polymorphism
SSCP	Single-strand conformation polymorphism
STAT1	Signal transducer and activator of transcription 1
SUMO	Small ubiquitin-like modifier
TAB2	TAK1 (transforming growth factor-β-activated kinase 1)-binding protein 2
TBL1	Transducin-β-like protein 1
TBLR1	TBL1-related protein

(Continued on p. 66)

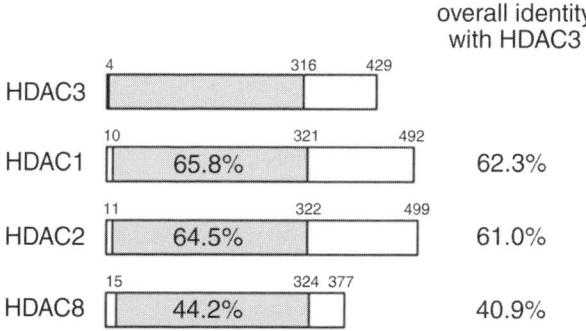

overall identity
with HDAC3

Fig. 1. Schematic representation of the relationship between the different human class I HDACs. HDAC3, HDAC1, HDAC2, and HDAC8 sequences were obtained from GeneBank accession numbers U75697, U50079, U31814, and AF230097, respectively. Percentages refer to the amino acid sequence identities as calculated by the LASERGENE Navigator sequence analysis program. The putative HDAC catalytic domains are shaded.

(HDAC1, HDAC2, HDAC3, and HDAC8), HDAC3 shares more similarity with HDAC1 and HDAC2 than with HDAC8 (Fig. 1). Uniquely, HDAC3 lacks a small segment corresponding to the extreme N termini of HDAC1, HDAC2, and HDAC8. Regions that correspond to the C termini of HDAC1 (residues 399–482) and HDAC2 (residues 400–488) also are absent in HDAC3, and the last 34 residues of HDAC3 have no similarity to any known proteins. These observations suggest that the two ends of the HDAC3 protein possess unique functions that are distinct from other class I HDACs.

Like all other class I HDACs, the HDAC domain in human HDAC3 (residues 4–316) possesses homology to the HDAC domains in human class II HDACs (HDAC4, HDAC5, HDAC6, HDAC7, HDAC9, and HDAC10) and to HDAC11, but the homology does not extend outside the conserved HDAC domains. Also similar to other class I HDACs, no significant homology exists between HDAC3 and the class III enzymes (SIRT1–7).

Both HDAC3 mRNA and protein are ubiquitously expressed in a wide variety of human cell lines and tissues *(4,7,8)*. In addition to humans, HDAC3 has been identified (and in most cases cloned) in many different organisms including mouse *(19,20)*, rat *(21)*, *Drosophila (22)*, and *Caenorhabditis elegans (23,24)*. As expected for a protein with critical biological functions, human and mouse HDAC3 are nearly identical, and the conservation extends to lower organisms. Phylogenetic analysis suggests that the existence of HDAC3 may even extend to single-cell organisms *(18)*. In yeast, HOS1, HOS2, and HOS3 share similarity with RPD3

Acronyms and Abbreviations *(Continued)*	
TCP-1	T-complex protein 1
TEL	Translocation-ETS-leukemia (or ETV6)
TFII-I	Transcription factor II-I
THAP7	Thanatos-associated protein 7
TNF-α	Tumor necrosis factor-α
TR/RXR	Thyroid hormone receptor/retinoid X receptor
TriC	TCP-1 ring complex
WD	Tryptophan, aspartic acid
YY1	Yin yang 1

Table 1
HDAC3 Identity Between Humans and Other Species

Species	Identity (%)
Mus musculus (NP034541)	99.8
Rattus norvegicus (NP445900)	99.5
Drosophila melanogaster (NP651978)	66.7
Caenorhabditis elegans (NP493026)	55.1
Saccharomyces cerevisiae RPD3/HOS2 (NP014069/NP011321)	58.1/52.4

and HDA1 *(25,26)*. Besides RPD3, human HDAC3 displays significant homology to yeast HOS2 (Table 1).

Isolation and a detailed analysis of human HDAC3 genomic clones showed that HDAC3 is a single-copy gene that spans over 13 kb and contains 15 exons ranging in size from 56 to 657 bp *(27)*. Fluorescence *in situ* hybridization (FISH) unambiguously localized the HDAC3 gene to chromosome 5q31, a region of the genome implicated in many human disorders including asthma, inherited deafness, acute myelogenous leukemia, large cell lymphoma, and myelodysplastic syndrome (*see* http://ncbi.nlm. nih.gov/Omim/getmap.cgi?l604417). Identical FISH results were obtained using human HDAC3 cDNA probes *(20,28)*. Further high-resolution physical mapping localized human HDAC3 exactly between the CD14 and GRIA1 genes within the 5q31.1 subband *(29)*. Using *in situ* hybridization, the mouse HDAC3 gene was localized to chromosome 18B3, which is syntenic with the distal portion of human chromosome 5q *(30)*. Single-strand conformation polymorphism (SSCP) analysis together with the NCBI Map Manager program confirmed the location of the mouse HDAC3 gene at chromosome 18 *(20)*.

The initial cloning of human HDAC3 uncovered cDNAs with different 5′ ends that potentially encode two additional HDAC3s with slightly different N termini *(4)*. Whether these two different forms of HDAC3 mRNA are caused by alternative splicing or other posttranscriptional modifications and whether they are expressed as protein products in the cell is not known at this time. Another isoform of human HDAC3, in which exon 3 is alternatively spliced from the rest of the transcript, was later identified by Gray et al. *(31)*.

The genomic region of human HDAC3 contains seven mapped single-nucleotide polymorphisms (SNPs) near its locus, one of which falls within the coding region. A G-to-C substitution at nucleotide 849 that results in an arginine to proline change in residue 265 of the HDAC3 protein has been reported *(32)*. Because Arg265 of HDAC3 is conserved in HDAC1 and HDAC2, and this position is occupied by proline in HDAC8 and most class II HDACs, it was speculated that this SNP might be functionally relevant to the HDAC3 protein.

To facilitate the identification of structural-functional motifs in HDAC3, Yang et al. *(33)* constructed a series of HDAC3 deletion mutants and assayed for their histone deacetylation activities, abilities to repress transcription, nuclear/cytoplasmic localization, and abilities to oligomerize. The results indicated that some activities reside in independent, nonoverlapping domains within HDAC3 (Fig. 2). An HDAC3 point mutant reveals that the conserved HDAC domain within HDAC3 is required for deacetylase activity *(34)*. However, it is not known whether the HDAC domain alone is sufficient for enzymatic activity. Clearly, small deletions in the extreme C terminus of HDAC3 outside of the conserved HDAC domain significantly reduced enzymatic and transcriptional repression activity, suggesting that the nonconserved portion of HDAC3 contributes to the overall activity of the protein *(33,35)*. It also is possible that HDAC3 activity is highly sensitive to structural conformation and that deletion of the extreme C terminus of HDAC3 changes the natural conformation of the protein, rendering it inactive. To clarify the exact function of the HDAC domain, it would be useful to perform experiments involving swapping HDAC domains between HDAC3 and other HDACs.

In most cell types, HDAC3 is located both in the nucleus and cytoplasm, and its subcellular distribution is regulated by competing nuclear import and export signals. Although a sequence present at position 29 to 41 of HDAC3 (LALTHSLVLHYGL) resembles the canonical nuclear

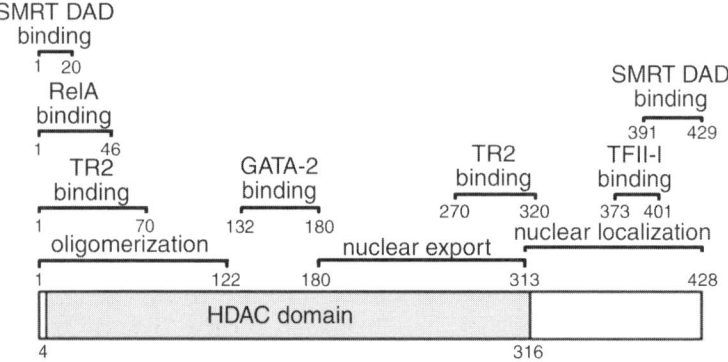

Fig. 2. Schematic diagram of the HDAC3 protein with multiple functional domains indicated. In the case of protein binding regions, the amino acid residues indicate only the minimal essential sequences. In most cases, additional sequences are required for efficient protein-protein interactions. For abbreviations, *see* Acronyms and Abbreviations, pp. 62, 64.

export signal, the actual functional nuclear export signal resides between residues 180 and 313 *(33)*. In addition, residues 313 to 428 of HDAC3 are crucial for nuclear localization. HDAC3 can self-associate into dimers and trimers in vitro and in vivo. Analysis of the same deletion mutants for elucidation of import/export domains revealed that the N terminus of HDAC3 (residues 1–122), a region essential for cell viability *(35)*, is necessary and sufficient for HDAC3 oligomerization. Therefore, the HDAC3 protein can be divided roughly into three parts, with the N-terminal portion important for oligomerization, the middle part for nuclear export, and the C-terminal segment for nuclear localization.

TARGETS OF HDAC3

Immediately after the identification of HDAC3, two questions became obvious: (1) Why is there more than one HDAC? and (2) Does HDAC3 uniquely deacetylate a subset of histones or certain lysines on histones differently from those of HDAC1 and HDAC2? Using an immunoprecipitated HDAC3 complex and purified nucleosomes, Emiliani et al. concluded that HDAC3 deacetylates histone H4 more efficiently than HDAC1 *(7)*. In a similar study, HDAC3 immunocomplexes completely deacetylated H2A, H4K5, and H4K12, but only partially deacetylated H3, H2B, H4K8, and H4K16 *(36)*. Interestingly, compared with immunoprecipitated HDAC1, HDAC3 immunoprecipitated from HeLa cells preferentially deacetylated H4K5, H4K12, and H2AK5. These studies provided reasonable evidence that HDAC3 has substrate specificity and might possess unique functions that are not shared with HDAC1 and other HDACs.

However, it is known that immunoprecipitated HDAC3 complexes contain many other proteins with HDAC activity *(37–39)*, thereby complicating the interpretation of these earlier results. In fact, in a study with homozygous chicken HDAC3-deficient DT40 cells, the acetylation levels of H4K8 and H4K12 remained intact compared with wild-type cells, suggesting that histone H4 might not be a major target of HDAC3 *(35)*. Also, in an in vitro reconstituted chromatin system, an HDAC3-containing protein complex selectively deacetylated histone H3, whereas a complex containing HDAC1/2 deacetylated both histones H3 and H4 *(40)*.

Using chromatin immunoprecipitation (ChIP) assays with *hos2Δ*, *rpd3Δ*, and *hos2Δrpd3Δ* mutant yeast strains, it was found that disruption of HOS2 and RPD3 resulted in a preferential hyperacetylation of all lysines tested on histones H3 and H4 in the *ERG11* gene *(41)*. Hyperacetylation owing to disruption of HOS2 is especially pronounced for H4K16. Unlike *Saccharomyes cerevisiae*, depletion of HDAC3 with RNAi in HeLa cells had no effect on the overall acetylation status of histones H3 or H4 or the acetylation of H4K8 or H4K12 *(42)*. However, expression of HDAC1 or HDAC3 siRNA (but not HDAC2 siRNA) increased the acetylation of H3K9 and H3K18. HDAC3 siRNA increased the acetylation of H3K9 to a greater extent than did HDAC1 siRNA, whereas the reverse was true for H3K18. Although these divergent results are quite confusing, they do support the general conclusion that the function of HDAC3 is not redundant. The possibility that HDAC3 targets specific lysines in certain histones warrants a more comprehensive investigation.

Consistent with the predicted function for HDACs, HDAC3 represses transcription when targeted to promoters and serves as a corepressor of multiple nuclear hormone receptors *(4,43)*. It is reasonable to say that some of the chief targets of HDAC3 are nuclear hormone receptor-regulated genes. Overexpression of HDAC3 by transient transfection can repress many cellular and viral promoters, as determined by reporter assays. Presumably, many more target genes regulated by HDAC3 under physiological conditions in the cell remain to be determined. In one study, Zhang et al. found that the growth/differentiation factor 11 (Gdf11) gene was downregulated by overexpression of HDAC3 but not by any other HDACs tested *(42)*. Importantly, depletion of HDAC3 with RNAi in HeLa cells resulted in activation of the *Gdf11* promoter.

Paradoxically, HDAC3 also is required for transcriptional activation of at least one class of retinoic acid response elements *(44)*. Furthermore, silencing of HDAC3 using RNAi markedly decreased interferon-γ (IFN-γ)-driven gene activation, and overexpression of HDAC3 enhanced signal transducer and activator of infection 1 (STAT1)-dependent transcriptional activity *(45)*. In a search for genes whose acetylation state is altered upon deletion of HOS2, Wang et al. found that within the yeast genome, HOS2 preferentially associates with the coding regions of genes with high transcriptional activity *(41)*. Furthermore, HOS2 is important for activation of *GAL1* and *INO1* genes in vivo. It was hypothesized that HOS2 is required for gene activation by reverting disrupted chromatin to the original permissive state required for efficient transcription. Because HOS2 possesses significant homology to HDAC3 and is directly required for gene activation, the assumption that HDAC3 is targeted to genes for repression may be oversimplified. Clearly, there is a definite need to decipher human HDAC3 target genes in more detail and to determine how these genes are regulated by HDAC3.

HDAC3 INTERACTING PROTEINS

One of the biggest challenges in the study of HDAC3, as in the study of other HDACs, is to understand the exact mechanisms by which HDAC3 changes gene expression and how it affects the functions of the transcriptional machinery. Early in the studies of HDACs, the identification and characterization of HDAC1/2 binding proteins were tremendously useful in elucidating the mechanisms of action and functions of these two HDACs. Following similar strategies, Wen et al. isolated a large HDAC3-containing multisubunit complex using anti-HDAC3 immunoaffinity chromatography (Table 2) *(34,46)*. The purified endogenous HDAC3 complex from HeLa cells contained nuclear receptor corepressor (NCoR) and silencing mediator for retinoid and thyroid receptors (SMRT) proteins. In parallel, NCoR and SMRT were identified in an anti-Flag affinity-purified complex from nuclear extracts of a cell line expressing Flag-tagged HDAC3 *(47)*. Further evidence that HDAC3 stably associates with SMRT and NCoR came from the purification of SMRT/NCoR complexes using anti-SMRT/NCoR affinity chromatography *(47–51)*. HDAC3 and SMRT were also copurified through multiple conventional chromatographic steps and coeluted from gel-filtration columns as 1 to 2-MDa complexes. The yeast analog of the mammalian HDAC3/SMRT/NCoR complex, SET3C, contains HOS2 and a large protein with the SANT domain, SNT1, reminiscent of NCoR/SMRT *(52)*.

Originally, NCoR and SMRT were identified in yeast two-hybrid screens using unliganded thyroid hormone receptor (TR) and retinoic acid receptor (RAR), respectively, as bait *(53,54)*. They associated with and served as effective corepressors not only for DNA-bound, unliganded nuclear hormone receptors, but also for many other transcription factors including Rev-Erb, chicken ovalbumin upstream promoter transcription factor (COUP-TF), DAX1, MAD, and Pit-1 *(55,56)*. Although NCoR/SMRT have been reported to partner with HDAC1, -2, -4, -5, and -7

Table 2
HDAC3 Protein Complexes

Reference	Protein source	Purification method	Proteins identified
34,46	HeLa whole cell extract	Anti-HDAC3 immunoaffinity	HDAC3 NCoR/SMRT TFII-I
47	Nuclear extract from Flag-HDAC3 HeLa stable cell line	Anti-Flag immunoaffinity	HDAC3 NCoR/SMRT TBL1/TBLR1 GPS2
48,49	HeLa nuclear extract	Conventional chromatography followed by anti-SMRT immunoaffinity	HDAC3 SMRT TBL1
49,51	HeLa nuclear extract	Conventional chromatography followed by anti-NCoR immunoaffinity	HDAC3 NCoR TBL1/TBLR1 IR10 GPS2
50	HeLa nuclear extract	Conventional chromatography followed by anti-NCoR immunoaffinity	HDAC3 N-CoR SWI/SNF related BAF170 BAF155 Splicing factors KAP-1 BAF47
52	Extract from HOS2-TAP transformed yeast cells	TAP	HOS2 SNT1 YIL112 SET3 SIF2 HST1 CPR1 TriC complex

(38,39,50,57–61), HDAC3 appears to form the most stable complex with NCoR/SMRT. Therefore, it is reasonable to predict that HDAC3 is the main component recruited by DNA binding factors that utilize NCoR or SMRT to repress transcription. Indeed, microinjection of antibodies against HDAC3 led to the relief of NCoR/SMRT-dependent repression by

Pit-1 and TR/RXR *(46,49)*, and knockdown of HDAC3 by siRNA markedly inhibited repression by TR and Rev-Erb *(43,51)*. Furthermore, using ChIP, it was demonstrated that HDAC3-containing SMRT and NCoR complexes are actively recruited by unliganded TR *(43,49)*. Together, these results impart an unsophisticated model whereby SMRT and NCoR function as platforms for recruitment of HDAC3 to deacetylate chromatin and consequently repress transcription.

TBL1, a transducin-β like protein that contains six WD-40 repeats, and a TBL1-related protein (TBLR1) are components commonly found associated with the HDAC3/SMRT/NCoR complex *(47–49,51)*. TBL1 and TBLR1 are equally represented in both immunopurified HDAC3 and NCoR complexes *(47)*. Although it has been suggested that TBL1 possesses histone binding activity *(48,51)*, at this time, the exact functional role of TBL1 in the HDAC3/NCoR/SMRT complex remains to be determined. However, it is intriguing that mutation of the human TBL1 gene is associated with X-linked late-onset sensorineural deafness *(62)* and deafness is one of the phenotypes in mice with a deleted TRβ gene *(63)*. Also, the *DFNA1* gene responsible for the autosomal dominant, fully penetrant and nonsyndromic sensorineural progressive hearing loss in a large Costa Rican family was localized to chromosome 5q31, the same region as the HDAC3 gene *(64,65)*.

In the immunoaffinity purification using anti-HDAC3, in addition to NCoR/SMRT, the transcription factor TFII-I copurified with HDAC3 *(34)*. TFII-I was originally isolated as a basal transcription factor that binds to and activates transcription from the initiator element *(66)*. Subsequent studies, however, suggest that TFII-I is an inducible factor that selectively regulates gene expression when activated by a variety of extracellular signals *(67)*. Immunoprecipitation of a TFII-I complex revealed HDAC activity, and HDAC3 was demonstrated to regulate TFII-I transcriptional activity negatively *(34)*. In a separate study, Tussie-Luna et al. discovered that TFII-I and a related protein, hMusTRD1/BEN, physically and functionally interact with HDAC3 *(68)*. Interestingly, a TFII-I-binding protein, PIASxβ which is involved in the small ubiquitin-like modifier (SUMO) pathway, also interacts with HDAC3 and relieves the transcriptional repression exerted by HDAC3 upon TFII-I-mediated gene activation. Together, these two studies suggest that HDAC3 is a key regulator of TFII-I activity.

Results from several studies, mostly relying on overexpression coupled with coimmunoprecipitation, suggest that HDAC3 binds HDAC4, -5, -7, -9, and -10 *(37–39,69–71)*. It was proposed that class II HDACs, particularly HDAC4, -5, and -7, are strictly dependent on their ability to interact with SMRT/NCoR and HDAC3 proteins in order to exhibit HDAC activity *(39)*. However, it is important to note that isolation of endogenous HDAC3 or NCoR/SMRT complexes containing high HDAC activity did not yield any class II HDACs, implying that the interactions of HDAC3 with HDAC4, -5, and -7 could be transient or that only a very small fraction of HDAC3/NCoR/SMRT complexes might associate with class II HDACs under physiological conditions. Until successful purification of endogenous class II HDAC complexes, it will be difficult to assess the exact contribution of HDAC3 to class II enzymatic activity. Conceivably, association with HDAC3 is only one of many mechanisms by which some class II HDAC activities could be regulated. In addition to class II HDACs, HDAC3 has also been reported to interact with HDAC1 in vitro, although the significance of this interaction is entirely unknown at this time *(72,73)*.

Besides proteins that copurified with the HDAC3/NCoR/SMRT complex, a long list of proteins has been reported to associate with HDAC3 without participating in a stable multisubunit complex. Proteins that bind HDAC3 and, in some cases, recruit deacetylase activity as a negative regulator of transcription include YY1 *(4)*, RIP140 *(74,75)*, TR2 *(76,77)*, PPAR-γ *(78,79)*, ER-α *(80)*, cyclin D1 *(81,81a)*, TEL *(82)*, ICSBP *(83)*, AML-MTG16 fusion *(84)*, GATA-1 *(85)*, GATA-2 *(86)*, Rb *(87)*, RbAp48 *(88)*, RBP1 *(87,89)*, Suv39H1 *(90)*, c-Jun *(91)*, JDP2 *(92)*, RelA *(93)*, and Hsp70 *(36)*. In the case of the HDAC3-TR2 interaction, the HDAC-interacting domain is located in the zinc finger DNA binding region of the nuclear receptor; and the receptor-interacting domains of HDAC3 were mapped to residues 1 to 70 and 270 to 320 of HDAC3 (Fig. 2) *(77,94)*. Unlike HDAC3-TR2, the interaction of HDAC3 with GATA-2 requires residues 132 to 180 of HDAC3 *(86)*.

Most of the HDAC3-interacting proteins associate with other HDACs in addition to HDAC3. For example, YY1, RBP1, RbAp48, Suv39H1, and Hsp70 bind HDAC1 and HDAC2, in addition to partnering with HDAC3. As mentioned before, NCoR/SMRT, which partners with HDAC3, also forms separate complexes with HDAC1, -2, -4, -5, and -7. In conclusion, it is clear at this point that many proteins function through interaction with HDAC3 and that HDAC3 is a major player in transcriptional repression. Efforts in the field should now be directed toward the identification of developmental and signaling pathways that could be activated or repressed by the different repressor/corepressor-HDAC3 complexes.

HDAC3 IN SIGNALING PATHWAYS

GPS2 (G protein pathway suppressor 2) cDNA was originally isolated from yeast as a suppressor of lethal G-protein subunit-activating mutations in the pheromone response pathway *(95)*. When overexpressed in mammalian cells, GPS2 potently suppressed RAS- and mitogen-activated protein kinase-mediated signals and interfered with JNK activity. Human

GPS2 has the ability to bind to the HTLV-1 oncoprotein Tax, and suppress Tax activation of JNK1 *(96)*. GPS2 also binds the acetyltransferase p300 and facilitates its recruitment into complexes with the papillomavirus E2 protein for transcriptional activation *(97)*. The E6 protein of papillo-mavirus might attenuate the function of p300 by suppressing GPS2 *(98)*. Finally, GPS2 was reported to associate with p53 and augment p53-dependent transcription *(99)*. Interestingly, GPS2 is a stoichiometric subunit of the NCoR/HDAC3 complex *(47,51)*. A Gal4-GPS2 fusion protein was demonstrated to repress transcription, and high HDAC activity is associated with endogenous GPS2. GPS2 facilitates the assembly of a complete GPS2/TBL1/NCoR/HDAC3 complex, and the GPS2-containing NCoR/HDAC3 complex can actively suppress intra-cellular JNK activation. NCoR strongly potentiated GPS2-mediated JNK1 inhibition, and JNK inhibition by GPS2/NCoR is independent of JNK expression but may occur through modulation of JNK phosphory-lation by JNK-specific MAPKK. GPS2 therefore provides a connection between the NCoR/HDAC3 corepressor complex and the intracellular JNK signaling pathways.

HDAC3 also physically interacts with the N-terminal region of c-Jun and is dissociated by JNK-mediated phosphorylation *(91)*. At this time, it is not known whether the HDAC3/c-Jun complex shares components with the HDAC3/NCoR/GPS2 complex. However, it is tempting to spec-ulate that a regulatory circuit exists in which the release of HDAC3 from c-Jun by JNK phosphorylation allows HDAC3 to participate in the HDAC3/NCoR/GPS2 complex to suppress JNK signaling and conse-quently favors the reestablishment of HDAC3/c-Jun complexes.

Chen et al. showed that the RelA subunit of nuclear factor-κB (NF-κB) transcription factor interacts with HDAC3 *(93,100)*. HDAC3 inhibits tumor necrosis factor-α (TNF-α) activation of NF-κB by deacetylation of RelA, which enhances the RelA-IκBα interaction and consequently pro-motes nuclear export of the NF-κB complex. Although RelA was also found to interact with HDAC1 and HDAC2 *(101–103,103a)*, it appears that only HDAC3 is able to deacetylate RelA. Thus, in addition to regulat-ing the JNK pathway through GPS2, HDAC3 is a negative regulator of the NF-κB pathway by a distinct mechanism.

Finally, one of the HDAC3 interacting proteins, TBL1/ebi, is highly conserved in *Drosophila* and appears to be involved in the epidermal growth factor (EGF) receptor signaling pathway, suggesting that HDAC3 might also participate in this signaling pathway.

REGULATION OF HDAC3

As expected for an enzyme with important cellular functions, the activity of HDAC3, like that of all other HDACs, is highly regulated by multiple mechanisms. Expression of the human *HDAC3* gene can be induced by treatment of peripheral blood mononuclear cells (PBMCs) with PHA, PMA, and α-CD3 *(8)*. In addition, HDAC3 is expressed at higher levels in the embryonic form of biliary atresia compared with the perinatal form *(104)*. In nude mice bearing human ovarian carcinoma xenografts, treatment with Taxol (paclitaxel) increases expression of HDAC3 *(105)*. Furthermore, the expression of mouse HDAC3 is induced in HDAC1-deficient cells *(106)*. In contrast, treatment of PBMCs with granulocyte/macrophage colony-stimulating factor (GM-CSF) downregulated the levels of human HDAC3 mRNA *(8)*.

A splice variant of the HDAC3 transcript in which exon 3 is alternatively spliced from the mRNA has been reported, and this spliced transcript is upregulated by treatment of cells with HDAC inhibitors *(31)*. The expression of this novel HDAC3 splice variant is regulated by many kinase inhibitors and by osmotic shock in mouse IMCD cells but not in human Hep3B or CRL-1611 cells.

Like most HDACs, HDAC3 has no DNA binding activity; therefore, proteins that target HDAC3 to DNA or to histones can indirectly regulate the activity of HDAC3. As stated before, extensive evidence supports the idea that some repressors/corepressors target HDAC3 to DNA through NCoR/SMRT. Unexpectedly, however, SMRT and NCoR not only bind HDAC3 but can stimulate HDAC3 enzymatic activity *(46,47,107)*. To test the possibility that the interaction between HDAC3 and NCoR modifies the activity of HDAC3, Wen et al. *(46)* expressed HDAC3 together with various NCoR deletion mutants and examined its deacetylase activity. An NCoR fragment (residues 267–549) with high affinity for HDAC3 in vitro significantly increased the deacetylase activity of HDAC3, whereas NCoR fragments that do not bind or bind weakly to HDAC3 had no effect. It was concluded that the enzymatic activity of HDAC3 is specifically regulated by the availability of interacting NCoR. In more elaborate studies, the deacetylase-activating domain (DAD) was mapped to residues 395 to 489 of SMRT and residues 403 to 497 of NCoR *(107)*, with an essential eight-amino acid region (residues 420–427 of NCoR) identified as critical for interaction *(47)*. The DAD was found to be necessary and sufficient for HDAC3 enzymatic activation in reconstitution experiments using purified components. However, HDAC3 interacts with SMRT in vivo only after priming by cellular chaperones, including the TCP-1 ring complex (TRiC) *(108)*. Both the N and C termini of HDAC3 are required for interaction with the SMRT DAD (Fig. 2). Together, the results from these three independent laboratories provide sound evidence that NCoR and SMRT not only serve to recruit HDAC3 to DNA but also function as dynamic regulating cofactors.

In most cell types, HDAC3 is distributed in both the nucleus and cytoplasm, and the subcellular localization of HDAC3 is regulated by competing

nuclear import and export signals *(33)*. Treatment of HeLa cells with leptomycin B, an inhibitor of the CRM1/exportin1-related export pathway,
caused accumulation of HDAC3 in the nucleus. In CV1 cells, a significant
portion of nuclear HDAC3 was shifted into the cytoplasm together with
NCoR and the NCoR-interacting protein TAB2 upon stimulation with
interleukin-1β (IL-1β), which activates the NF-κB pathway *(109)*. The IL-
1β-induced cytoplasmic appearance of the HDAC3/NCoR/TAB2 complex
can be blocked by treatment with leptomycin B. Interestingly, the protein
folding inhibitor geldanamycin prevented formation of the HDAC3/TRiC
complex and also inhibited nuclear localization of HDAC3 *(108)*. It
appears, therefore, that an active CRM1 export pathway regulates the cytoplasmic localization of HDAC3 via an IL-1β signal-dependent mechanism, whereas the nuclear localization of HDAC3 may be regulated by the
TRiC multiprotein chaperone complex.

IκBα is an inhibitory protein that sequesters NF-κB dimers in the cytoplasm of unstimulated cells. In a surprising finding, cytoplasmic IκBα
was reported to associate with HDAC3 and sequester it in the cytoplasm
(110). RelA can disrupt the interaction between IκB and HDAC3. Thus, a
reciprocal regulatory process might exist in the HDAC3/NF-κB network
in which HDAC3 deacetylates RelA and negatively regulates NF-κB activation whereas IκB negatively regulates the DNA- and histone-related
activities of HDAC3 by sequestering HDAC3 to the cytoplasm.

BIOLOGICAL ROLES OF HDAC3

In the human virology arena, HDAC3 has been shown to regulate
cytomegalovirus infection by repression of the viral major immediate early
promoter in nonpermissive cells *(111)*. In yeast, loss of HOS2 affects
acetylation at ribosomal protein gene promoter regions, implying that
HDAC3 might be important in the control of ribosome biogenesis *(112)*.
Unfortunately, no HDAC3 animal knockout models are currently available, and our knowledge of the biological function of HDAC3 in vertebrates is extremely limited. Overexpression of HDAC3 in THP-1 or HeLa
cells led to increased cell size, aberrant nuclear morphology, and G2/M
cell cycle arrest, suggesting the involvement of HDAC3 in cell cycle control *(8,20)*. In HeLa cells, siRNA-mediated HDAC3 knockdown also
caused significant morphological changes and inhibited cell proliferation
(113). From these studies, it is clear that a critical concentration of HDAC3
is required for normal cell survival.

SUMMARY AND PERSPECTIVES

Given our current knowledge of HDAC3, it is indisputable that this factor (like other HDACs) is critically involved in gene regulation. Enormous

benefits can be gained from a thorough understanding of the mechanisms of action, functions, and regulation of HDAC3 activity.

Although the *HDAC3* gene has been cloned in many different organisms, research on nonhuman HDAC3 has certainly been lagging. The successful generation of mice harboring mutations or deletions of *HDAC3*, for example, will be tremendously helpful in addressing the biological function of HDAC3. Likewise, although much has been learned about the structure of class I HDACs based on the crystal structures of the bacterium *Aquifex aeolicus* HDAC-like protein and the human HDAC8 *(114,115,115a)*, currently there is no structural information for HDAC3. Therefore, structural studies on HDAC3, either alone or together with NCoR/SMRT will lay an essential foundation for future work.

Our past understanding of the biology of HDAC3 has often been extrapolated from our knowledge of HDAC1 and HDAC2. However, HDAC3 possesses many unique characteristics that are not shared by HDAC1/2 or other HDACs. Biochemically, HDAC3 forms several protein complexes that are not found with other HDACs. Remarkable progress has already been made in understanding the relationship between HDAC3 and NCoR/SMRT. The time is ripe to characterize other HDAC3-interacting proteins. For example, do these other proteins stimulate (similar to NCoR/SMRT) or antagonize HDAC3 activity? Also, does HDAC3 reciprocally modify the function of these HDAC3 binding proteins?

Currently, only a few cellular genes that are regulated by HDAC3 have been defined. A good start will be to couple siRNA (to deplete HDAC3 in a cell) with gene expression profiling to determine globally what genes are up- or downregulated in the absence of HDAC3. With regard to HDAC3 substrates, a key question is what nonhistone proteins are targets for HDAC3. Because HDAC3 is found in the cytoplasm, the possibility that some cytoplasmic proteins can serve as substrates for HDAC3 cannot yet be ruled out. In addition, there is an immediate need to systematically evaluate and obtain a comprehensive picture of deacetylation sites on histones by HDAC3. With the continuous development of site-specific antibodies that recognize particular histone acetylation and the ever-increasing usefulness of mass spectrometry to characterize acetylation of histones, the answer to this important question is on the horizon.

Finally, besides the need to increase our understanding of gene regulation in eukaryotic cells, a leading motivation for studying HDAC3, as with other HDACs, is the hope that a thorough understanding of HDAC will guide us into the development of better and more specific HDAC inhibitors for treatment of cancer and other diseases. Understanding how HDAC3 activity can be regulated will undoubtedly provide alternative and unique opportunities to target HDACs effectively.

UPDATE

The previous notion that HDAC3 possesses substrate specificity is now reinforced by the discovery of a precise order for lysine deacetylation in H4 tails by HDAC3 *(116)*. Interestingly, the HDAC3 H4 lysine substrate preference matches the H4 binding specificity of NCoR/SMRT. In addition, the DLK1 *(117)*, TNF *(118)*, osteocalcin *(119)*, and Bmall *(120)* genes have recently been reported to be repressed by HDAC3 in association with other cellular proteins.

The solution structure of the HDAC3 activation domain (DAD) from SMRT has recently been reported *(121)*. In one surprising case, a mutant of DAD that still interacted with HDAC3 failed to activate, giving evidence that simply binding to the DAD is insufficient to activate HDAC3. Reports of proteins that interact with HDAC3 continue to expand at a rapid pace including KLF6 *(117)*, MAPK11 (p38 β-isoform) *(118)*, PP4 *(122)*, SRY (a Y chromosome-encoded DNA binding protein) *(123)*, Runx2 *(119)*, THAP7 *(124)*, and the cytomegalovirus IE1 and IE2 *(125)*. The consequence of these interactions varies widely. For example, by binding to KLF6 and Runx2, HDAC3 is recruited to the DLK1 and osteocalcin promoters, respectively, to repress transcription. By physical association with SRY, HDAC3 deacetylates SRY and induces its cytoplasmic delocalization. Partnering with HDAC3, IE1 inhibits the activity of HDAC3. Likewise, the interaction between HDAC3 and PP4 results in a downregulation of HDAC3 activity.

In a differential gene expression profiling experiment, HDAC3 was found to be differentially expressed in umbilical cord blood HSPCs compared with their progenies *(126)*. Similarly, by comparing gene expression microarray data from the Stanford microarray database, Pilarsky et al. *(127)* found that HDAC3 is commonly upregulated in many solid tumors. Furthermore, using antibody microarrays Bartling et al. *(128)* found that HDAC3 protein is upregulated in squamous cell lung carcinoma, suggesting the potential role of HDAC3 as a marker for discriminating malignant from normal lung tissue. In addition, using immunoscreening of tumor-derived cDNA expression libraries, Shebzukhov et al. *(129)* identified HDAC3 as a serologically defined antigen in colon cancer. Finally, in an interesting new twist, two groups reported that HDAC3 protein expression levels are significantly downregulated following treatment with HDAC inhibitors, suggesting that the expression of HDAC3 itself is regulated by histone deacetylation *(130,131)*.

ACKNOWLEDGMENTS

I apologize to all investigators whose works were not cited in this article owing to space limitations. I am grateful to Xiang-Jiao Yang and Jiemin Wong for their constructive comments. HDAC-related research in my laboratory is supported by NIH grants (GM58486, GM64850, and CA109699) and an endowment from the Kaul Foundation.

REFERENCES

1. Taunton J, Hassig CA, Schreiber SL. A mammalian histone deacetylase related to the yeast transcriptional regulator Rpd3p. Science 1996;272:408–411.
2. Vidal M, Gaber RF. RPD3 encodes a second factor required to achieve maximum positive and negative transcriptional states in *Saccharomyces cerevisiae*. Mol Cell Biol 1991;11:6317–6327.
3. Yang WM, Inouye C, Zeng Y, Bearss D, Seto E. Transcriptional repression by YY1 is mediated by interaction with a mammalian homolog of the yeast global regulator RPD3. Proc Natl Acad Sci U S A 1996;93:12,845–12,850.
4. Yang WM, Yao YL, Sun JM, Davie JR, Seto E. Isolation and characterization of cDNAs corresponding to an additional member of the human histone deacetylase gene family. J Biol Chem 1997;272:28,001–28,007.
5. Ayer DE. Histone deacetylases: transcriptional repression with SINers and NuRDs. Trends Cell Biol 1999;9:193–198.
6. Ng HH, Bird A. Histone deacetylases: silencers for hire. Trends Biochem Sci 2000;25:121–126.
7. Emiliani S, Fischle W, Van LC, Al AY, Verdin E. Characterization of a human RPD3 ortholog, HDAC3. Proc Natl Acad Sci U S A 1998;95:2795–2800.
8. Dangond F, Hafler DA, Tong JK, et al. Differential display cloning of a novel human histone deacetylase (HDAC3) cDNA from PHA-activated immune cells. Biochem Biophys Res Commun 1998;242:648–652.
9. Zamore PD, Williamson JR, Lehmann R. The Pumilio protein binds RNA through a conserved domain that defines a new class of RNA-binding proteins. RNA 1997;3:1421–1433.
10. Zamore PD, Bartel DP, Lehmann R, Williamson JR. The PUMILIO-RNA interaction: a single RNA-binding domain monomer recognizes a bipartite target sequence. Biochemistry 1999;38:596–604.
11. Spassov DS, Jurecic R. The PUF family of RNA-binding proteins: does evolutionarily conserved structure equal conserved function? IUBMB Life 2003;55:359–366.
12. Wang X, McLachlan J, Zamore PD, Hall TM. Modular recognition of RNA by a human pumilio-homology domain. Cell 2002;110:501–512.
13. Edwards TA, Trincao J, Escalante CR, Wharton RP, Aggarwal AK. Crystallization and characterization of Pumilo: a novel RNA binding protein. J Struct Biol 2000;132:251–254.
14. Grozinger CM, Schreiber SL. Deacetylase enzymes: biological functions and the use of small-molecule inhibitors. Chem Biol 2002;9:3–16.
15. Thiagalingam S, Cheng KH, Lee HJ, Mineva N, Thiagalingam A, Ponte JF. Histone deacetylases: unique players in shaping the epigenetic histone code. Ann N Y Acad Sci 2003;983:84–100.

16. Verdin E, Dequiedt F, Kasler HG. Class II histone deacetylases: versatile regulators. Trends Genet 2003;19:286–293.

17. Yang XJ, Seto E. Collaborative spirit of histone deacetylases in regulating chromatin structure and gene expression. Curr Opin Genet Dev 2003;13:143–153.

18. Gregoretti IV, Lee YM, Goodson HV. Molecular evolution of the histone deacetylase family: functional implications of phylogenetic analysis. J Mol Biol 2004;338:17–31.

19. Mahlknecht U, Hoelzer D, Bucala R, Verdin E. Cloning and characterization of the murine histone deacetylase (HDAC3). Biochem Biophys Res Commun 1999;263:482–490.

20. Dangond F, Foerznler D, Weremowicz S, Morton CC, Beier DR, Gullans SR. Cloning and expression of a murine histone deacetylase 3 (mHdac3) cDNA and mapping to a region of conserved synteny between murine chromosome 18 and human chromosome 5. Mol Cell Biol Res Commun 1999;2:91–96.

21. Strausberg RL, Feingold EA, Grouse LH, et al. Generation and initial analysis of more than 15,000 full-length human and mouse cDNA sequences. Proc Natl Acad Sci U S A 2002;99:16,899–16,903.

22. Johnson CA, Barlow AL, Turner BM. Molecular cloning of *Drosophila melanogaster* cDNAs that encode a novel histone deacetylase dHDAC3. Gene 1998;221:127–134.

23. Lu X, Horvitz HR. lin-35 and lin-53, two genes that antagonize a *C. elegans* Ras pathway, encode proteins similar to Rb and its binding protein RbAp48. Cell 1998;95:981–991.

24. Shi Y, Mello C. A CBP/p300 homolog specifies multiple differentiation pathways in *Caenorhabditis elegans*. Genes Dev 1998;12:943–955.

25. Carmen AA, Rundlett SE, Grunstein M. HDA1 and HDA3 are components of a yeast histone deacetylase (HDA) complex. J Biol Chem 1996;271: 15,837–15,844.

26. Rundlett SE, Carmen AA, Kobayashi R, Bavykin S, Turner BM, Grunstein M. HDA1 and RPD3 are members of distinct yeast histone deacetylase complexes that regulate silencing and transcription. Proc Natl Acad Sci U S A 1996;93: 14,503–14,508.

27. Mahlknecht U, Emiliani S, Najfeld V, Young S, Verdin E. Genomic organization and chromosomal localization of the human histone deacetylase 3 gene. Genomics 1999;56:197–202.

28. Randhawa GS, Bell DW, Testa JR, Feinberg AP. Identification and mapping of human histone acetylation modifier gene homologues. Genomics 1998;51: 262–269.

29. Mahlknecht U, Bucala R, Hoelzer D, Verdin E. High resolution physical mapping of human HDAC3, a potential tumor suppressor gene in the 5q31 region. Cytogenet Cell Genet 1999;86:237–239.

30. Mahlknecht U, Bucala R, Verdin E. Assignment of the histone deacetylase gene (Hdac3) to mouse chromosome 18B3 by in situ hybridization. Cytogenet Cell Genet 1999;84:192–193.

31. Gray SG, Iglesias AH, Teh BT, Dangond F. Modulation of splicing events in histone deacetylase 3 by various extracellular and signal transduction pathways. Gene Expr 2003;11:13–21.

32. Wolfsberg TG, McEntyre J, Schuler GD. Guide to the draft human genome. Nature 2001;409:824–826.

33. Yang WM, Tsai SC, Wen YD, Fejer G, Seto E. Functional domains of histone deacetylase-3. J Biol Chem 2002;277:9447–9454.

34. Wen YD, Cress WD, Roy AL, Seto E. Histone deacetylase 3 binds to and regulates the multifunctional transcription factor TFII-I. J Biol Chem 2003;278: 1841–1847.

35. Takami Y, Nakayama T. N-terminal region, C-terminal region, nuclear export signal, and deacetylation activity of histone deacetylase-3 are essential for the viability of the DT40 chicken B cell line. J Biol Chem 2000;275:16,191–16,201.

36. Johnson CA, White DA, Lavender JS, O'Neill LP, Turner BM. Human class I histone deacetylase complexes show enhanced catalytic activity in the presence of ATP and co-immunoprecipitate with the ATP- dependent chaperone protein Hsp70. J Biol Chem 2002;277:9590–9597.

37. Grozinger CM, Hassig CA, Schreiber SL. Three proteins define a class of human histone deacetylases related to yeast Hda1p. Proc Natl Acad Sci U S A 1999; 96:4868–4873.

38. Fischle W, Dequiedt F, Fillion M, Hendzel MJ, Voelter W, Verdin E. Human HDAC7 histone deacetylase activity is associated with HDAC3 in vivo. J Biol Chem 2001;276:35,826–35,835.

39. Fischle W, Dequiedt F, Hendzel MJ, et al. Enzymatic activity associated with class II HDACs is dependent on a multiprotein complex containing HDAC3 and SMRT/N-CoR. Mol Cell 2002;9:45–57.

40. Vermeulen M, Carrozza MJ, Lasonder E, Workman JL, Logie C, Stunnenberg HG. In vitro targeting reveals intrinsic histone tail specificity of the Sin3/histone deacetylase and N-CoR/SMRT corepressor complexes. Mol Cell Biol 2004;24: 2364–2372.

41. Wang A, Kurdistani SK, Grunstein M. Requirement of Hos2 histone deacetylase for gene activity in yeast. Science 2002;298:1412–1414.

42. Zhang X, Wharton W, Yuan Z, Tsai SC, Olashaw N, Seto E. Activation of the growth-differentiation factor 11 gene by the histone deacetylase (HDAC) inhibitor trichostatin A and repression by HDAC3. Mol Cell Biol 2004;24: 5106–5118.

43. Ishizuka T, Lazar MA. The N-CoR/histone deacetylase 3 complex is required for repression by thyroid hormone receptor. Mol Cell Biol 2003;23:5122–5131.

44. Jepsen K, Hermanson O, Onami TM, et al. Combinatorial roles of the nuclear receptor corepressor in transcription and development. Cell 2000;102:753–763.

45. Klampfer L, Huang J, Swaby LA, Augenlicht L. Requirement of histone deactylase activity for signaling by STAT1. J Biol Chem 2004;279:30,358–30,368.

46. Wen YD, Perissi V, Staszewski LM, et al. The histone deacetylase-3 complex contains nuclear receptor corepressors. Proc Natl Acad Sci U S A 2000;97: 7202–7207.

47. Zhang J, Kalkum M, Chait BT, Roeder RG. The N-CoR-HDAC3 nuclear receptor corepressor complex inhibits the JNK pathway through the integral subunit GPS2. Mol Cell 2002;9:611–623.

48. Guenther MG, Lane WS, Fischle W, Verdin E, Lazar MA, Shiekhattar R. A core SMRT corepressor complex containing HDAC3 and TBL1, a WD40-repeat protein linked to deafness. Genes Dev 2000;14:1048–1057.

49. Li J, Wang J, Nawaz Z, Liu JM, Qin J, Wong J. Both corepressor proteins SMRT and N-CoR exist in large protein complexes containing HDAC3. EMBO J 2000;19:4342–4350.

50. Underhill C, Qutob MS, Yee SP, Torchia J. A novel nuclear receptor corepressor complex, N-CoR, contains components of the mammalian SWI/SNF complex and the corepressor KAP-1. J Biol Chem 2000;275:40,463–40,470.

51. Yoon HG, Chan DW, Huang ZQ, et al. Purification and functional characterization of the human N-CoR complex: the roles of HDAC3, TBL1 and TBLR1. EMBO J 2003;22:1336–1346.

52. Pijnappel WW, Schaft D, Roguev A, et al. The *S. cerevisiae* SET3 complex includes two histone deacetylases, Hos2 and Hst1, and is a meiotic-specific repressor of the sporulation gene program. Genes Dev 2001;15:2991–3004.

53. Horlein AJ, Naar AM, Heinzel T, et al. Ligand-independent repression by the thyroid hormone receptor mediated by a nuclear receptor co-repressor. Nature 1995;377:397–404.

54. Chen JD, Evans RM. A transcriptional co-repressor that interacts with nuclear hormone receptors. Nature 1995;377:454–457.

55. Jepsen K, Rosenfeld MG. Biological roles and mechanistic actions of co-repressor complexes. J Cell Sci 2002;115:689–698.

56. Urnov FD, Yee J, Sachs L, et al. Targeting of N-CoR and histone deacetylase 3 by the oncoprotein v-erbA yields a chromatin infrastructure-dependent transcriptional repression pathway. EMBO J 2000;19:4074–4090.

57. Heinzel T, Lavinsky RM, Mullen TM, et al. A complex containing N-CoR, mSin3 and histone deacetylase mediates transcriptional repression. Nature 1997;387:43–48.

58. Alland L, Muhle R, Hou H Jr, et al. Role for N-CoR and histone deacetylase in Sin3-mediated transcriptional repression. Nature 1997;387:49–55.

59. Kao HY, Downes M, Ordentlich P, Evans RM. Isolation of a novel histone deacetylase reveals that class I and class II deacetylases promote SMRT-mediated repression. Genes Dev 2000;14:55–66.

60. Huang EY, Zhang J, Miska EA, Guenther MG, Kouzarides T, Lazar MA. Nuclear receptor corepressors partner with class II histone deacetylases in a Sin3-independent repression pathway. Genes Dev 2000;14:45–54.

61. Nagy L, Kao HY, Chakravarti D, et al. Nuclear receptor repression mediated by a complex containing SMRT, mSin3A, and histone deacetylase. Cell 1997;89:373–380.

62. Bassi MT, Ramesar RS, Caciotti B, et al. X-linked late-onset sensorineural deafness caused by a deletion involving OA1 and a novel gene containing WD-40 repeats. Am J Hum Genet 1999;64:1604–1616.

63. Forrest D, Erway LC, Ng L, Altschuler R, Curran T. Thyroid hormone receptor beta is essential for development of auditory function. Nat Genet 1996;13: 354–357.

64. Leon PE, Raventos H, Lynch E, Morrow J, King MC. The gene for an inherited form of deafness maps to chromosome 5q31. Proc Natl Acad Sci U S A 1992;89:5181–5184.

65. Lynch ED, Lee MK, Morrow JE, Welcsh PL, Leon PE, King MC. Nonsyndromic deafness DFNA1 associated with mutation of a human homolog of the *Drosophila* gene diaphanous. Science 1997;278:1315–1318.

66. Roy AL, Meisterernst M, Pognonec P, Roeder RG. Cooperative interaction of an initiator-binding transcription initiation factor and the helix-loop-helix activator USF. Nature 1991;354:245–248.

67. Roy AL. Biochemistry and biology of the inducible multifunctional transcription factor TFII-I. Gene 2001;274:1–13.

68. Tussie-Luna MI, Bayarsaihan D, Seto E, Ruddle FH, Roy AL. Physical and functional interactions of histone deacetylase 3 with TFII-I family proteins and PIASxbeta. Proc Natl Acad Sci U S A 2002;99:12,807–12,812.

69. Grozinger CM, Schreiber SL. Regulation of histone deacetylase 4 and 5 and transcriptional activity by 14-3-3-dependent cellular localization. Proc Natl Acad Sci U S A 2000;97:7835–7840.

70. Zhou X, Richon VM, Rifkind RA, Marks PA. Identification of a transcriptional repressor related to the noncatalytic domain of histone deacetylases 4 and 5. Proc Natl Acad Sci U S A 2000;97:1056–1061.

71. Tong JJ, Liu J, Bertos NR, Yang XJ. Identification of HDAC10, a novel class II human histone deacetylase containing a leucine-rich domain. Nucleic Acids Res 2002;30:1114–1123.

72. Taplick J, Kurtev V, Kroboth K, Posch M, Lechner T, Seiser C. Homo-oligomerisation and nuclear localisation of mouse histone deacetylase 1. J Mol Biol 2001;308:27–38.

73. Li J, Staver MJ, Curtin ML, et al. Expression and functional characterization of recombinant human HDAC1 and HDAC3. Life Sci 2004;74:2693–2705.

74. Wei LN, Hu X, Chandra D, Seto E, Farooqui M. Receptor-interacting protein 140 directly recruits histone deacetylases for gene silencing. J Biol Chem 2000;275:40,782–40,787.

75. Wei LN, Farooqui M, Hu X. Ligand-dependent formation of retinoid receptors, receptor-interacting protein 140 (RIP140), and histone deacetylase complex is mediated by a novel receptor-interacting motif of RIP140. J Biol Chem 2001;276:16,107–16,112.

76. Franco PJ, Farooqui M, Seto E, Wei LN. The orphan nuclear receptor TR2 interacts directly with both class I and class II histone deacetylases. Mol Endocrinol 2001;15:1318–1328.

77. Li G, Franco PJ, Wei LN. Identification of histone deacetylase-3 domains that interact with the orphan nuclear receptor TR2. Biochem Biophys Res Commun 2003;310:384–390.

78. Fajas L, Egler V, Reiter R, et al. The retinoblastoma-histone deacetylase 3 complex inhibits PPARgamma and adipocyte differentiation. Dev Cell 2002;3:903–910.

79. Fajas L, Egler V, Reiter R, Miard S, Lefebvre AM, Auwerx J. PPARgamma controls cell proliferation and apoptosis in an RB-dependent manner. Oncogene 2003;22:4186–4193.

80. Liu XF, Bagchi MK. Recruitment of distinct chromatin-modifying complexes by tamoxifen-complexed estrogen receptor at natural target gene promoters in vivo. J Biol Chem 2004;279:15,050–15,058.

81. Lin HM, Zhao L, Cheng SY. Cyclin D1 is a ligand-independent co-repressor for thyroid hormone receptors. J Biol Chem 2002;277:28,733–28,741.

81a. Fu M, Rao M, Bouras T, et al. Cyclin D1 inhibits peroxisome proliferators-activated receptor γ-mediated adipogenesis through histone deacetylase recruitment. J Biol Chem 2005;280:16,934–16,941.

82. Wang L, Hiebert SW. TEL contacts multiple co-repressors and specifically associates with histone deacetylase-3. Oncogene 2001;20:3716–3725.

83. Kuwata T, Gongora C, Kanno Y, et al. Gamma interferon triggers interaction between ICSBP (IRF-8) and TEL, recruiting the histone deacetylase HDAC3 to the interferon-responsive element. Mol Cell Biol 2002;22:7439–7448.

84. Hoogeveen AT, Rossetti S, Stoyanova V, et al. The transcriptional corepressor MTG16a contains a novel nucleolar targeting sequence deranged in t (16;21)-positive myeloid malignancies. Oncogene 2002;21:6703–6712.

85. Watamoto K, Towatari M, Ozawa Y, et al. Altered interaction of HDAC5 with GATA-1 during MEL cell differentiation. Oncogene 2003;22:9176–9184.

86. Ozawa Y, Towatari M, Tsuzuki S, et al. Histone deacetylase 3 associates with and represses the transcription factor GATA-2. Blood 2001;98:2116–2123.

87. Lai A, Lee JM, Yang WM, et al. RBP1 recruits both histone deacetylase-dependent and -independent repression activities to retinoblastoma family proteins. Mol Cell Biol 1999;19:6632–6641.

88. Nicolas E, Ait-Si-Ali S, Trouche D. The histone deacetylase HDAC3 targets RbAp48 to the retinoblastoma protein. Nucleic Acids Res 2001;29: 3131–3136.

89. Lai A, Kennedy BK, Barbie DA, et al. RBP1 recruits the mSIN3-histone deacetylase complex to the pocket of retinoblastoma tumor suppressor family proteins found in limited discrete regions of the nucleus at growth arrest. Mol Cell Biol 2001;21:2918–2932.

90. Vaute O, Nicolas E, Vandel L, Trouche D. Functional and physical interaction between the histone methyl transferase Suv39H1 and histone deacetylases. Nucleic Acids Res 2002;30:475–481.

91. Weiss C, Schneider S, Wagner EF, Zhang X, Seto E, Bohmann D. JNK phosphorylation relieves HDAC3-dependent suppression of the transcriptional activity of c-Jun. EMBO J 2003;22:3686–3695.

92. Jin C, Li H, Murata T, et al. JDP2, a repressor of AP-1, recruits a histone deacetylase 3 complex to inhibit the retinoic acid-induced differentiation of F9 cells. Mol Cell Biol 2002;22:4815–4826.

93. Chen L, Fischle W, Verdin E, Greene WC. Duration of nuclear NF-kappaB action regulated by reversible acetylation. Science 2001;293:1653–1657.

94. Franco PJ, Li G, Wei LN. Interaction of nuclear receptor zinc finger DNA binding domains with histone deacetylase. Mol Cell Endocrinol 2003;206:1–12.

95. Spain BH, Bowdish KS, Pacal AR, et al. Two human cDNAs, including a homolog of Arabidopsis FUS6 (COP11), suppress G-protein- and mitogen-activated protein kinase-mediated signal transduction in yeast and mammalian cells. Mol Cell Biol 1996;16:6698–6706.

96. Jin DY, Teramoto H, Giam CZ, Chun RF, Gutkind JS, Jeang KT. A human suppressor of c-Jun N-terminal kinase 1 activation by tumor necrosis factor alpha. J Biol Chem 1997;272:25,816–25,823.

97. Peng YC, Breiding DE, Sverdrup F, Richard J, Androphy EJ. AMF-1/Gps2 binds p300 and enhances its interaction with papillomavirus E2 proteins. J Virol 2000;74:5872–5879.

98. Degenhardt YY, Silverstein SJ. Gps2, a protein partner for human papillomavirus E6 proteins. J Virol 2001;75:151–160.

99. Peng YC, Kuo F, Breiding DE, Wang YF, Mansur CP, Androphy EJ. AMF1 (GPS2) modulates p53 transactivation. Mol Cell Biol 2001;21:5913–5924.

100. Chen LF, Greene WC. Regulation of distinct biological activities of the NF-kappaB transcription factor complex by acetylation. J Mol Med 2003;81: 549–557.

101. Ashburner BP, Westerheide SD, Baldwin AS, Jr. The p65 (RelA) subunit of NF-kappaB interacts with the histone deacetylase (HDAC) corepressors HDAC1 and HDAC2 to negatively regulate gene expression. Mol Cell Biol 2001;21:7065–7077.

102. Zhong H, May MJ, Jimi E, Ghosh S. The phosphorylation status of nuclear NF-kappa B determines its association with CBP/p300 or HDAC-1. Mol Cell 2002;9:625–636.

103. Kiernan R, Bres V, Ng RW, et al. Post-activation turn-off of NF-kappa B-dependent transcription is regulated by acetylation of p65. J Biol Chem 2003; 278:2758–2766.

103a. Gao Z, Chiao P, Zhang X, et al. Coactivators and corepressors of NF-κB in IκBα gene promoter. J Biol Chem 2005;280:21,091–21,098.

104. Zhang DY, Sabla G, Shivakumar P, et al. Coordinate expression of regulatory genes differentiates embryonic and perinatal forms of biliary atresia. Hepatology 2004;39:954–962.

105. Bani MR, Nicoletti MI, Alkharouf NW, et al. Gene expression correlating with response to paclitaxel in ovarian carcinoma xenografts. Mol Cancer Ther 2004;3:111–121.

106. Lagger G, O'Carroll D, Rembold M, et al. Essential function of histone deacetylase 1 in proliferation control and CDK inhibitor repression. EMBO J 2002;21:2672–2681.

107. Guenther MG, Barak O, Lazar MA. The SMRT and N-CoR corepressors are activating cofactors for histone deacetylase 3. Mol Cell Biol 2001;21: 6091–6101.

108. Guenther MG, Yu J, Kao GD, Yen TJ, Lazar MA. Assembly of the SMRT-histone deacetylase 3 repression complex requires the TCP-1 ring complex. Genes Dev 2002;16:3130–3135.

109. Baek SH, Ohgi KA, Rose DW, Koo EH, Glass CK, Rosenfeld MG. Exchange of N-CoR corepressor and Tip60 coactivator complexes links gene expression by NF-kappaB and beta-amyloid precursor protein. Cell 2002;110:55–67.

110. Viatour P, Legrand-Poels S, van Lint C, et al. Cytoplasmic IkappaBalpha increases NF-kappaB-independent transcription through binding to histone deacetylase (HDAC) 1 and HDAC3. J Biol Chem 2003;278:46,541–46,548.

111. Murphy JC, Fischle W, Verdin E, Sinclair JH. Control of cytomegalovirus lytic gene expression by histone acetylation. EMBO J 2002;21:1112–1120.

112. Robyr D, Suka Y, Xenarios I, et al. Microarray deacetylation maps determine genome-wide functions for yeast histone deacetylases. Cell 2002;109:437–446.

113. Glaser KB, Li J, Staver MJ, Wei RQ, Albert DH, Davidsen SK. Role of class I and class II histone deacetylases in carcinoma cells using siRNA. Biochem Biophys Res Commun 2003;310:529–536.

114. Finnin MS, Donigian JR, Cohen A, et al. Structures of a histone deacetylase homologue bound to the TSA and SAHA inhibitors. Nature 1999;401:188–193.

115. Somoza JR, Skene, RJ, Katz, BA, et al. Structural snapshots of human HDAC8 provide insights into the class I histone deacetylases. Structure 2004;12: 1325–1334.

115a. Vannini A, Volpari C, Filocamo G, et al. Crystal structure of a eukaryotic zinc-dependent histone deacetylase, human HDAC8, complexed with a hydroxamic acid inhibitor. Proc Natl Acad Sci U S A 2004;101:15,064–15,069.

116. Hartman HB, Yu J, Alenghat T, Ishizuka T, Lazar MA. The histone-binding code of nuclear receptor co-repressors matches the substrate specificity of histone deacetylase 3. EMBO Rep 2005;6:445–451.

117. Li D, Yea S, Li S, et al. Kruppel-like factor-6 promotes preadipocyte differentiation through histone deacetylase 3-dependent repression of DLK1. J Biol Chem 2005;280:26,941–26,952.

118. Mahlknecht U, Will J, Varin A Hoelzer D, Herbein G. Histone deacetylase 3, a class I histone deacetylase, suppress MAPK11-mediated activating transcription

factor-2 activation and represses TNF gene expression. J Immunol 2004;173: 3979–3990.

119. Schroeder TM, Kahler RA, Li X, Westendorf JJ. Histone deacetylase 3 interacts with runx2 to repress the osteocalcin promoter and regulate osteoblast differentiation. J Biol Chem 2004;279:41,998–42,007.

120. Yin L, Lazar MA. The orphan nuclear receptor Rev-erbalpha recruits the N-CoR/ histone deacetylase 3 corepressor to regulate the circadian Bmall gene. Mol Endocrinol 2005;19:1452–1459.

121. Cordina A, Love JD, Li Y, Lazar MA, Neuhaus D, Schwabe JW. Structural insights into the interaction and activation of histone deacetylase 3 by nuclear receptor corepressors. Proc Natl Acad Sci U S A 2005;102:6009–6014.

122. Zhang X, Ozawa Y, Lee H, et al. Histone deacetylase 3 (HDAC3) activity is regulated by interaction with protein serine/threonine phosphatase 4. Genes Dev 2005;19:827–839.

123. Thevenet L, Mejean C, Moniot B, et al. Regulation of human SRY subcellular distribution by its acetylation/deacetylation. EMBO J 2004;23:3336–3345.

124. Macfarlan T, Kutney S, Altman B, Montross R, Yu J, Chakravarti D. Human THAP7 is a chromatin-associated, histone tail-binding protein that represses transcription via recruitment of HDAC3 and nuclear hormone receptor corepressor. J Biol Chem 2005;280:7346–7358.

125. Nevels M, Paulus C, Shenk T. Human cytomegalovirus immediate-early 1 protein facilities viral replication by antagonizing histone deacetylation. Proc Natl Acad Sci U S A 2004;101:17,234–17,239.

126. He X, Gonzaler V, Tsang A, Thompson J, Tsang TC, Harris DT. Differential gene expressionprofiling og CD34+ CD133+ umbilical cord blood hematopoietic stem progenitor cells. Stem Cells Dev 2005;14:188–198.

127. Pilarsky C, Wenzig M, Saeger HD, Grutzmann R. Identification and validation of commonly overexpressed genes in solid tumors by comparison of microarray data. Neoplasia 2004;6:744–750.

128. Bartling B, Hofmann HS, Boettger T, et al. Comparative application of antibody and gene array for expression profiling in human squamous cell lung carcinoma. Lung Cancer 2005;49:145–154.

129. Shebzukhov YV, Koroleva EP, Khlgatian SV, et al. Antibody response to a non-conserved C-terminal part of human histone deacetylase 3 in colon cancer patients. Int J Cancer 2005; in press.

130. Liu HL, Chen Y, Cui GH, Zhou JF. Curcumin, a potent anti-tumor reagent, is a novel histone deacetylase inhibitor regulating B-NHL cell line Raji proliferation. Acta Pharmacol Sin 2005;26:603–609.

131. Xu Y, Voelter-Mahlknecht S, Mahlknecht U. The histone eacetylase inhibitor suberoylanilide hydroxamic acid down-regulates expression levels of Bcr-abl, c-Myc and HDAC3 in chronic myeloid leukemia cell lines. Int J Mol Med 2005;15:169–172.

4 The Biology of HDAC8, a Unique Class I Histone Deacetylase

David Waltregny, MD, PhD
and Vincent Castronovo, MD, PhD

CONTENTS

SUMMARY

HDAC8 is a class I member of the histone deacetylases family, although lying phylogenetically close to the evolutionary boundary between class I and class II HDACs. After a comprehensive review of the current understanding of the biology of HDAC8 and its gene, we present recent evidence indicating that this HDAC is selectively expressed by cells showing

From: *Cancer Drug Discovery and Development*
Histone Deacetylases: Transcriptional Regulation and Other Cellular Functions
Edited by: E. Verdin © Humana Press Inc., Totowa, NJ

smooth muscle cell differentiation, including smooth muscle, myofibro-blastic, and myoepithelial cells. The possible involvement of HDAC8 in the regulation of the smooth muscle cytoskeleton is also presented and discussed.

Key Words: Histone deacetylase, transcription, cytoskeleton, smooth muscle, actin, contractility.

HDAC8: THE FOURTH IDENTIFIED CLASS I HDAC

In 2000, database searches of expressed sequence tags showing high similarity with class I human histone deacetylases (HDACs; HDAC1–3) led three independent groups to clone a cDNA encoding a novel human histone deacetylase *(1–3)*. This fourth identified class I HDAC was called HDAC8 because at that time seven human HDACs had already been discovered, falling into class I (HDAC1–3) and class II (HDAC4–7).

HDAC8 mRNA encodes 377 amino acid residues with a predicted molecular mass of 45,240 Daltons *(1–3)*. It possesses no apparent hydrophobic leader sequence but contains a stretch of basic region from Arg[164] to Lys[168] (RLRRK), which may serve as a nuclear localization signal *(1)*.

Sequence Comparisons Reveal Significant Differences Between HDAC8 and Other Class I HDACs

Amino acid sequence comparisons have indicated that HDAC8 is most similar to HDAC3 *(1,2)*, with 34% amino acid identity and 54% similarity, when one considers conservative amino acid substitutions *(2)*. HDAC8 contains a shorter C-terminal extension relative to the other class I members *(2)* and in fact constitutes the second shortest human HDAC, after HDAC11 (347 amino acid residues) *(4)*. In this respect, HDAC8 is similar to the HDAC-like protein (HDLP) from the hyperthermophilic bacterium *Aquifex aeolicus*, an enzyme with no known function that shares approx 31% sequence identity with HDAC8 *(5)*.

Phylogenetic tree analyses have placed HDAC8 close to the evolutionary boundary between the class I and class II HDACs *(1,3)*. In fact, HDAC8 seems to have diverged from other class I human HDACs early in evolution, and it may, therefore, represent a key point that distinguishes class I and class II HDACs in humans *(1)*.

The first 34 N-terminal amino acids of HDAC8 considerably differ from those of HDAC1 to 3, as do the last 30 C-terminal amino acids *(3)*. In addition, a distinct stretch of mainly acidic amino acids at position 83 to 95 in HDAC8, possibly involved in protein-protein interactions, is absent in HDAC1 to 3 *(3)*. The sequence conservation is, however, higher at the catalytic domain. Indeed, as in most HDACs *(5)*, HDAC8 has nine conserved blocks and two histidine residues (His^{142} and His^{143}) that are presumably important for its catalytic activity *(1–3)*.

Compared with other class I HDACs, HDAC8 lacks a 50- to 111-amino acid C-terminal domain that extends from the catalytic domain *(6)*. In HDAC1 to 3, the C-terminal domains participate in the recruitment of the enzymes to protein complexes that modulate their enzymatic activities and localization *(7,8)*. In addition, the activities of these class I HDACs are regulated by posttranslational modifications to the C-terminal extension, such as phosphorylation *(9,10)* and sumoylation *(11)*. Given these differences, it has been suggested that HDAC8 either does not require to be recruited to protein complexes to function, or its recruitment utilizes entirely different regions of the protein surface *(6)*.

Unlike Other Class I HDACs, HDAC8 Can Be Phosphorylated in the N-Terminus by Cyclic AMP-Dependent Protein Kinase

Several potential posttranslational modification sites of HDAC8 have been identified. They include a putative *N*-glycosylation site (NWS) at Asn^{136}, a cyclic AMP-dependent protein kinase (PKA) phosphorylation site (KRAS) at Ser^{39}, and two potential casein kinase II phosphorylation sites at Ser^{63} and Ser^{83} *(1)*. However, unlike other class I members, HDAC8 is not phosphorylated by CK2 *(10)*. In fact, HDAC8 can be phosphorylated by PKA, a serine-threonine kinase, both in vitro and in vivo, with consequent reduction of its deacetylase activity *(12)*. In contrast to HDAC1 and HDAC2, which are phosphorylated on C-terminal residues, HDAC8 is phosphorylated in the N terminus at Ser^{39}, a nonconserved residue among class I HDACs *(12)*. Thus, HDAC8 phosphorylation may have consequences distinct from those resulting from the phosphorylation of other class I HDAC enzymes *(12)*. In agreement with this suggestion, phosphorylation of HDAC1 and HDAC2 increases their deacetylation activity *(9,10,13)*, whereas phosphorylation of HDAC8 by PKA reduces HDAC8's activity *(12)*. It is currently unknown whether HDAC8 phosphorylation levels are modulated by phosphatases.

Analysis of Human HDAC8's Crystal Structure Sheds Light on Potential Differences in Substrate Specificity Across the HDAC Family

The three-dimensional structures of HDAC8, including crystal structures of HDAC8 complexed with four structurally diverse hydroxamate HDAC inhibitors, have been recently described *(6)*. The structure of HDAC8 has been shown to set strong constraints on how catalysis occurs in this family of enzymes (HDAC classes I and II) and has led to a proposed mechanism of deacetylation reaction *(6)* that is similar to the mechanism suggested for HDLP *(5)*.

HDAC8 comprises a single α/β domain that includes an eight-stranded parallel β-sheet sandwiched between 13 α-helices *(6)*. Comparisons of the structures of HDAC8 and HDLP, coupled with analysis of the sequence alignments of the class I HDACs and HDLP, have revealed that HDAC8 is structurally and, as a consequence, functionally unique in several important aspects *(6)*.

Among others, a presumably important feature that distinguishes HDAC8 from HDLP and HDAC1 to 3 is the size and composition of the N-terminal L1 loop (residues 30–36). The L1 loop in HDAC8, as in HDLP, lines a large portion of one face of the active site pocket and extends to the protein surface but is two residues shorter than its counterpart in HDLP, resulting in a wider active site pocket with a larger surface opening. In fact, a comparison of the structures of four HDAC8 inhibitor complexes has revealed considerable structural differences in the protein surface in the vicinity of the opening to the active site, mainly mediated by the L1 loop, suggesting that this region is highly malleable and able to accommodate binding to a variety of different ligands, such as acetylated lysines presented in different structural contexts. HDAC8 flexibility may contrast with the more conformationally static active sites of the other class I human HDACs, as suggested by extrapolations of structural comparisons between HDAC8 and HDLP and sequence alignments of HDAC8 with HDAC1 to 3 *(6)*.

The HDAC8 Gene Is Localized to the Long Arm of Chromosome X

The HDAC8 gene is organized into 11 exons over a total length of 242.7 kb *(3)*. Fluorescence *in situ* hybridization studies and linkage analysis after radiation hybrid mapping have localized the HDAC8 gene to the long arm of chromosome X, at position q21.3 or q13 *(2,3)*. HDAC8 is thus, like HDAC6, an X-linked HDAC.

EXPRESSION OF HDAC8 IS RESTRICTED TO CELLS SHOWING SMOOTH MUSCLE DIFFERENTIATION IN NORMAL HUMAN TISSUES

Expression Profile of HDAC8 Transcript Suggests That HDAC8 Is a Ubiquitous HDAC

Initial data on HDAC8 expression have been generated through the analysis of its transcript expression. The abundance and distribution of HDAC8 mRNA has indeed been examined by Northern blot, real-time quantitative reverse transcriptase-polymerase chain reaction (RT-PCR), and serial analysis of gene expression (SAGE) in various human tissues and cells *(1,2,4)*. It has been suggested that HDAC8 mRNA is ubiquitously expressed since this transcript could be detected in all normal human tissues examined *(1–3)*. Intriguingly, different authors have observed HDAC8 transcript to be expressed at the highest levels in different organs, including normal human brain *(1,3)*, pancreas *(1,4)*, kidney *(3,4)*, prostate *(3)*, and liver *(2)*. Nevertheless, the expression profile of HDAC8 mRNA has been found to be distinctly different from that of HDAC1 to 3 transcripts *(3)*.

Two HDAC8 mRNA Species But Only One HDAC8 Protein Can Be Detected in Various Cells and Tissues

Interestingly, two HDAC8 mRNA species (1.7–2.0 and 2.2–2.4 kb) have been detected with variable relative abundance of the longer vs shorter mRNA in various human normal tissues and cancer cell lines *(1–3)*. The two different mRNA species detected by Northern blot have been suggested to represent tissue-specific splice variants of HDAC8 *(3)*. Cloning and sequence analysis of the larger transcript (2.4 kb) from a HeLa cell cDNA library has revealed that it encodes a product resulting in a fusion of 22 extraneous amino acid residues after Gly^{234} of HDAC8, followed by a stop codon *(2)*. It is not known at this time whether this truncation is the result of alternative splicing and whether this larger transcript is actually translated into protein. Nevertheless, it is expected that if this transcript is effectively translated in cells, the truncation would delete many of the residues predicted to be important for HDAC enzyme activity *(2)*.

Despite the possible existence of two HDAC8 mRNA species, an apparently unique HDAC8 protein is detected by Western blot analysis. Tagged HDAC8 has been transiently expressed into various eukaryotic cells, including HEK293 *(1,3)*, Rat-2 *(1)*, NIH-3T3 *(1,14)*, HeLa *(2,12)*, Cos7 *(15)*, and Sf9 cells *(2)*. In Western blots using anti-tag antibodies, exogenously expressed HDAC8 migrates as a single protein band with an observed molecular mass of around 49 kDa *(1–3,14)*. Western blots performed with the use of specific anti-HDAC8 antibodies and protein extracts from various cell lines or tissues have also yielded a single band with an expected slightly lighter apparent molecular weight of ±45 kDa *(1,12,14,16)*.

HDAC8 Is Exclusively Expressed by Normal Human Cells Showing Smooth Muscle Differentiation

Recent data have shed considerable light on the distribution of HDAC8 in normal human tissues. Indeed, the results of a screening of HDAC expression profiles in human prostate tissues have initially suggested that

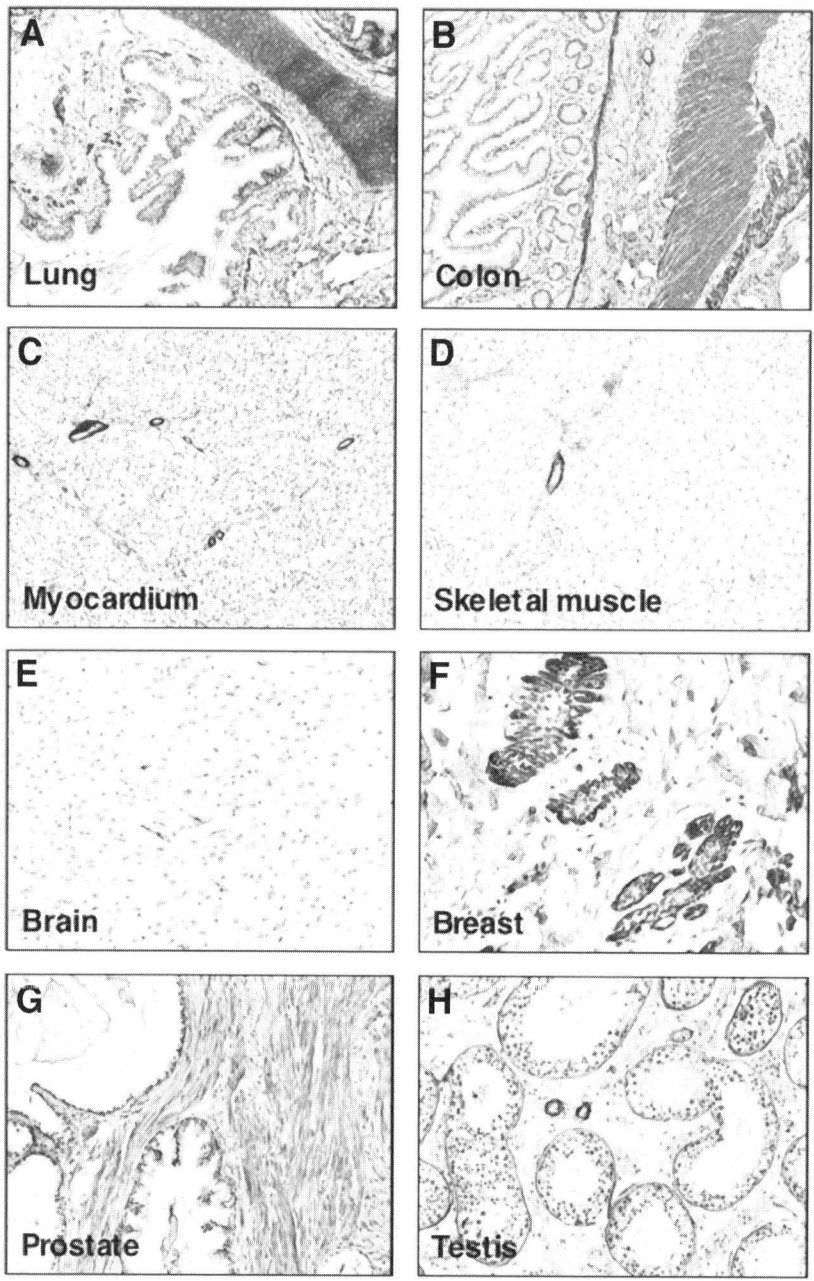

HDAC8, rather than being detected in all cell types, is exclusively expressed by some prostate stromal cells as well as by cells present in vascular walls *(16)*. Further extensive investigations of HDAC8 expression by immunohistochemistry in normal human tissues have demonstrated that HDAC8 is exclusively expressed by normal human cells showing smooth muscle differentiation in vivo, including vascular and visceral smooth muscle cells, myoepithelial cells, and myofibroblasts *(14)* (Fig. 1). Unexpectedly, the enzyme has been found to be predominantly cytosolic, both in human tissues and in in vitro grown primary human vascular smooth muscle cells (HSMCs), where it displays a cytoskeleton-like pattern of distribution reminiscent of actin stress fibers *(14)*. These latter cells exhibit substantially higher amounts of HDAC8 than primary human fibroblasts and HeLa cervix epithelial cells *(14)*.

In all tissues and organs that have been tested, smooth muscle and myoepithelial cells coexpress HDAC8 and two major components of the smooth muscle contractile apparatus, smooth muscle α-actin (α-SMA) and smooth muscle myosin heavy chain (SMMHC) *(14,17–20)*. HDAC8 is expressed by myofibroblasts that reside in some, but not all, myofibroblast-containing normal human tissues, including lung alveolar septae myofibroblasts, prostate stromal cells, reticular cells of the spleen, external theca cells of the ovary, testis peritubular myoid cells, and intestine subepithelial myofibroblasts. Interestingly, these HDAC8-positive myofibroblastic cells also uniquely coexpress α-SMA and smooth muscle myosin *(14,16,21–27)*. At the opposite, HDAC8-negative myofibroblasts, such as reticular cells of the thymus, stromal cells of the breast,

---

Fig. 1. HDAC8 is a marker of smooth muscle differentiation in normal human tissues. Formalin-fixed, paraffin-embedded normal human tissue sections were subjected to detection of HDAC8 by an immunoperoxidase technique, as previously described *(14)*. Anti-HDAC8 immunoreactivity, appearing as a brown staining, was mainly detected in the cytosol of cells showing smooth muscle differentiation, including visceral and vascular smooth muscle cells, myofibroblasts, and myoepithelial cells. **(A)** In the lung, smooth muscle cells from bronchial walls displayed strong anti-HDAC8 reactivity. **(B)** Strong diffuse anti-HDAC8 reactivity was observed in the cytosol of smooth muscle cells from colon muscularis mucosae and from arterial and capillary walls, as well as in intestinal subepithelial myofibroblasts located in the lamina propria. **(C–E)** Cardiomyocytes, skeletal muscle cells, and neuronal cells did not exhibit any detectable level of HDAC8 expression, whereas vascular smooth muscle cells harbored strong anti-HDAC8 immunoreactivity. **(F)** Strong diffuse cytoplasmic anti-HDAC8 immunoreactivity was found in myoepithelial cells lining mammary glands. **(G,H)** HDAC8 was expressed in a subset of myofibroblastic cells, including prostatic myofibroblasts **(G)** and testis peritubular myoid cells. **(H)** Sections were counterstained with hematoxylin. Original magnification: A, B, C, D and E: ×100; in A to E; ×200 in F to H.

periacinar stellate cells of the pancreas, perisinusoidal stellate (Ito) cells of the liver, and mesangial cells of the kidney may express neither α-SMA nor SMMHC *(16–19,28–34)*, suggesting that coexpression of HDAC8, α-SMA, and SMMHC may distinguish subsets of myofibroblasts residing in specific normal human tissues *(14)*.

Expression profiling data have thus unveiled HDAC8 as a novel biological marker of the smooth muscle phenotype and have further suggested a specific involvement for this HDAC in smooth muscle differentiation *(14)*.

HDAC8 IS A PREDOMINENTLY CYTOSOLIC HDAC THAT COLOCALIZES AND ASSOCIATES WITH THE SMOOTH MUSCLE ACTIN CYTOSKELETON

HDAC8 Is a Predominantly Cytoplasmic HDAC In Vivo

Based on the results of human HDAC8 cDNA transfection studies coupled with immunofluorescence analysis in various cell lines, it has been inferred that HDAC8, like other class I HDACs, is a predominantly nuclear HDAC *(1,3)*. The recently reported predominent cytoplasmic localization of HDAC8 in smooth muscle differentiated cells, in both vitro and in vivo, has therefore contrasted with a previous observation showing that a N-terminally myc-tagged HDAC8 construct transiently transfected into NIH-3T3 cells is expressed only in the cell nucleus *(1)* (Fig. 2). These differences in protein subcellular localization may have been the result of an improper folding of the N-terminally tagged protein construct, possibly hindering its localization to the cytoplasm. Indeed, other groups have shown that overexpression of C-terminally V5- or HA-tagged human HDAC8 in HEK293 or NIH-3T3 cells, respectively, leads to its concentration in nuclear regions as well as in the cytosol *(3,14,35)*. This subcellular distribution of exogenous HDAC8 is in fact similar to that of the endogenously expressed enzyme in these cells, as revealed by nuclear and cytoplasmic fractionation and Western blot analysis as well as by immunocytochemistry experiments *(14)*. It has thus been concluded that HDAC8 is a predominantly cytosolic HDAC *(14)*. This observation is not unprecedented for a class I HDAC since HDAC3 can also be cytoplasmic and contains a nuclear export signal in its central portion *(8,36)*. Whether HDAC8 also possesses an active nuclear export motif remains to be determined. At this time, one cannot exclude the possibility that HDAC8 may have a variable localization within the cell (cytosol versus nucleus), depending on the cell type and/or possible posttranslational modifications of the protein, such as phosphorylation *(12)*. In line with this possibility, it has been observed, using cellular fractionation coupled with Western blot

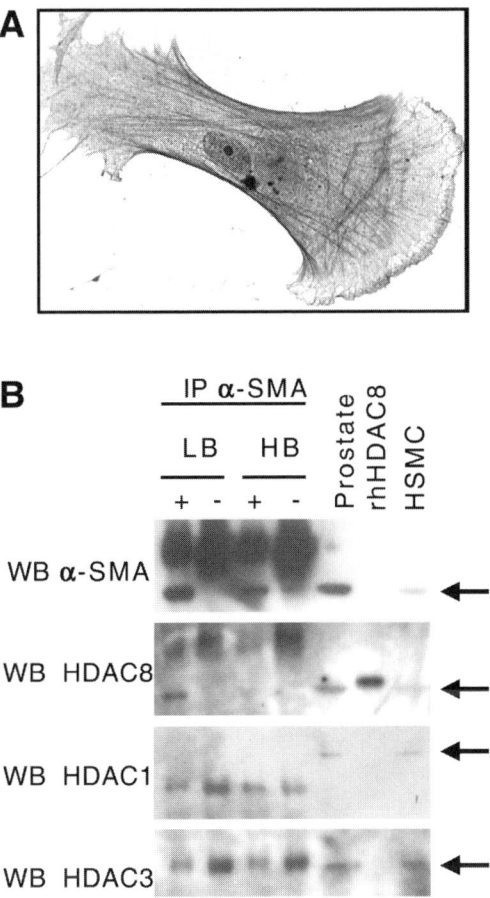

Fig. 2. HDAC8 is a predominently cytosolic HDAC that associates with the smooth muscle actin cytoskeleton. (**A**) HDAC8 expression was investigated in primary human smooth muscle cells (HSMCs) from umbilical cord vein by immunoperoxidase. Anti-HDAC8 immunostaining presented a cytoskeleton-like pattern of distribution reminiscent of actin stress fibers. (**B**) Normal human prostate tissues were lysed either in ice-cold low-stringency buffer (LB) or in high-stringency buffer (HB). Protein lysates were immunoprecipitated with a monoclonal antibody against smooth muscle α-actin (α-SMA) or with IgG2a (negative control). Whole extracts and immunocomplexes were subjected to immunoblot analysis using antibodies directed against α-SMA, HDAC8, HDAC1, and HDAC3. In protein lysates from normal human prostate tissues, HDAC8 coimmunoprecipitated with the smooth muscle isoform of α-actin, whereas neither HDAC1 nor HDAC3 were detected in the α-SMA-containing immunocomplexes. rhHDAC8, recombinant human HDAC8. (higher apparent molecular weight is because of the presence of a C-terminal V5/His[6] tag); Original magnification: ×630 in A.

experiments, that the human cancer colon cell line SW620 expresses endogenous HDAC8 mainly in its nuclear compartment *(1)*.

HDAC8 Colocalizes and Associates With α-SMA

Recent evidence has suggested that HDAC8 is not randomly distributed within the cytoplasm of smooth muscle cells. Indeed, HDAC8 is expressed in the cytoplasm of these cells according to a filamentous-like pattern reminiscent of stress fibers that is suggestive of a cytoskeletal association *(14)*. In addition, double immunofluorescence staining experiments coupled with confocal microscopy analysis have shown that epitope-tagged HDAC8 overexpressed in NIH-3T3 cells forms cytoplasmic stress fibers-like structures that colocalize with α-SMA. Recently, it has been demonstrated that the protein product resulting from inversion *(16)*, a frequent chromosomal translocation found in acute myeloid leukemia (AML), which fuses the first 165 amino acids of core binding factor β (CBF-β) to the tail region of SMMHC, specifically associates with HDAC8 through a domain present in the SMMHC portion of the CBF-β-SMMHC fusion protein *(15)*. Moreover, it has been shown previously that, in NIH-3T3 cells transfected with full-length CBF-β/SMMHC plasmid cDNA, the fusion protein is present in cytoplasm stress fiber-like structures colocalizing with actin filaments *(37)*. Collectively, these data have suggested that HDAC8 may associate with, and possibly regulate, smooth muscle acto-myosin complexes *(14)*. In agreement with this idea, coimmunoprecipitation studies have recently demonstrated that HDAC8 associates with α-SMA, both in vitro and in vivo *(38)*. In protein lysates from both primary human smooth muscle cells and human prostate tissues, HDAC8 associates with the smooth muscle isoform of α-actin, whereas no interaction is found between HDAC8 and the ubiquitously expressed β-actin isoform *(38)*. In addition, neither HDAC1 nor HDAC3 are detected in the α-SMA-containing immunocomplexes, further suggesting that HDAC8 uniquely and specifically interacts with the smooth muscle cytoskeleton *(38)*. HDAC8 therefore represents the first example of an actin cytoskeleton-interacting HDAC. Whether HDAC8 interacts directly or indirectly with α-SMA and whether any smooth muscle cytoskeletal protein may be a target of HDAC8's deacetylase activity remain to be elucidated.

ARE HISTONES THE PHYSIOLOGICAL SUBSTRATES OF HDAC8 IN VIVO?

Princeps observations have indicated that HDAC activities are constrained to the nucleus for deacetylation of nucleosomal histones. Most

HDACs can indeed function as transcriptional corepressors and often form large multisubunit protein complexes with different sets of transcriptional repressors, such as the Sin3/HDAC and Mi-2/nucleosome remodeling and deacetylase complex (NuRD)/HDAC complexes *(39–45)*. However, it has recently become clear that a number of nonhistone nuclear proteins, including the tumor suppressor p53 *(46–52)*, are also substrates for HDACs, which regulate their activity by deacetylation. In addition, some HDACs, such as HDAC6 (a class II HDAC) and SIRT2 (a class III HDAC), are predominantly expressed in the cell cytoplasm. These HDACs can deacetylate cytoskeletal acetylated α-tubulin *(35,53–56)*, with concomitant destabilization of dynamic microtubules *(35)*. Finally, recent reports have suggested a previously unrecognized HDAC location in the cell. It has indeed been demonstrated that SIRT3, a human silent information regulator 2 (SIR2) homolog, is a mitochondrial NAD-dependent deacetylase, suggesting that this sirtuin may deacetylate a substrate localized within this organelle *(57,58)*. Furthermore, a recent phylogenetic analysis of bacterial HDAC relatives has suggested that all three HDAC classes precede the evolution of histone proteins, raising the possibility that the primary activity of some "histone deacetylase" enzymes is directed against non-histone substrates *(59)*. It is thus expected that HDACs might exert, within the cell, much broader biological activities than the exclusive control of gene transcription.

Currently Known Interactors of HDAC8

Up to now, few data have been available on the potential interactions of HDAC8 with known transcriptional regulators. In initial coimmuno-precipitation studies, in contrast to other class I HDACs, no molecular interaction has been detected between HDAC8 and other characterized HDAC transcriptional cofactors such as YY1, Sin3a, and retinoblastoma-associated protein 48 (RbAp48) *(2)*. It was shown that the murine homolog of MTG16, eight twenty-one (ETO) 2—a target of t(16;21) in acute leukemia—interacts with the corepressors nuclear receptor corepressor (NCoR) and silencing mediator for retinoid and thyroid receptors (SMRT) as well as with HDAC8 but fails to bind Sin3A *(60)*. More recently, it has been demonstrated that the leukemogenic protein product resulting from inversion(16) specifically associates with HDAC8. This interaction between HDAC8 and the inv(16) fusion protein is not mediated by AML1 or Sin3A and does not occur through the CBF-β portion of the fusion protein but, unexpectedly, through a domain present in its C-terminal SMMHC portion *(15)*. In fact, this C-terminal myosin heavy chain portion of inv(16) contains an assembly competence domain (ACD), a domain required for multimerization of SMMHC *(61,62)*, that is both necessary and sufficient for trichostatin A

(TSA)-sensitive transcriptional repression mediated by inv(16) protein and is sufficient for association with HDAC8 *(15)*.

Histone Deacetylase Activity of HDAC8 In Vitro

Besides the possible association of HDAC8 with known corepressors, contradictory and variable results have been reported with respect to the capacity of HDAC8 to deacetylate histones. Hu et al. *(1)* have shown that N-terminally myc-tagged HDAC8 immunoprecipitated from HEK293 cells exhibits TSA and butyrate-inhibitable deacetylase activity toward [3H]acetate-labeled histones. In addition, they have observed in cotransfection experiments that HDAC8 is able to repress a viral SV40 early promoter activity. These authors have also intriguingly found that HDAC8, expressed as a C-terminal hexahistidine-tagged fusion protein in *E. coli* and further purified as a recombinant enzyme, is also active toward all tritiated acetylated core histones, in the absence of cofactors and without the further posttranslational modifications that occur in eukaryotic cells *(1)*. Thus, unlike most other HDACs, it has been proposed that HDAC8 may be uniquely expressed and purified from *E. coli* while retaining its enzymatic activity *(1)*. Unlike bacterial HDACs *(5)*, the addition of Zn^{2+} may completely inhibit recombinant human HDAC8 histone deacetylase activity in vitro *(1)*.

Buggy et al. *(2)* have shown that purified flag-tagged human HDAC8 from transfected insect Sf9 cells is able to deacetylate a radioacetylated histone H4 peptide, corresponding to the N-terminal 20 residues of human histone H4 and all core histones (H2A, H2B, H3, and H4), in a reaction inhibited by both sodium butyrate and TSA. Matsuyama et al. *(35)* have also observed that recombinant human His^6-tagged HDAC8 protein, produced using the baculoviral expression system in Sf9 insect cells and affinity purified using nickel-nitriloacetic acid columns, is catalytically active toward [3H]acetate-labeled histones as well as a 20-mer peptide (1–20) containing acetylated Lys^{16} of histone H4, in a TSA-inhibitable manner.

More recently, Lee et al. *(12)* have reported that phosphorylation of HDAC8 by PKA decreases its deacetylase activity, with consequent hyperacetylation of histones H3 and H4. Indeed, treatment of HeLa cells with forskolin (a potent activator of adenyl cyclase, the enzyme that catalyzes the conversion of ATP to cAMP), induces phosphorylation of transfected FLAG-tagged HDAC8 by PKA and negates the capacity of overexpressed HDAC8 to deacetylate H3 and H4.

Van den Wyngaert et al. *(3)* have created HEK293 clones constitutively overexpressing C-terminally V5-tagged HDAC8 approx five- to sixfold above untransfected cells. Total cell extracts from HDAC8 stably transfected cells have shown increased global deacetylation activity compared with the empty vector-transfected control cells. However, no change in the level of histone acetylation has been observed between the HDAC8-transfected and control cells *(3)*. In addition, as opposed to other studies *(1,12)*, immuno-precipitated HDAC8 has shown no significant deacetylase activity *(3)*.

Thus, overall, most but not all studies reported to date support the notion that HDAC8, either immunoprecipitated from eukaryotic cells or produced as a recombinant protein using various systems, exhibits deacetylase activity toward histones or histone peptides, as assessed by specific in vitro deacetylase assays.

Does HDAC8 Exert a Cytosolic Deacetylase Activity?

The question of whether histones are the true physiological substrates needs to be definitely answered. Interestingly, Hu et al. *(63)* have recently identified a potent HDAC8-selective inhibitor compound, SB-379872-A, that is not capable of increasing cellular histone acetylation or the activity of an early SV40 promoter in SW620 and Rat-2 cells, respectively, sug-gesting either that proteins other than histones may be the physiological substrate of HDAC8 or that HDAC8 is unimportant for histone deacetylation in these cells *(63)*.

In line with these observations, the analysis of HDAC8 structure has recently provided evidence that, thanks to a shorter L1 loop, the active site pocket of HDAC8 may be, as opposed to HDLP and HDAC1-3, wider and more malleable. This particular organization of HDAC8 may increase its flexibility, which in turn could enable the binding, and presumably deacetylation, of various acetylated lysines presented in different structural contexts *(6)*.

Probably one of the most compelling arguments that support the claim according to which HDAC8 may deacetylate other substrate(s) than his-tones in vivo is derived from the findings showing the predominent cytoso-lic localization of the enzyme and its ability to bind the actin cystoskeleton in smooth muscle differentiated cells from human tissues *(14,38)*. Alternatively, HDAC8 may shuttle in and out of the nucleus upon certain, yet unknown, conditions, in a scenario similar to that of class II HDACs during the myogenic process *(64,65)*, and be sequestered by the actin cytoskeleton in the cytosol.

HDAC8 REGULATES SMOOTH MUSCLE
CYTOSKELETON DYNAMICS

The demonstration that HDAC8 specifically colocalizes and associates with the smooth muscle actin cytoskeleton has suggested potential new functions for this enzyme in normal human cells showing smooth muscle differentiation *(14)*. The possible involvement of HDAC8 in the regulation of the smooth muscle cytoskeleton has been recently investigated using

RNA interference in primary HSMCs *(38)*. A striking reduction in cell size with decreased spreading has been observed in HDAC8-silenced HSMCs, whereas mock- and HDAC6 small interfering RNA (siRNA)-transfected HSMCs have exhibited no obvious modification in cell shape or size at any time before or after reseeding *(38)*. HDAC8 silencing-induced alterations of smooth muscle cell shape are readily detectable only after trypsinization and replating of the cells *(38)*. This observation has suggested that HDAC8, possibly through its interaction with α-SMA cytoskeletal protein, regulates the dynamics of smooth muscle cytoskeleton rather than its statics and may be involved in mechanisms responsible for the attachment/spreading of these cells *(38)*. This involvement may account, at least in part, for the reduced capability of HDAC8-silenced HSMCs to contract type I collagen lattices. Indeed, it has been further shown that HDAC8 is necessary for conferring the capacity to HSMCs to contract type I collagen lattices *(38)*. Thus, HDAC8 may exert its effects through a predominant cytosolic deacetylase activity possibly affecting the function of smooth muscle cytoskeletal proteins. Further studies are needed to address this issue.

REFERENCES

1. Hu E, Chen Z, Fredrickson T, et al. Cloning and characterization of a novel human class I histone deacetylase that functions as a transcription repressor. J Biol Chem 2000;275:15,254–15,264.
2. Buggy JJ, Sideris ML, Mak P, Lorimer DD, McIntosh B, Clark JM. Cloning and characterization of a novel human histone deacetylase, HDAC8. Biochem J 2000;350:199–205.
3. Van den Wyngaert I, de Vries W, Kremer A, et al. Cloning and characterization of human histone deacetylase 8. FEBS Lett 2000;478:77–83.
4. De Ruijter AJ, Van Gennip AH, Caron HN, Kemp S, Van Kuilenburg AB. Histone deacetylases (HDACs): characterization of the classical HDAC family. Biochem J 2003;370:737–749.
5. Finnin MS, Donigian JR, Cohen A, et al. Structures of a histone deacetylase homologue bound to the TSA and SAHA inhibitors. Nature 1999;401:188–193.
6. Somoza JR, Skene RJ, Katz BA, et al. Structural snapshots of human HDAC8 provide insights into the class I histone deacetylases. Structure (Camb) 2004;12:1325–1334.
7. Ayer DE. Histone deacetylases: transcriptional repression with SINers and NuRDs. Trends Cell Biol 1999;9:193–198.
8. Yang WM, Tsai SC, Wen YD, Fejer G, Seto E. Functional domains of histone deacetylase-3. J Biol Chem 2002;277:9447–9454.
9. Pflum MK, Tong JK, Lane WS, Schreiber SL. Histone deacetylase 1 phosphorylation promotes enzymatic activity and complex formation. J Biol Chem 2001;276:47,733–47,741.
10. Tsai SC, Seto E. Regulation of histone deacetylase 2 by protein kinase CK2. J Biol Chem 2002;277:31,826–31,833.

11. David G, Neptune MA, DePinho RA. SUMO-1 modification of histone deacety-lase 1 (HDAC1) modulates its biological activities. J Biol Chem 2002;277: 23,658–23,663.

12. Lee H, Rezai-Zadeh N, Seto E. Negative regulation of histone deacetylase 8 activity by cyclic AMP-dependent protein kinase A. Mol Cell Biol 2004;24: 765–773.

13. Galasinski SC, Resing KA, Goodrich JA, Ahn NG. Phosphatase inhibition leads to histone deacetylases 1 and 2 phosphorylation and disruption of corepressor interactions. J Biol Chem 2002;277:19,618–19,626.

14. Waltregny D, de Leval L, Glénisson W, et al. Expression of HDAC8, a class I his-tone deacetylase, is restricted to cells showing smooth muscle differentiation in normal human tissues. Am J Pathol 2004;165:553–564.

15. Durst KL, Lutterbach B, Kummalue T, Friedman AD, Hiebert SW. The inv(16) fusion protein associates with corepressors via a smooth muscle myosin heavy-chain domain. Mol Cell Biol 2003;23:607–619.

16. Waltregny D, North BJ, Van Mellaert F, de Leval J, Verdin E, Castronovo V. Screening of histone deacetylase (HDAC) expression in human prostate cancer reveals distinct class I HDAC profiles between epithelial and stromal cells. Eur J Histochem 2004;48:273–290.

17. Skalli O, Ropraz P, Trzeciak A, Benzonana G, Gillessen D, Gabbiani G. A mon-oclonal antibody against alpha-smooth muscle actin: a new probe for smooth muscle differentiation. J Cell Biol 1986;103:2787–2796.

18. Longtine JA, Pinkus GS, Fujiwara K, Corson JM. Immunohistochemical local-ization of smooth muscle myosin in normal human tissues. J Histochem Cytochem 1985;33:179–184.

19. Benzonana G, Skalli O, Gabbiani G. Correlation between the distribution of smooth muscle or non muscle myosins and alpha-smooth muscle actin in normal and pathological soft tissues. Cell Motil Cytoskelet 1988;11:260–274.

20. Gugliotta P, Sapino A, Macri L, Skalli O, Gabbiani G, Bussolati G. Specific demonstration of myoepithelial cells by anti-alpha smooth muscle actin antibody. J Histochem Cytochem 1988;36:659–663.

21. Amsterdam A, Lindner HR, Groschel-Stewart U. Localization of actin and myosin in the rat oocyte and follicular wall by immunofluorescence. Anat Rec 1977;187:311–328.

22. Leslie KO, Mitchell JJ, Woodcock-Mitchell JL, Low RB. Alpha smooth muscle actin expression in developing and adult human lung. Differentiation 1990;44: 143–149.

23. Walles B, Groschel-Stewart U, Kannisto P, Owman C, Sjoberg NO, Unsicker K. Immunocytochemical demonstration of contractile cells in the human ovarian follicle. Experientia 1990;46:682–683.

24. Schmitt-Graff A, Desmouliere A, Gabbiani G. Heterogeneity of myofibroblast phenotypic features: an example of fibroblastic cell plasticity. Virchows Arch 1994;425:3–24.

25. Zhang HY, Gharaee-Kermani M, Zhang K, Karmiol S, Phan SH. Lung fibroblast alpha-smooth muscle actin expression and contractile phenotype in bleomycin-induced pulmonary fibrosis. Am J Pathol 1996;148:527–537.

26. Jostarndt-Fogen K, Djonov V, Draeger A. Expression of smooth muscle markers in the developing murine lung: potential contractile properties and lineal descent. Histochem Cell Biol 1998;110:273–284.

27. Powell DW, Mifflin RC, Valentich JD, Crowe SE, Saada JI, West AB. Myofibroblasts. I. Paracrine cells important in health and disease. Am J Physiol 1999;277:C1–C9.

28. Ramadori G, Veit T, Schwogler S, et al. Expression of the gene of the alpha-smooth muscle-actin isoform in rat liver and in rat fat-storing (ITO) cells. Virchows Arch B Cell Pathol Incl Mol Pathol 1990;59:349–357.

29. Nouchi T, Tanaka Y, Tsukada T, Sato C, Marumo F. Appearance of alpha-smooth-muscle-actin-positive cells in hepatic fibrosis. Liver 1991;11:100–105.

30. Schmitt-Graff A, Kruger S, Bochard F, Gabbiani G, Denk H. Modulation of alpha smooth muscle actin and desmin expression in perisinusoidal cells of normal and diseased human livers. Am J Pathol 1991;138:1233–1242.

31. Rockey DC, Boyles JK, Gabbiani G, Friedman SL. Rat hepatic lipocytes express smooth muscle actin upon activation in vivo and in culture. J Submicrosc Cytol Pathol 1992;24:193–203.

32. Elger M, Drenckhahn D, Nobiling R, Mundel P, Kriz W. Cultured rat mesangial cells contain smooth muscle alpha-actin not found in vivo. Am J Pathol 1993;142:497–509.

33. Lazard D, Sastre X, Frid MG, Glukhova MA, Thiery JP, Koteliansky VE. Expression of smooth muscle-specific proteins in myoepithelium and stromal myofibroblasts of normal and malignant human breast tissue. Proc Natl Acad Sci U S A 1993;90:999–1003.

34. Apte MV, Haber PS, Applegate TL, et al. Periacinar stellate shaped cells in rat pancreas: identification, isolation, and culture. Gut 1998;43:128–133.

35. Matsuyama A, Shimazu T, Sumida Y, et al. In vivo destabilization of dynamic microtubules by HDAC6-mediated deacetylation. EMBO J 2002;21:6820–6831.

36. Takami Y, Nakayama T. N-terminal region, C-terminal region, nuclear export signal, and deacetylation activity of histone deacetylase-3 are essential for the viability of the DT40 chicken B cell line. J Biol Chem 2000;275:16,191–16,201.

37. Wijmenga C, Gregory PE, Hajra A, et al. Core binding factor beta-smooth muscle myosin heavy chain chimeric protein involved in acute myeloid leukemia forms unusual nuclear rod-like structures in transformed NIH 3T3 cells. Proc Natl Acad Sci U S A 1996;93:1630–1635.

38. Waltregny D, Glénisson W, Tran SL, et al. Histone deacetylase HDAC8 associates with smooth muscle alpha-actin and is essential for smooth muscle contractility. FASEB J 2005;19:966–968.

39. Nagy L, Kao HY, Chakravarti D, et al. Nuclear receptor repression mediated by a complex containing SMRT, mSin3A, and histone deacetylase. Cell 1997;89:373–380.

40. Alland L, Muhle R, Hou H Jr, et al. Role for N-CoR and histone deacetylase in Sin3-mediated transcriptional repression. Nature 1997;387:49–55.

41. Koipally J, Renold A, Kim J, Georgopoulos K. Repression by Ikaros and Aiolos is mediated through histone deacetylase complexes. EMBO J 1999;18:3090–3100.

42. Johnson CA, Turner BM. Histone deacetylases: complex transducers of nuclear signals. Semin Cell Dev Biol 1999;10:179–188.

43. Khochbin S, Wolffe AP. The origin and utility of histone deacetylases. FEBS Lett 1997;419:157–160.

44. Knoepfler PS, Eisenman RN. Sin meets NuRD and other tails of repression. Cell 1999;99:447–450.
45. Zhang Y, Ng HH, Erdjument-Bromage H, Tempst P, Bird A, Reinberg D. Analysis of the NuRD subunits reveals a histone deacetylase core complex and a connection with DNA methylation. Genes Dev 1999;13:1924–1935.
46. Vaziri H, Dessain SK, Ng Eaton E, et al. hSIR2(SIRT1) functions as an NAD-dependent p53 deacetylase. Cell 2001;107:149–159.
47. Langley E, Pearson M, Faretta M, et al. Human SIR2 deacetylates p53 and antagonizes PML/p53-induced cellular senescence. EMBO J 2002;21:2383–2396.
48. Luo J, Su F, Chen D, Shiloh A, Gu W. Deacetylation of p53 modulates its effect on cell growth and apoptosis. Nature 2000;408:377–381.
49. Luo J, Nikolaev AY, Imai S, et al. Negative control of p53 by Sir2alpha promotes cell survival under stress. Cell 2001;107:137–148.
50. Avalos JL, Celic I, Muhammad S, Cosgrove MS, Boeke JD, Wolberger C. Structure of a Sir2 enzyme bound to an acetylated p53 peptide. Mol Cell 2002;10:523–535.
51. Smith J. Human Sir2 and the 'silencing' of p53 activity. Trends Cell Biol 2002;12:404–406.
52. Zeng L, Zhang Y, Chien S, Liu X, Shyy JY. The role of p53 deacetylation in p21Waf1 regulation by laminar flow. J Biol Chem 2003;278:24,594–24,599.
53. Haggarty SJ, Koeller KM, Wong JC, Grozinger CM, Schreiber SL. Domain-selective small-molecule inhibitor of histone deacetylase 6 (HDAC6)-mediated tubulin deacetylation. Proc Natl Acad Sci U S A 2003;100:4389–4394.
54. Hubbert C, Guardiola A, Shao R, et al. HDAC6 is a microtubule-associated deacetylase. Nature 2002;417:455–458.
55. North BJ, Marshall BL, Borra MT, Denu JM, Verdin E. The human Sir2 ortholog, SIRT2, is an NAD+-dependent tubulin deacetylase. Mol Cell 2003;11:437–444.
56. Zhang Y, Li N, Caron C, et al. HDAC-6 interacts with and deacetylates tubulin and microtubules in vivo. EMBO J 2003;22:1168–1179.
57. Onyango P, Celic I, McCaffery JM, Boeke JD, Feinberg AP. SIRT3, a human SIR2 homologue, is an NAD-dependent deacetylase localized to mitochondria. Proc Natl Acad Sci U S A 2002;99:13,653–13,658.
58. Schwer B, North BJ, Frye RA, Ott M, Verdin E. The human silent information regulator (Sir)2 homologue hSIRT3 is a mitochondrial nicotinamide adenine dinucleotide-dependent deacetylase. J Cell Biol 2002;158:647–657.
59. Gregoretti I, Lee YM, Goodson HV. Molecular evolution of the histone deacetylase family: functional implications of phylogenetic analysis. J Mol Biol 2004;338:17–31.
60. Amann JM, Nip J, Strom DK, et al. ETO, a target of t(8;21) in acute leukemia, makes distinct contacts with multiple histone deacetylases and binds mSin3A through its oligomerization domain. Mol Cell Biol 2001;21:6470–6483.
61. Kummalue T, Lou J, Friedman AD. Multimerization via its myosin domain facilitates nuclear localization and inhibition of core binding factor (CBF) activities by the CBFβ-smooth muscle myosin heavy chain myeloid leukemia protein. Mol Cell Biol 2002;22:8278–8291.
62. Sohn RL, Vikstrom KL, Strauss M, Cohen C, Szent-Gyorgyi AG, Leinwand LA. A 29 residue region of the sarcomeric myosin rod is necessary for filament formation. J Mol Biol 1997;266:317–330.

63. Hu E, Dul E, Sung CM, et al. Identification of novel isoform-selective inhibitors within class I histone deacetylases. J Pharmacol Exp Ther 2003;307:720–728.

64. McKinsey TA, Zhang CL, Lu J, Olson EN. Signal-dependent nuclear export of a histone deacetylase regulates muscle differentiation. Nature 2000;408:106–111.

65. McKinsey TA, Zhang CL, Olson EN. Activation of the myocyte enhancer factor-2 transcription factor by calcium/calmodulin-dependent protein kinase-stimulated binding of 14-3-3 to histone deacetylase 5. Proc Natl Acad Sci U S A 2000; 97:14,400–14,405.

II CLASS II HISTONE DEACETYLASES

5 Regulation of Muscle Gene Expression by Histone Deacetylases

Timothy A. McKinsey, PhD
and Eric N. Olson, PhD

From: *Cancer Drug Discovery and Development*
Histone Deacetylases: Transcriptional Regulation and Other Cellular Functions
Edited by: E. Verdin © Humana Press Inc., Totowa, NJ

SUMMARY

Histone deacetylases (HDACs) repress gene expression by deacetylating lysine residues in core histones, which promotes chromatin condensation and thereby limits access of basal transcriptional machinery to gene regulatory elements. In the past 5 years, HDACs have emerged as key regulators of gene expression in muscle. In this chapter, we discuss the initial findings linking HDACs to the control of striated muscle cell differentiation and growth. In addition, we describe work that established roles for a subset of HDACs as signal integrators that couple cues emanating from the cell surface to muscle-specific genes in the nucleus, and we speculate on the potential to manipulate these regulatory cascades with small molecules as a means to treat cardiac and skeletal myopathies.

Key Words: Histone deacetylase, transcription, muscle differentiation, muscle hypertrophy, MEF2, MyoD.

HISTONE ACETYLATION AND CHROMATIN STRUCTURE

In eukaryotes, histone-dependent packaging of genomic DNA into chromatin is a central mechanism for gene regulation. The basic unit of chromatin is the nucleosome, which comprises 146 bp of DNA wrapped around a histone octamer that consists of two copies each of histones H2A, H2B, H3, and H4. Nucleosomes interact to create a highly compact structure that limits access of genomic DNA to transcription factors, thereby repressing gene expression (1).

Histone tails are unstructured, protrude from the nucleosome, and are thought to help establish intranucleosome and internucleosome interactions. Residues within histone tails are subject to diverse posttranslational modifications, including phosphorylation, acetylation, methylation, and ubiquitination, which together establish a "histone code" that governs the higher order structure of chromatin and thus gene expression (2).

Histone acetyltransferases (HATs) and histone deacetylases (HDACs) act in an opposing manner to control the acetylation state of nucleosomal histones. Acetylation of the conserved amino-terminal histone tails by

HATs is thought to result in relaxation of nucleosomal structure by weakening the interaction of the positively charged histone tails with the negatively charged phosphate backbone of DNA, allowing access of transcriptional activators and gene induction. Deacetylation of nucleosomal histones by HDACs results in transcriptional repression.

The many mammalian HDACs fall into three classes on the basis of structural and biochemical characteristics *(3)*. The detailed distinctions among classes I, II, and III HDACs are well described elsewhere in this book. Briefly, class I HDACs are comprised primarily of a catalytic domain, whereas class II HDACs contain amino-terminal extensions of approx 500 residues that harbor binding sites for other transcriptional regulators and signal transduction machinery. Class III HDACs are unique in that they require nicotinamide adenine dinucleotide (NAD) for catalytic activity. As detailed below, members of each HDAC class have been shown to repress muscle gene expression, albeit through unique mechanisms.

TRANSCRIPTIONAL CONTROL OF SKELETAL MUSCLE DIFFERENTIATION

The notion that HDACs regulate muscle gene expression initially stemmed from studies of skeletal muscle. The formation of skeletal muscle involves a series of steps in which multipotential mesodermal precursor cells become committed to a muscle cell fate and then proliferate as myoblasts until they encounter an environment lacking mitogens, at which point they exit the cell cycle and differentiate. The process of differentiation is accompanied by fusion of mononucleate myoblasts to form multinucleate muscle fibers, transcriptional activation of hundreds of muscle-specific genes, and repression of genes associated with cell proliferation (Fig. 1).

Members of the myoblast determination gene (MyoD) family of basic helix-loop-helix (bHLH) proteins—MyoD, myogenic factor 5 (Myf5), myogenin, and MRF4—act at multiple steps in the myogenic pathway to control the establishment of the myogenic lineage and the activation of differentiation genes *(4)*. These factors activate muscle transcription as heterodimers with ubiquitous bHLH proteins known as E proteins and bind E boxes (CANNTG) in the regulatory regions of muscle-specific genes. Each of the myogenic bHLH proteins can activate the complete skeletal muscle differentiation program when expressed in fibroblasts and certain other cell types.

Activation of muscle gene expression by myogenic bHLH proteins is dependent on their association with members of the myocyte enhancer factor 2 (MEF2) family of MADS (MCM1, agamous, deficiens, serum response factor)-box transcription factors, which bind a conserved A/T-rich

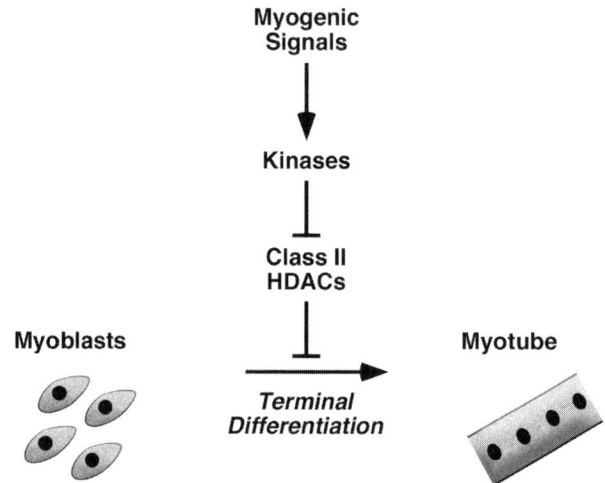

Fig. 1. Control of myoblast differentiation by myogenic signals impinging on class II HDACs. Proliferating, undifferentiated myoblasts exit the cell cycle and fuse to form multinucleated myotubes in response to myogenic signals, which activate kinases that impinge on class II HDACs. Phosphorylation of class II HDACs derepresses the muscle differentiation program, allowing for activation of muscle structural genes.

sequence in muscle gene control regions *(5)*. MEF2 factors cannot activate muscle genes alone, but they potentiate the muscle-inducing activity of MyoD family proteins and are essential for myoblast differentiation in vivo and in vitro.

INHIBITION OF SKELETAL MUSCLE DIFFERENTIATION BY CLASS II HDAC-MEF2 INTERACTIONS

Investigators began focusing on potential roles for HDACs in the control of skeletal muscle differentiation following the discovery that MEF2 can physically associate with class II HDACs 4, 5, 7, and 9. MEF2-HDAC interactions were initially uncovered by yeast two-hybrid screens for MEF2 binding partners *(6,7)* and have now been confirmed employing a variety of independent biochemical techniques *(8–12)*. Binding of class II HDACs to MEF2 is mediated by 18 conserved amino acids in the amino-terminal extensions of HDAC4, -5, -7, and -9 (Fig. 2). Class I and III HDACs lack this domain and fail to associate directly with or regulate the activity of MEF2.

Class II HDACs bind sequences in MEF2 at the junction of the MADS/MEF2 domains *(13)*. Of note, the transcriptional coactivators p300

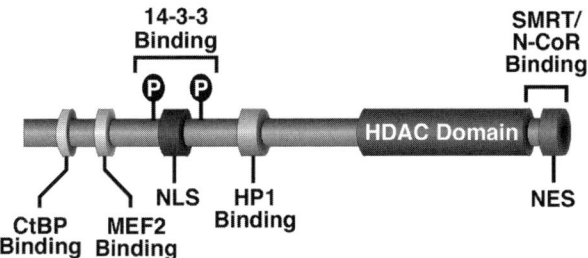

Fig. 2. Schematic diagram of a class II HDAC. The structure of class II HDACs is shown, with binding sites for other transcriptional activators and repressors and for the 14-3-3 protein. CtBP, carboxy-terminal binding protein; HP1, heterochromatin protein 1; MEF2, myocyte enhancer factor 2; NES, nuclear export sequence; NLS, nuclear localization sequence; SMRT/NCoR, silencing mediator for retinoid and thyroid receptors/nuclear receptor corepressor.

and glucocorticoid receptor interacting protein (GRIP), which possess HAT activity, bind to the same region of MEF2 *(14,15)*. Thus, MEF2 functions as either a transcriptional activator or repressor, depending on the type of chromatin-modifying enzymes to which it is bound. Association of HDAC or HAT with MEF2 does not appear to alter its DNA binding properties significantly *(13)*, and the crystal structure of MEF2 bound to DNA is fully consistent with the formation of a ternary complex of MEF2, a HAT or HDAC, and MEF2 target genes *(16)*. More recent crystal structure analysis has revealed that the HDAC/HAT binding site of MEF2 exhibits remarkable structural similarity to the peptide-binding cleft of the major histocompatibility complex, with a hydrophobic groove consisting of a β-sheet floor and two α-helical rims *(17)*. Class II HDACs appear to form an amphipathic α-helix to bind the hydrophobic groove on MEF2, establishing a triple-helical interaction.

Given the ability of class II HDACs to associate with MEF2 and the key role of MEF2 factors in muscle gene regulation, it was hypothesized that these interactions may be relevant to muscle differentiation. Indeed, HDACs 4, 5, and 7, which are expressed in undifferentiated myoblasts, act as potent inhibitors of C2 skeletal muscle cell differentiation, and also efficiently block MyoD-dependent conversion of fibroblasts into muscle *(11,13)*. The effect of class II HDACs on MyoD function is mediated indirectly via MEF2, since MyoD-dependent transcription is unaffected unless an E-box is present in tandem with a MEF2 binding site. Consistent with this, class II HDACs do not directly interact with MyoD, and class II HDAC mutants lacking the MEF2 binding domain fail to inhibit myogenesis efficiently *(13)*.

The repressive effects of class II HDACs on MEF2 transcriptional activity and muscle differentiation are mediated not only by intrinsic deacetylase activity but also by corepressors, which tether to the amino termini of class II HDACs. These corepressors include carboxy-terminal binding protein (CtBP) and heterochromatin protein 1 (HP1) (Fig. 2) *(18,19)*. Class II HDACs also associate with class I HDACs *(18,20)*, and it has been proposed that this interaction is essential for class II HDAC-mediated transcriptional repression *(20)*. The ability of class II HDACs to associate with corepressors and other HDACs probably accounts for the potent antimyogenic activity of MEF2-interacting transcription repressor (MITR), a deacetylase domain-deficient splice variant of HDAC9 *(21)*.

INHIBITION OF SKELETAL MUSCLE DIFFERENTIATION BY CLASS I HDAC-MyoD INTERACTIONS

Studies have also suggested roles for class I HDACs in the control of MyoD function. Whereas we showed that class II HDACs could indirectly affect MyoD activity via MEF2, class I HDACs (HDAC1 in particular) appear to target MyoD directly. HDAC activity can be recruited to MyoD via a corepressor complex containing nuclear receptor corepressor (NCoR) *(22)*. In addition, there is evidence that HDAC1 directly associates with MyoD *(23)*. Overexpression of either NCoR or HDAC1 blocks MyoD-mediated transcription and muscle differentiation. HDAC1 appears to regulate MyoD target gene expression through deacetylation of nucleosomal histones as well as MyoD itself, which results in reduced activity of the transcription factor *(23–25)*.

CONVERTING MyoD AND MEF2 FROM REPRESSORS TO ACTIVATORS OF SKELETAL MYOGENESIS

The expression of HDACs that bind MEF2 and MyoD in myoblasts provides a potential explanation for the paradoxical findings that these transcription factors are present in undifferentiated muscle cells, but their target genes are not expressed. This model is based on the assumption that MEF2 and MyoD are bound to target sites in regions of repressed chromatin in undifferentiated myoblasts (Fig. 3). Although initial in vivo footprinting experiments argued otherwise *(26)*, more recent work employing the highly sensitive chromatin immunoprecipitation technique support the hypothesis. Specifically, Mal and Harter *(27)* demonstrated that MyoD recruits HDAC1 to the *myogenin* promoter, and we have provided evidence that MEF2 tethers class II HDACs to the same regulatory region *(13,18)*, the net result being deacetylation of local histones. Interestingly, nucleosomes within the *myogenin* promoter are also methylated on lysine-9, which has been associated with transcriptional repression in

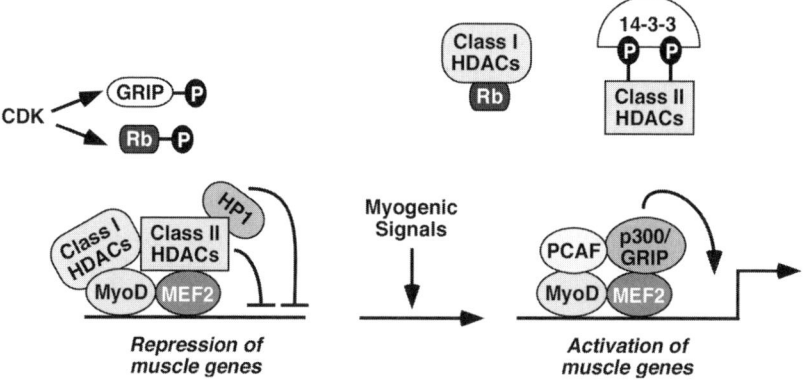

Fig. 3. Differential association of myoblast determination gene (MyoD) and myocyte enhancer factor (MEF2) with chromatin remodeling enzymes during skeletal muscle differentiation. Muscle structural genes are repressed in proliferating, undifferentiated myoblasts, at least in part, by the association of MyoD and MEF2 with class I and II HDACs, respectively. Class II HDACs also recruit heterochromatin protein 1 (HP1), which further represses downstream target genes by histone methylation. Cyclin-dependent kinase (CDK) phosphorylates retinoblastoma (Rb) protein and glucocorticoid receptor interacting protein (GRIP) in undifferentiated cells. In response to myogenic signals, class II HDACs are phosphorylated, which creates docking sites for 14-3-3 and stimulates nuclear export, allowing for the docking of p300/GRIP on MEF2 and transcriptional activation. Association of class I HDACs with hypophosphorylated Rb allows for association of MyoD with p300/CBP-associated factor (PCAF) and transcriptional activation.

other systems. This posttranslational modification appears to be regulated by recruitment of the histone methyltransferase suppressor of variegation (SUVAR) by class II HDACs bound by HP1. Thus, MEF2 and MyoD function as transcriptional repressors in undifferentiated myoblasts by recruiting multiple negatively acting chromatin-modifying enzymes to muscle gene-regulatory elements.

How is HDAC-mediated repression of MyoD and MEF2 overcome in myoblasts? In both cases, the bound HDACs are replaced with HATs, thus transforming MyoD and MEF2 from transcriptional repressors to transcriptional activators (Fig. 3). With regard to MEF2, class II HDACs are shuttled from the nucleus to the cytoplasm during muscle differentiation, thereby freeing MEF2 to associate with HATs and activate downstream target genes *(28)*. All MEF2-binding class II HDACs harbor two conserved serine residues that are targets for phosphorylation, and phosphoryl transfer to these serines creates a docking site for the intracellular chaperone protein 14-3-3 *(29–31)* (Fig. 2). Binding of 14-3-3 to phospho-HDACs results in dissociation of HDACs from MEF2 and activation of a cryptic nuclear export sequence (NES) at the extreme carboxy terminus of all class II HDACs (Fig. 2), with resulting export of the 14-3-3/HDAC complexes from the nucleus to the cytoplasm *(32,33)*. HDAC5, HDAC7, and MITR all undergo phosphorylation-dependent release from MEF2, although MITR lacks an NES and thus is retained in the nucleus *(21)*. Despite possessing the same regulatory serines as other class II HDACs, HDAC4 is localized to the cytoplasm of myoblasts and translocated to the nucleus of differentiated myotubes *(34)*. The nature of this differential regulation remains unknown. The signaling pathways that govern class II HDAC phosphorylation are complex and are discussed below.

Analogously, MyoD associates with HDAC1 in undifferentiated myoblasts and the HAT p300/cyclic AMP-responsive element binding protein (CBP)-associated factor (PCAF) during skeletal muscle differentiation *(25)* (Fig. 3). However, the mechanism for neutralization of MyoD-bound HDAC is different from that observed for MEF2-bound HDAC. The retinoblastoma (Rb) tumor suppressor protein positively regulates muscle differentiation, and it appears to do so by competing with MyoD for binding to HDAC1 *(35)*. Rb is phosphorylated in undifferentiated myoblasts by cyclin-dependent kinases (CDKs), and this posttranslational modification prohibits binding to HDAC1. During muscle differentiation, CDKs are inactivated, leading to hypophosphorylation of Rb. In this state, Rb effectively displaces HDAC1 from MyoD, allowing it to associate with PCAF and activate muscle gene expression. Remarkably, approx 70% of total HDAC1 can be found complexed with hypophosphorylated Rb in myotubes. CDK activity in proliferating myoblasts was also recently shown to block MEF2 function by prohibiting binding of the GRIP coactivator to the MADS/MEF2 domain of the transcription factor *(36)*.

DIFFERENTIAL EFFECTS OF HDAC INHIBITORS ON SKELETAL MUSCLE

Given the ability of HDAC1 to repress MyoD activity as well as the ability of class II HDACs to block MEF2 target gene expression, one would predict that pharmacological inhibitors of HDACs would stimulate muscle gene expression via these transcription factors and thus enhance myogenesis *(37)*. Paradoxically, however, HDAC inhibitors, including the hydroxamic acid trichostatin A (TSA) and the short-chain fatty acid butyrate, have been shown to block muscle differentiation in cultured myoblasts and frog embryos *(38)*. A potential explanation for these results was provided by the discovery that TSA, butyrate, and another recently characterized HDAC inhibitor, valproic acid, can either stimulate or inhibit muscle differentiation, depending on when and for how long they are added to cells *(39)*. Skeletal muscle differentiation is induced in cell culture by removing growth medium from proliferating myoblasts and replacing it with low-serum-containing medium. Myoblasts fail to differentiate when treated with HDAC inhibitors at the time of serum withdrawal. However, exposure of growing myoblasts to HDAC inhibitors followed by removal of the inhibitor before serum withdrawal results in enhanced muscle differentiation.

What is the molecular basis for the temporally restricted effects of HDAC inhibitors on the muscle differentiation program? The data suggest that HDACs can either stimulate or block myogenesis depending on the protein to which they are bound. For example, association of HDAC1 with MyoD in proliferating myoblasts results in repression of MyoD-dependent gene expression and inhibition of myogenesis. Thus, addition of HDAC inhibitors to myoblasts should stimulate muscle gene expression by relieving MyoD from the repressive effects of HDAC1. In contrast, association of HDAC1 with hypophosphorylated Rb promotes muscle differentiation by blocking the E2F-dependent genes that stimulate proliferation. Thus, inhibition of Rb-bound HDAC, which exists only after serum withdrawal, should result in impaired ability to exit the cell cycle and thus a failure to differentiate (Fig. 3).

HDAC inhibitors also promote fusion of myoblasts with preexisting myotubes *(39)*. The fusigenic activity of HDAC inhibitors appears to be mediated by follistatin, a protein that binds members of the transforming growth factor-β (TGF-β) superfamily of secreted proteins. Exposure of myoblasts to HDAC inhibitors results in upregulation of follistatin expression. In turn, follistatin binds to and suppresses the activity of myostatin, a TGF-β family member that negatively regulates muscle mass *(40)*. Thus, it has been suggested that HDAC inhibitors may be useful in treating individuals with defects in muscle regeneration *(39)*.

CLASS II HDACS AND MUSCLE FIBER TYPE

Work with the arrested development of righting response (ADR) mouse suggests that in certain contexts, activation of MEF2 may be coupled to signal-dependent proteolysis of class II HDACs and that this mode of regulation has important implications for muscle fiber type determination. The ADR mouse contains mutations in the *chloride channel 1 (CLCN1)* gene that lead to the development of nondystrophic myotonia characterized by increased numbers of slow/oxidative skeletal muscle fibers and a lack of fast/glycolytic fibers. Previous studies demonstrated that MEF2 plays a central role in the regulation of slow fiber-specific genes and in the transformation from the fast to the slow phenotype *(41–43)*. Consistent with these findings, MEF2 transcriptional activity was dramatically elevated in the muscles of ADR mice, and this activation appeared to be post-translationally regulated, since there was no change in the level of MEF2 protein in ADR muscles compared with those in wild-type controls *(44)*. Remarkably, the protein levels for HDAC4, -5, and -7 were found to be dramatically decreased in ADR muscles, without a concomitant reduction in the expression of mRNA transcripts for these HDACs. These results suggest that under certain conditions, activation of MEF2-responsive genes involves signal-dependent degradation of class II HDACs. Of note, HDAC7 has been shown to undergo ubiquitin/proteasome-dependent degradation in cultured fibroblasts *(45)*. It will be of interest to determine the potential involvement of the ubiquitin/proteasome pathway in governing skeletal muscle fiber type.

CLASS III HDACs IN SKELETAL MUSCLE

In mammals, seven homologs of the *Saccharomyces cerevisiae* HDAC silent information regulator (Sir)2 have been identified and are referred to as class III HDACs *(46)*. Sir2 HDACs uniquely require NAD for activity. In yeast, Sir2 governs life span extension in response to caloric restriction. In vitro studies have revealed a role for mammalian Sir2α in the control of skeletal muscle differentiation. Sir2α is recruited to muscle gene regulatory elements through association with MyoD, resulting in histone hypoacetylation and transcription repression *(47)*. The repressive actions of Sir2α appear to be overcome by changes in metabolic state that normally accompany muscle differentiation. Specifically, in cells undergoing differentiation, the levels of NAD are reduced such that Sir2α catalytic activity is diminished. Sir2α is also abundantly expressed in the heart *(48)*. Thus it will be of interest to determine whether this metabolic sensor controls transcriptional responses to stress in the myocardium (*see* the next section).

HDACs IN THE HEART

Adult cardiac myocytes respond to stress by hypertrophic growth, during which cells increase in size without dividing, assemble additional sarcomeres to maximize force generation, and activate a fetal cardiac gene program *(49–52)*. Cardiac hypertrophy is often associated with increased risk of morbidity and mortality, and thus studies aimed at understanding the molecular mechanisms of cardiomyocyte hypertrophy could have a significant impact on human health.

A variety of stimuli elicit a hypertrophic response, including hypertension, myocardial infarction, and abnormal contractile proteins. At the cell surface, humoral factors such as angiotensin II and endothelin-1 trigger cardiac hypertrophy by activating diverse downstream signaling pathways, including those involving the calcium/calmodulin-dependent phosphatase calcineurin, calcium/calmodulin-dependent protein kinase

(CaMK), mitogen-activated protein kinases, and protein kinase C (PKC). Despite our understanding of the signaling pathways that contribute to hypertrophic growth, the terminal steps in the pathways that lead to reactivation of fetal cardiac genes are only now being defined *(53)*.

Recent data suggest that signal-dependent nuclear export of class II HDACs serves as a final common end point for cardiac hypertrophic signaling cascades. Given the fact that class II HDACs are abundantly expressed in the heart *(54,55)* and that MEF2 transcriptional activity is upregulated in response to cardiac hypertrophic signals *(56)*, it was hypothesized that these chromatin-modifying enzymes may negatively control pathological cardiac gene expression. Consistent with this notion, HDAC5 undergoes nuclear export in response to a plethora of hypetrophic agonists *(57,58)*, and nonphosphorylatable mutants of class II HDACs block hypertrophy in response to diverse pathological signals when they are overexpressed in cultured cardiac myocytes *(59–61)*. Furthermore, targeted disruption of the gene encoding either HDAC5 or HDAC9 results in extreme hypersensitivity to pathologic signals in the heart and triggers spontaneous cardiac hypertrophy with age *(59,61)* (Fig. 4).

Given the apparent role of class II HDACs as nuclear integrators of hypertrophic signaling networks, there has been interest in identifying the signaling molecules that impinge on these transcriptional regulators. Therapeutic strategies designed to sustain the repressive function of class II HDACs by blocking signal-dependent nuclear export of these factors could provide clinical benefit in the treatment of pathologic cardiac remodeling. Early studies demonstrated that CaMK is a potent class II HDAC kinase *(28)*. CaMK phosphorylates class II HDACs, triggering 14-3-3-dependent nuclear export of the factors *(12,29,34)*. CaMK targeting of class II HDACs provides a mechanism for coupling increases in cytosolic calcium in stressed myocardium to pathological changes in gene expression. However, an important issue that had not been resolved was whether CaMK was the sole kinase responsible for regulating HDAC nuclear export and hypertrophy or whether multiple kinases might converge on the regulatory HDAC phosphorylation sites, such that different HDAC kinases might be activated in response to different stimuli.

We recently showed that PKC signaling leads to the phosphorylation of the same sites in HDAC5 that are phosphorylated by CaMK *(57)*. The PKC family includes at least 12 different isoforms, many, but not all, of which are expressed at appreciable levels in the myocardium *(62)*. Our results demonstrated that direct activation of PKC by phorbol ester is sufficient to induce nuclear export of HDAC5 and that hypertrophic agonists stimulate nuclear export of HDAC5 in cardiac myocytes through a signaling pathway that depends on PKC activation. We also showed that a

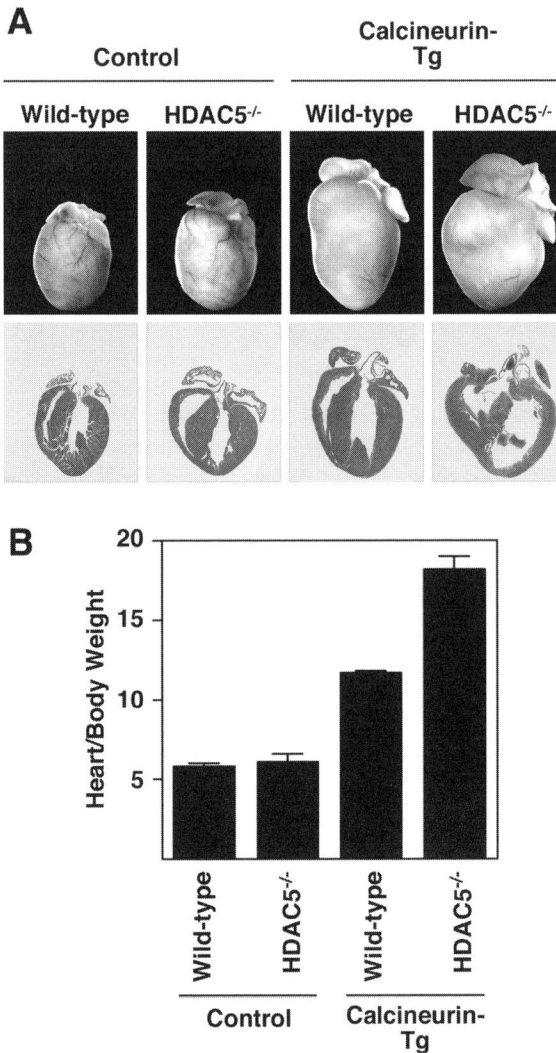

Fig. 4. Exaggerated cardiac hypertrophy of histone deacetylase 5 (HDAC5) knock-out mice in response to calcineurin signaling. (**A**) The hearts of adult mice. HDAC5$^{-/-}$ mice have normal hearts in the absence of stress. In the presence of a cardiac-specific transgene encoding activated calcineurin (Cn-Tg), the heart undergoes dramatic hypertrophic growth. The hypertrophic response is exaggerated in the HDAC5$^{-/-}$ background. (**B**) Heart weight/body weight ratios.

protein kinase D (PKD), a downstream effector of PKC, could associate with and phosphorylate HDAC5 (Fig. 5). Importantly, small-molecule inhibitors of PKC/PKD, but not CaMK, abolished agonist-mediated

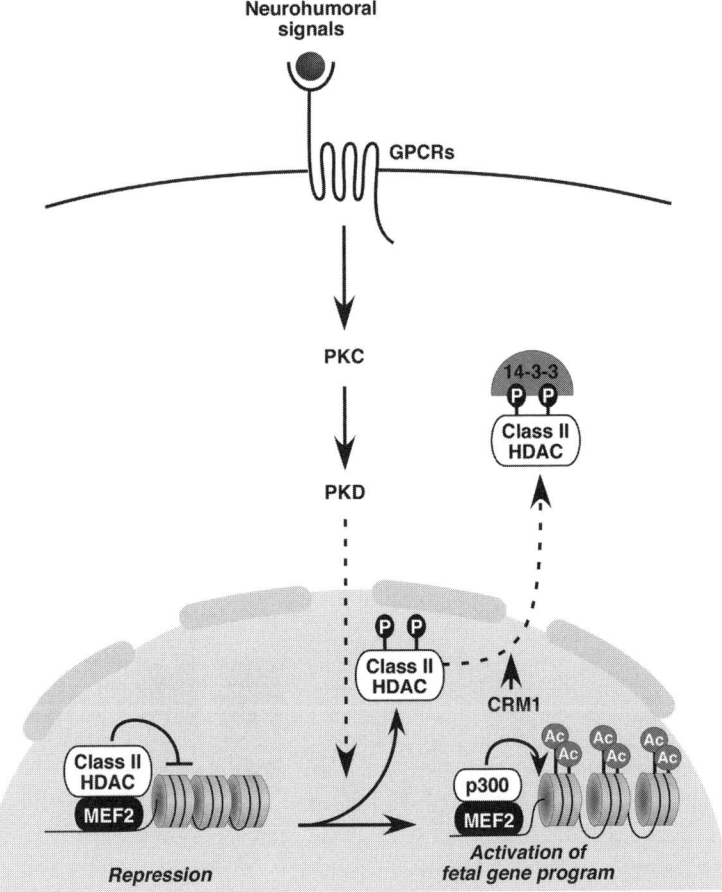

Fig. 5. Activation of the fetal gene program and cardiac hypertrophy by signaling to class II histone deacetylases (HDACs). Neurohumoral agonists acting through G-protein-coupled receptors (GPCRs) activate protein kinase C (PKC), which activates protein kinase D (PKD), which phosphorylates class II HDACs. Phospho-HDACs interact with 14-3-3 and are exported from the nucleus by the nuclear exportin protein CRM1 (chromosomal region maintenance I). Release of class II HDACs from myocyte enhancer factor 2 (MEF2) allows for binding of p300 to MEF2, acetylation of histones and nucleosome relaxation, and activation of fetal cardiac genes.

nuclear export of HDAC5 in cardiac myocytes, suggesting a predominant role for this pathway in the control of HDAC5 in the heart. Nonetheless, it remains possible that CaMK regulates HDACs in response to a subset of cardiac hypertrophic stimuli or that CaMK crosstalks with the PKC/PKD pathway.

PARADOXICAL BLOCKADE OF CARDIAC HYPERTROPHY BY HDAC INHIBITORS

Given the potent antihypertrophic activity of class II HDACs, it was hypothesized that these inhibitors, which are general antagonists of both class I and class II HDACs, would stimulate pathologic cardiac growth. Paradoxically, treatment of cardiomyocytes with three independent HDAC inhibitors (TSA, sodium butyrate, and *Helminthosporium carbonum* [HC]-toxin) repressed the increases in cell size, protein synthesis, and fetal gene expression normally evoked by hypertrophic agonists in vitro *(63–66)*.

In retrospect, the observed inability of HDAC inhibitors to override class II HDAC-mediated repression of hypertrophy is not surprising, because class II HDAC catalytic activity is not required to repress the hypertrophic program *(59)*. However, the antihypertrophic action of HDAC inhibitors remains paradoxical. The simplest interpretation of the data is that one or more HDACs play a positive role in the control of cardiac hypertrophy. Since the inhibitors used our studies antagonize the action of multiple HDACs, the identity of the putative prohypertrophic HDAC(s) remains unclear. However, a class I HDAC is a likely candidate, since class II HDACs suppress hypertrophy, and class III HDACs are resistant to inhibition by TSA.

The mechanism for HDAC inhibitor-mediated repression of cardiac hypertrophy remains unknown. We envision at least three possibilities (Fig. 6). First, HDAC inhibitors may stimulate expression of genes that encode repressors of cardiac growth. Second, HDAC inhibitors may repress expression of procardiac growth genes. Third, HDAC inhibitors may suppress cardiac hypertrophic signaling cascades, a hypothesis for which we have supporting evidence (B.C. Harrison and T.A. McKinsey, unpublished data).

HDAC inhibitors are in clinical development for treatment of cancer *(67)*. Thus, the discovery that HDAC inhibitors repress cardiac hypertrophy in the face of stress may ultimately impact on the treatment of heart failure in humans. Recently, inhibitors of the class III HDAC Sir2 were shown to stimulate cardiomyocyte apoptosis *(68)*. Given this finding, and the fact that class II HDACs repress pathological hypertrophy, future efforts to develop HDAC inhibitors as therapeutics for the heart will need to focus on specific inhibition of class I HDACs.

POTENTIAL ROLES OF CLASS II HDACs IN HEART DEVELOPMENT

Whereas mice lacking either HDAC5 or HDAC9 display normal cardiac structure and function at birth, a high percentage of HDAC5/9 double

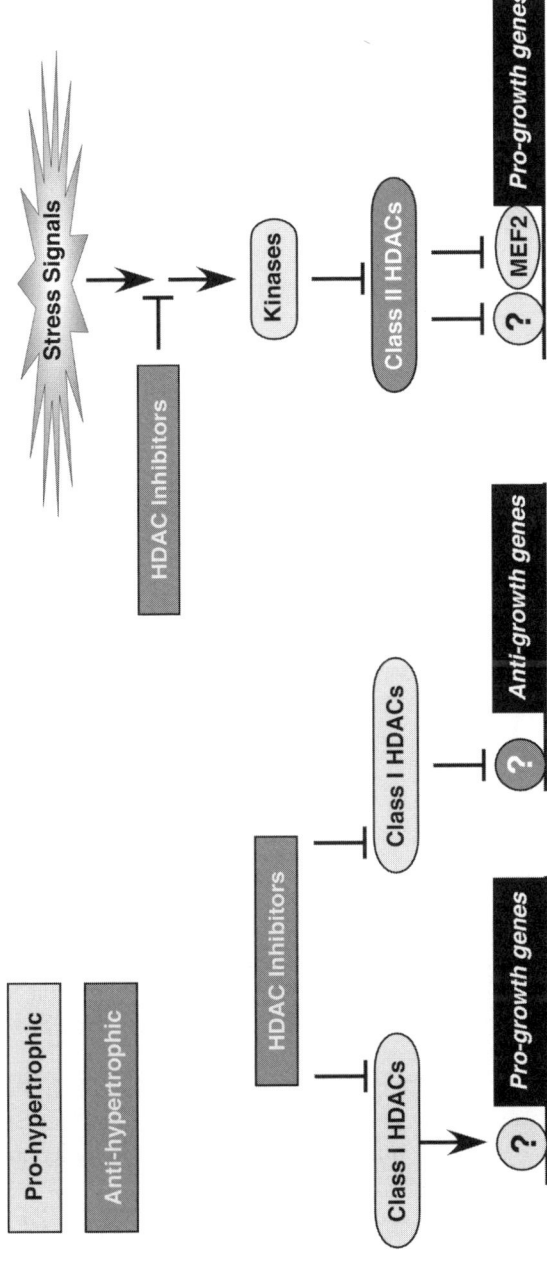

Fig. 6. Potential mechanisms of action of histone deacetylases (HDACs) and HDAC inhibitors in stress signaling in cardiac myocytes. Stress signals activate pro-hypertrophic kinases that inactivate class II HDACs, leading to activation of myocyte enhancer factor 2 (MEF2) and prohypertrophic genes. Other transcription factors may also be regulated by class II HDACs. Class I HDACs may repress expression of antigrowth genes or potentially may activate progrowth genes. HDAC inhibitors may act on class I HDACs or potentially may perturb stress signaling.

mutants die during embryogenesis and the perinatal period from ventricular septal defects and thin ventricular walls, which typically arise from
abnormalities in growth and maturation of cardiomyocytes. Both HDAC5
and HDAC9 are expressed in the developing myocardial chambers and
interventricular septum during embryogenesis *(21,61)*. Given the interaction between class II HDACs and MEF2, and the central role of MEF2 in
the control of cardiomyocyte differentiation *(69)*, the cardiac developmental defects in double mutants may result from superactivation of MEF2,
with consequent precocious differentiation and cell cycle withdrawal of
cardiomyocytes, causing hypocellularity of the myocardium. In addition,
class II HDACs have also been shown to modulate the activities of other
transcription factors involved in myocardial growth, such as the retinoic
acid receptor, serum response factor (SRF), and myocardin *(70–73)*. The
absence of HDACs 5 and 9 may therefore affect the activities of other cardiac transcriptional activators and repressors, thereby perturbing the pre-
cisely regulated programs of gene expression required for cardiac
development.

HDACs IN SMOOTH MUSCLE

In contrast to striated muscles, little is known about the roles of HDACs
in the control of gene expression in nonstriated smooth muscle. Dynamic
changes in histone acetylation have been observed at smooth muscle-specific gene regulatory elements during differentiation *(74)*, and these modifications are sensitive to histone deacetylase activity *(75)*. As mentioned
at the end of previous section, class II HDACs have been shown to associate with and repress the activity of the SRF and myocardin transcription
factors *(70,73)*. In addition to their roles in cardiac development, SRF and
myocardin function as master regulators of smooth muscle cell differentiation (reviewed in ref. *76*). Thus, although definitive experimental proof is
lacking, it seems likely that class II HDACs will prove to regulate gene
expression in smooth muscle via interactions with these and as-yet-uniden-
tified factors. The class I HDAC HDAC8 has also been reported to be
highly specific for developing smooth muscle cells, suggesting its involvement in smooth muscle gene expression *(77)*.

Expression of class II HDAC7 is highly enriched in endothelial cells
that line blood vessels (S. Chang and E.N. Olson, unpublished data), and
targeted disruption of HDAC7 in mice leads to embryonic lethality owing
to severely impaired vasculogenesis. Thus, class II HDACs may serve dual
roles in the control of blood vessel formation, by regulating SRF and
myocardin in the outer smooth muscle layer of the vessel and by coordinating gene expression in the inner endothelial cell layer. The target(s) of
HDAC7 in endothelial cells remains unknown, although MEF2 is an

obvious candidate. MEF2 is required for vascular development *(78)* and mediates endothelial cell survival *(79)*. In addition, genetic studies in humans implicate MEF2 in protection from coronary artery disease and myocardial infarction *(80)*. Studies to determine the interplay between HDAC7 and MEF2 in the control of these developmental and pathophysiological processes are forthcoming.

THERAPEUTIC IMPLICATIONS IN MUSCLE AND BEYOND

The diverse roles of HDACs in muscle gene expression during development and disease offer interesting opportunities for therapeutic modulation of muscle growth and function via the control of HDAC activity and subcellular localization. In but one example of such an approach, HDAC inhibitors are currently being tested in human clinical trials for cancer, and therapeutic benefit and tolerability have been reported. Based on studies in animal models and cultured cells, such inhibitors might be expected to exert salutary effects in the settings of heart failure or skeletal muscle wasting disorders.

Given the multiplicity of HDACs, there has been great interest in identifying specific functions of each HDAC as well as the small-molecule inhibitors that can selectively modulate the activities of individual HDAC isoforms. The generation of mice lacking individual HDAC genes will facilitate the identification of such inhibitors and promises to continue to reveal unexpected functions of HDACs in vivo.

ACKNOWLEDGMENTS

Work in the laboratory of Eric Olson is supported by grants from the NIH, the Donald W. Reynolds Cardiovascular Clinical Research Center, the Robert A. Welch Foundation, the Muscular Dystrophy Association, and the Texas Advanced Technology Program.

REFERENCES

1. Fischle W, Wang Y, Allis CD. Histone and chromatin cross-talk. Curr Opin Cell Biol 2003;15:172–183.
2. Strahl BD, Allis CD. The language of covalent histone modifications. Nature 2000;403:41–45.
3. Verdin E, Dequiedt F, Kasler HG. Class II histone deacetylases: versatile regulators. Trends Genet 2003;19:286–293.
4. Arnold HH, Winter B. Muscle differentiation: more complexity to the network of myogenic regulators. Curr Opin Genet Dev 1998;8:539–544.
5. Black BL, Olson EN. Transcriptional control of muscle development by myocyte enhancer factor-2 (MEF2) proteins. Annu Rev Cell Dev Biol 1998;14:167–196.

6. Sparrow DB, Miska EA, Langley E, et al. MEF-2 function is modified by a novel co-repressor, MITR. EMBO J 1999;18:5085–5098.

7. Lu J, McKinsey TA, Nicol RL, Olson EN. Signal-dependent activation of the MEF2 transcription factor by dissociation from histone deacetylases. Proc Natl Acad Sci U S A 2000;97:4070–4075.

8. Miska EA, Karlsson C, Langley E, Nielsen SJ, Pines J, Kouzarides T. HDAC4 deacetylase associates with and represses the MEF2 transcription factor. EMBO J 1999;18:5099–5107.

9. Wang AH, Bertos NR, Vezmar M, et al. HDAC4, a human histone deacetylase related to yeast HDA1, is a transcriptional corepressor. Mol Cell Biol 1999;19: 7816–7827.

10. Lemercier C, Verdel A, Galloo B, Curtet S, Brocard MP, Khochbin S. mHDA1/HDAC5 histone deacetylase interacts with and represses MEF2A transcriptional activity. J Biol Chem 2000;275:15,594–15,599.

11. Dressel U, Bailey PJ, Wang SC, Downes M, Evans RM, Muscat GE. A dynamic role for HDAC7 in MEF2-mediated muscle differentiation. J Biol Chem 2001;276:17,007–17,013.

12. Kao HY, Verdel A, Tsai CC, Simon C, Juguilon H, Khochbin S. Mechanism for nucleocytoplasmic shuttling of histone deacetylase 7. J Biol Chem 2001;276: 47,496–47,507.

13. Lu J, McKinsey TA, Zhang CL, Olson EN. Regulation of skeletal myogenesis by association of the MEF2 transcription factor with class II histone deacetylases. Mol Cell 2000;6:233–244.

14. Youn HD, Grozinger CM, Liu JO. Calcium regulates transcriptional repression of myocyte enhancer factor 2 by histone deacetylase 4. J Biol Chem 2000;275: 22,563–22,567.

15. Chen SL, Loffler KA, Chen D, Stallcup MR, Muscat GE. The coactivator-associated arginine methyltransferase is necessary for muscle differentiation: CARM1 coactivates myocyte enhancer factor-2. J Biol Chem 2002;277:4324–4333.

16. Santelli E, Richmond TJ. Crystal structure of MEF2A core bound to DNA at 1.5 A resolution. J Mol Biol 2000;297:437–449.

17. Han A, Pan F, Stroud JC, Youn HD, Liu JO, Chen L. Sequence-specific recruitment of transcriptional co-repressor Cabin1 by myocyte enhancer factor-2. Nature 2003;422:730–734.

18. Zhang CL, McKinsey TA, Lu JR, Olson EN. Association of COOH-terminal-binding protein (CtBP) and MEF2-interacting transcription repressor (MITR) contributes to transcriptional repression of the MEF2 transcription factor. J Biol Chem 2001;276:35–39.

19. Zhang CL, McKinsey TA, Olson EN. Association of class II histone deacetylases with heterochromatin protein 1: potential role for histone methylation in control of muscle differentiation. Mol Cell Biol 2002;22:7302–7312.

20. Fischle W, Dequiedt F, Hendzel MJ, et al. Enzymatic activity associated with class II HDACs is dependent on a multiprotein complex containing HDAC3 and SMRT/N-CoR. Mol Cell 2002;9:45–57.

21. Zhang CL, McKinsey TA, Olson EN. The transcriptional corepressor MITR is a signal-responsive inhibitor of myogenesis. Proc Natl Acad Sci U S A 2001;98:7354–7359.

22. Bailey P, Downes M, Lau P, et al. The nuclear receptor corepressor N-CoR regulates differentiation: N-CoR directly interacts with MyoD. Mol Endocrinol 1999;13:1155–1168.

23. Mal A, Sturniolo M, Schiltz RL, Ghosh MK, Harter ML. A role for histone deacetylase HDAC1 in modulating the transcriptional activity of MyoD: inhibition of the myogenic program. EMBO J 2001;20:1739–1753.

24. Sartorelli V, Puri PL, Hamamori Y, et al. Acetylation of MyoD directed by PCAF is necessary for the execution of the muscle program. Mol Cell 1999;4:725–734.

25. Polesskaya A, Duquet A, Naguibneva I, et al. CREB-binding protein/p300 activates MyoD by acetylation. J Biol Chem 2000;275:34,359–34,364.

26. Mueller PR, Wold B. In vivo footprinting of a muscle specific enhancer by ligation mediated PCR. Science 1989;246:780–786.

27. Mal A, Harter ML. MyoD is functionally linked to the silencing of a muscle-specific regulatory gene prior to skeletal myogenesis. Proc Natl Acad Sci U S A 2003;100:1735–1739.

28. McKinsey TA, Zhang CL, Lu J, Olson EN. Signal-dependent nuclear export of a histone deacetylase regulates muscle differentiation. Nature 2000;408: 106–111.

29. McKinsey TA, Zhang CL, Olson EN. Activation of the myocyte enhancer factor-2 transcription factor by calcium/calmodulindependent protein kinase-stimulated binding of 14-3-3 to histone deacetylase 5. Proc Natl Acad Sci U S A 2000;97:14,400–14,405.

30. Grozinger CM, Schreiber SL. Regulation of histone deacetylase 4 and 5 and transcriptional activity by 14-3-3-dependent cellular localization. Proc Natl Acad Sci U S A 2000;97:7835–7840.

31. Wang AH, Kruhlak MJ, Wu J, et al. Regulation of histone deacetylase 4 by binding of 14-3-3 proteins. Mol Cell Biol 2000;20:6904–6912.

32. McKinsey TA, Zhang CL, Olson EN. Identification of a signal-responsive nuclear export sequence in class II histone deacetylases. Mol Cell Biol 2001;21: 6312–6321.

33. Wang AH, Yang XJ. Histone deacetylase 4 possesses intrinsic nuclear import and export signals. Mol Cell Biol 2001;21:5992–6005.

34. Miska EA, Langley E, Wolf D, Karlsson C, Pines J, Kouzarides T. Differential localization of HDAC4 orchestrates muscle differentiation. Nucleic Acids Res 2001;29:3439–3447.

35. Puri PL, Iezzi S, Stiegler P, et al. Class I histone deacetylases sequentially interact with MyoD and pRb during skeletal myogenesis. Mol Cell 2001;8:885–897.

36. Lazaro JB, Bailey PJ, Lassar AB. Cyclin D-cdk4 activity modulates the subnuclear localization and interaction of MEF2 with SRC-family coactivators during skeletal muscle differentiation. Genes Dev 2002;16:1792–1805.

37. McKinsey TA, Zhang CL, Olson EN. Signaling chromatin to make muscle. Curr Opin Cell Biol 2002;14:763–772.

38. Iezzi S, Cossu G, Nervi C, Sartorelli V, Puri PL. Stage-specific modulation of skeletal myogenesis by inhibitors of nuclear deacetylases. Proc Natl Acad Sci U S A 2002;99:7757–7762.

39. Iezzi S, Di Padova M, Serra C, et al. Deacetylase inhibitors increase muscle cell size by promoting myoblast recruitment and fusion through induction of follistatin. Dev Cell 2004;6:673–684.

40. McPherron AC, Lawler AM, Lee SJ. Regulation of skeletal muscle mass in mice by a new TGF-beta superfamily member. Nature 1997;387:83–90.

41. Wu H, Naya FJ, McKinsey TA, et al. MEF2 responds to multiple calcium-regulated signals in the control of skeletal muscle fiber type. EMBO J 2000;19: 1963–1973.

42. Wu H, Rothermel B, Kanatous S, et al. Activation of MEF2 by muscle activity is mediated through a calcineurin-dependent pathway. EMBO J 2001;20: 6414–6423.
43. Dunn SE, Simard AR, Bassel-Duby R, Williams RS, Michel RN. Nerve activity-dependent modulation of calcineurin signaling in adult fast and slow skeletal muscle fibers. J Biol Chem 2001;276:45,243–45,254.
44. Wu H, Olson EN. Activation of the MEF2 transcription factor in skeletal muscles from myotonic mice. J Clin Invest 2002;109:1327–1333.
45. Li X, Song S, Liu Y, Ko SH, Kao HY. Phosphorylation of the histone deacetylase 7 modulates its stability and association with 14-3-3 proteins. J Biol Chem 2004;279:34,201–34,208.
46. Blander G, Guarente L. The Sir2 family of protein deacetylases. Annu Rev Biochem 2004;73:417–435.
47. Fulco M, Schiltz RL, Iezzi S, et al. Sir2 regulates skeletal muscle differentiation as a potential sensor of the redox state. Mol Cell 2003;12:51–62.
48. Afshar G, Murnane JP. Characterization of a human gene with sequence homology to *Saccharomyces cerevisiae* SIR2. Gene 1999;234:161–168.
49. Chien KR. Stress pathways and heart failure. Cell 1999;98:555–558.
50. Molkentin JD, Dorn IG. Cytoplasmic signaling pathways that regulate cardiac hypertrophy. Annu Rev Physiol 2001;63:391–426.
51. Olson EN, Schneider MD. Sizing up the heart: development redux in disease. Genes Dev 2003;17:1937–1956.
52. Marks AR. A guide for the perplexed: towards an understanding of the olecular basis of heart failure. Circulation 2003;107:1456–1459.
53. Frey N, Olson EN. Cardiac hypertrophy: the good, the bad, and the ugly. Annu Rev Physiol 2003;65:45–79.
54. Grozinger CM, Hassig CA, Schreiber SL. Three proteins define a class of human histone deacetylases related to yeast Hda1p. Proc Natl Acad Sci U S A 1999;96:4868–4873.
55. Verdel A, Khochbin S. Identification of a new family of higher eukaryotic histone deacetylases. Coordinate expression of differentiation-dependent chromatin modifiers. J Biol Chem 1999;274:2440–2445.
56. Passier R, Zeng H, Frey N, et al. CaM kinase signaling induces cardiac hypertrophy and activates the MEF2 transcription factor in vivo. J Clin Invest 2000;105:1395–1406.
57. Vega RB, Harrison BC, Meadows E, et al. Protein kinases C and D mediate agonist-dependent cardiac hypertrophy through nuclear export of histone deacetylase 5. Mol Cell Biol 2004;24:8374–8385.
58. Harrison BC, Roberts CR, Bush E, Kronlage JM, Hood DB, McKinsey TA. The CRM1 nuclear export receptor controls of pathological cardiac gene expression. Mol Cell Biol 2004;24:10,636–10,649.
59. Zhang CL, McKinsey TA, Chang S, Antos CL, Hill JA, Olson EN. Class II histone deacetylases act as signal-responsive repressors of cardiac hypertrophy. Cell 2002;110:479–488.
60. Bush E, Fielitz J, Melvin L, et al. A small molecular activator of cardiac hypertrophy uncovered in a chemical screen for modifiers of the calcineurin signaling pathway. Proc Natl Acad Sci U S A 2004;101:2870–2875.
61. Chang S, McKinsey TA, Zhang CL, Richardson JA, Hill J, Olson EN. Histone deacetylases 5 and 9 govern responsiveness of the heart to a subset of stress signals and play redundant roles in heart. Mol Cell Biol 2004;24:8467–8476.

62. Das DK. Protein kinase C isozymes signaling in the heart. J Mol Cell Cardiol 2003;35:887–889.
63. Antos CL, McKinsey TA, Dreitz M, et al. Dose-dependent blockade to cardiomyocyte hypertrophy by histone deacetylase inhibitors. J Biol Chem 2003;278: 28,930–28,937.
64. Kook H, Lepore JJ, Gitler AD, et al. Cardiac hypertrophy and histone deacetylase-dependent transcriptional repression mediated by the atypical homeodomain protein Hop. J Clin Invest 2003;112:863–871.
65. Davis FJ, Pillai JB, Gupta M, Gupta MP. Concurrent opposite effects of an inhibitor of histone deacetylases, trichostatin-A, on the expression of cardiac {alpha}-myosin heavy chain and tubulins: implication for gain in cardiac muscle contractility. Am J Physiol Heart Circ Physiol 2005;288:H1477–H1490.
66. Hamamori Y, Schneider MD. HATs off to Hop: recruitment of a class I histone deacetylase incriminates a novel transcriptional pathway that opposes cardiac hypertrophy. J Clin Invest 2003;112:824–826.
67. Piekarz R, Bates S. A review of depsipeptide and other histone deacetylase inhibitors in clinical trials. Curr Pharm Des 2004;10:2289–2298.
68. Alcendor RR, Kirshenbaum LA, Imai S, Vatner SF, Sadoshima J. Silent information regulator 2alpha, a longevity factor and class III histone deacetylase, is an essential endogenous apoptosis inhibitor in cardiac myocytes. Circ Res 2004;95: 971–980.
69. Lin Q, Schwarz J, Bucana C, Olson EN. Control of mouse cardiac morphogenesis and myogenesis by transcription factor MEF2C. Science 1997;276: 1404–1407.
70. Davis FJ, Gupta M, Camoretti-Mercado B, Schwartz RJ, Gupta MP. Calcium/ calmodulin-dependent protein kinase activates serum response factor transcription activity by its dissociation from histone deacetylase, HDAC4. Implications in cardiac muscle gene regulation during hypertrophy. J Biol Chem 2003; 278:20,047–20,058.
71. Fischle W, Dequiedt F, Hendzel MJ, et al. Enzymatic activity associated with class II HDACs is dependent on a multiprotein complex containing HDAC3 and SMRT/N-CoR. Mol Cell 2002;9:45–57.
72. Wu XY, Li H, Park EJ, Chen JD. SMRTe inhibits MEF2C transcriptional activation by targeting HDAC4 and 5 to nuclear domains. J Biol Chem 2001;276: 24,177–24,185.
73. Cao D, Wang Z, Zhang C, et al. Modulation of smooth muscle gene expression by association of histone acetyltransferases and deacetylases with Myocardin. Mol Cell Biol 2005;25:364–376.
74. Manabe I, Owens GK. Recruitment of serum response factor and hyperacetylation of histones at smooth muscle-specific regulatory regions during differentiation of a novel P19-derived in vitro smooth muscle differentiation system. Circ Res 2001;88:1127–1134.
75. Qiu P, Li L. Histone acetylation and recruitment of serum responsive factor and CREB-binding protein onto SM22 promoter during SM22 gene expression. Circ Res 2002;90:858–865.
76. Wang DZ, Olson EN. Control of smooth muscle development by the myocardin family of transcriptional coactivators. Curr Opin Genet Dev 2004;14:558–566.
77. Waltregny D, De Leval L, Glenisson W, et al. Expression of histone deacetylase 8, a class I histone deacetylase, is restricted to cells showing smooth muscle differentiation in normal human tissues. Am J Pathol 2004;165:553–564.

78. Lin Q, Lu J, Yanagisawa H, et al. Requirement of the MADS-box transcription factor MEF2C for vascular development. Development 1998;125:4565–4574.
79. Hayashi M, Kim SW, Imanaka-Yoshida K, et al. Targeted deletion of BMK1/ERK5 in adult mice perturbs vascular integrity and leads to endothelial failure. J Clin Invest 2004;113:1138–1148.
80. Wang L, Fan C, Topol SE, Topol EJ, Wang Q. Mutation of MEF2A in an inherited disorder with features of coronary artery disease. Science 2003;302: 1578–1581.

6 The Class IIa Histone Deacetylases

Functions and Regulation

Herbert G. Kasler, PhD
and Eric Verdin, MD

CONTENTS

SUMMARY

Posttranslational modifications of histone proteins in chromatin play a critical role in the control of gene expression in eukaryotes. Histone deacetylases (HDACs) catalyze the deacetylation of lysine residues in the histone amino-terminal tails and are found in large multiprotein transcriptional compressor complexes. Human HDACs are grouped into three classes based on their similarity to known yeast factors. Class I HDACs are similar to the

From: *Cancer Drug Discovery and Development*
Histone Deacetylases: Transcriptional Regulation and Other Cellular Functions
Edited by: E. Verdin © Humana Press Inc., Totowa, NJ

Acronyms and Abbreviations

BCL6	B-cell lymphoma 6
B-MyB	B-myeloblastosis virus
BTB/POZ	Bric-a-brac, tramtrack, and broad complex/ Pox virus and zinc finger
BCOR	BCL-6 interacting corepressor
Cam	Calmodulin
CRM1	Chromosome region maintenance 1
CtBP	COOH-terminal binding protein
DAG	Diacylglycerol
Erk	Extracellular signal-related kinase
ETO	Eight twenty-one
Eu-HMTase1	Eukaryotic histone methyltransferase
GPS2	G protein pathway suppressor 2
HAST	*Hda*1p-affected subtelomeric
Hos 1/3, Hos2	Hda One Similar 2
Hox	Homeobox
HP1	Heterochromatin protein 1
Hst1	Homolog of SIR2
IP_3	Inositol triphosphate
Mad	MAX dimerization protein 1
MADS	MCM1, agamous, deficiens, and serum response factor
MAX	MYC associated factor X
MCM1 (in the MADS definition)	Mini-chromosome maintenance
MEF2	Myocyte enhancer-binding factor 2
MRF	Muscle regulatory factor 4
MyoD	Myogenic differentiation
MYST family	MOZ, YBF2/SAS 3, SAS 2, and Tip60
NCoR	Nuclear receptor corepressor
NES	Nuclear export signal
NLS	Nuclear localization signal
NR	Nuclear receptor
PKC	Protein kinase C
PKD	Protein kinase D
PLCg	Phospholipase c-γ
PLZF	Promyelocytic leukemia zinc finger
RanBP2	RAs-related nuclear protein, binding protein 2
REA	Repressor of estrogen activity
Rpx2	Rathkee pouch homeobox 2
Runx2	Runt-related transcription factor 2
SMRT	Silencing mediator for retinoid and thyroid receptors
STAT3	Signal transducer and activator of transcription 3

(Continued on p. 132)

yeast transcriptional repressor yRPD3, whereas class II HDACs are related to yHDA1 and class III HDAs to ySIR2. In this review, we focus on the structure and function of class IIa HDACs. These recently discovered enzymes have been implicated as important regulators of gene expression during cell differentiation and development.

Key Words: HDAC, muscle, thymus, pkd, differentiation, mef2.

INTRODUCTION

The directed acetylation and deacetylation of lysine residues in the N-terminal tails of histone octamer subunits provide a rapid, reversible means for the modification of gene expression levels. In all known cases, removal of acetyl groups from histones by histone deacetylases (HDACs) represses gene transcription at the affected loci, and the addition of acetyl groups activates transcription.

Class IIa HDACs, which include HDACs 4, 5, 7, and 9, are defined by a large, functionally important noncatalytic N-terminal domain. This domain mediates both the recruitment of class IIa HDACs to specific promoters and the signal-dependent shuttling of the class IIa HDACs between the nucleus and the cytoplasm. The combination of these two functionalities in the N-terminal domain of class IIa HDACs defines them as signal-dependent repressors of specific sets of genes. Thus they have important roles in the developmentally regulated expression of genes that are involved in the differentiation and function of muscle, immune, and neural cells. Because of the extensive functional characterization of their shared N-terminal domain and also the rapidly emerging phenotypic data from mutant animals, class IIa HDACS are perhaps the best understood of the HDACs. The purpose of this chapter is to outline what is currently known about the structure, function, phylogeny, and regulation of this family of versatile, important developmental gene regulators.

PHYLOGENY, GENOMIC STRUCTURE, AND EXPRESSION PATTERNS OF CLASS IIa HDACs

Phylogenetic Distribution and Conservation

In the less than 10 years since the first HDAC was identified, the family has expanded to include 18 known members in three major families in humans. Representatives of all the families are also found in all genetically characterized organisms. A recent taxonomic study, based on homology within the catalytic domain, identified class II HDACs in all eukaryotic and the vast majority of prokaryotic organisms, including the archaebacteria (1). Thus, class II HDACs represent the most broadly distributed family.

Acronyms and Abbreviations *(Continued)*

SUV39H1	Suppressor of variegation 3-9 homolog 1
Tat	Transactivator of transcription
TBL-1	Transducin β-like protein
TIP60	Tat-interacting protein, 60 kilodaltons
ZEBRA	*Bam*hI fragment Z Epstein-Barr replication activator

Interestingly, class IIa HDACs appear to occur only in metazoans, and the full family of four known class IIa HDACs seems to be unique to vertebrates.

Within the vertebrates, the available data indicate that class IIa HDACs are well conserved. The possible exception is HDAC7, for which no cDNA sequence has yet been submitted from fish or amphibians. Discontiguous MEGABLAST searches querying the unassembled shotgun sequences of the zebrafish (*Danio rario*) genome yielded multiple strong alignments with the N termini of HDACs 4, 5, and 9, but not HDAC7. Similarly, MEGABLAST queries of the genome of the frog *Xenopus tropicalis* yielded alignments with the N termini of HDACs 4, 5, and 9 but not HDAC7. These data suggest that the absence of HDAC7 cDNAs reflects their absence from the genomes of these organisms.

For each of the class IIa HDACs, conservation of protein sequence is quite high between all species for which a cDNA has been isolated. For example, HDAC4 sequences of humans and the puffer fish (*Tetraodon nigroviridis*) have a 73% identity and 83% similarity. HDAC7 of humans and chickens (*Gallus gallus*) is 66% identical and 75% similar. Importantly, in all available comparisons, extensive regions of exact identity are punctuated by shorter heterologous linkers, suggesting that the functionally important regions of these proteins are nearly identical. This hypothesis is supported by the finding that all currently functionally characterized regions of these proteins fall within the blocks of identity or near-identity.

The reason for the different numbers of HDACs between vertebrates and other organisms is unclear. The duplication and divergence of these molecules may be somehow tied to the evolution of the vertebrate body plan. The invertebrates *Caenorhabtidis elegans* and *Drosophila melanogaster* have only one class IIa HDAC each. As an alternative hypothesis, the adaptive radiation of the class IIa HDACs might be associated with the evolution of deuterostomal development. Unfortunately, there are not yet enough data from the sea urchin (*Strongylocentrotus purpuratus*) genome project to distinguish between these possibilities. The latest sea urchin build (1.1) appears to show two different class IIa HDAC genes.

Conservation between human HDAC4 and the fruit fly dHDAC4 is less than among vertebrates, at 37% identity and 54% similarity. However, several functionally important regions in the N-terminal domain are conserved (Fig. 1B). The class IIa HDAC of nematode, ce-HDA 7, is 30% identical and 50% similar to human HDAC4. Although this level of conservation is only slightly lower than that between human and fruit fly HDAC4, there is a strikingly lower degree of conservation in regions that have been functionally characterized, most notably in the region that interacts with myocyte enhancer factor 2 (MEF2) transcription factors (Fig. 1C). The lack of conservation in ce-HDA 7 is probably not owing to a corresponding difference in nematode MEF2, which is 90% identical to human MEF2 in the N-terminal MADS/MEF2 region that interacts with the class IIa HDACs. Interestingly, deletion of dHDAC4 or dMEF2 results in segmentation defects in fruit flies, while RNAi-mediated suppression of ce-HDA 7 or ce-MEF2 has no effect in nematode (2–4), suggesting that the biologic function of both molecules is conserved between human and fruit fly but divergent or vestigial in nematode.

Genomic Structure and Isoforms

Table 1 lists the details of the genomic loci of the four human class IIa HDACs. All four genes are composed of 24 to 27 exons, corresponding almost exactly to homologous segments within the coding regions of the four genes (Fig. 1A). Whereas the mapping of exons to coding sequences within the four class IIa HDAC loci is nearly identical, the loci themselves vary greatly in size, ranging from only 16.4 kb for HDAC7 to 500 kb for HDAC9. Human HDAC4, the best conserved family member, has only one known isoform, encoding a protein of 1084 amino acids. HDAC5 has two characterized isoforms, of which one incorporates all the exons corresponding to HDAC4. The other lacks exons 14 and 15, leading to an in-frame deletion of 85 residues from positions 693 to 768. Interestingly, this deletion would disrupt the catalytic domain, producing a molecule that might be functionally similar to the MEF2-interacting transcriptional repressor (MITR) isoform of HDAC9 (see next paragraph). Like HDAC5, HDAC7 has two known isoforms. Variant 1 incorporates sequences homologous to all but the first two short coding exons of HDAC4, omitting the first residue of the binding site for the transcriptional repressor C-terminal binding protein (CtBP). Variant 2 differs from variant 1 in the loss of exon 7 and the first three residues of exon 8, leading to an in-frame deletion of 40 residues, from positions 227 to 367. This results in the loss of a short block of conserved sequence ($Rx_4d/exSx_5LxTx_3LPxIs/tLGLxA$) that has yet to have a functional significance ascribed to it.

With five known variants, HDAC9 is the most complex class IIa HDAC. Variants 4 and 5 encode proteins of 1066 and 1069 amino acids, respectively, that contain all the exons associated with HDAC4. They differ from one another in that variant 4 lacks a short segment (89–91 LQQ) at the

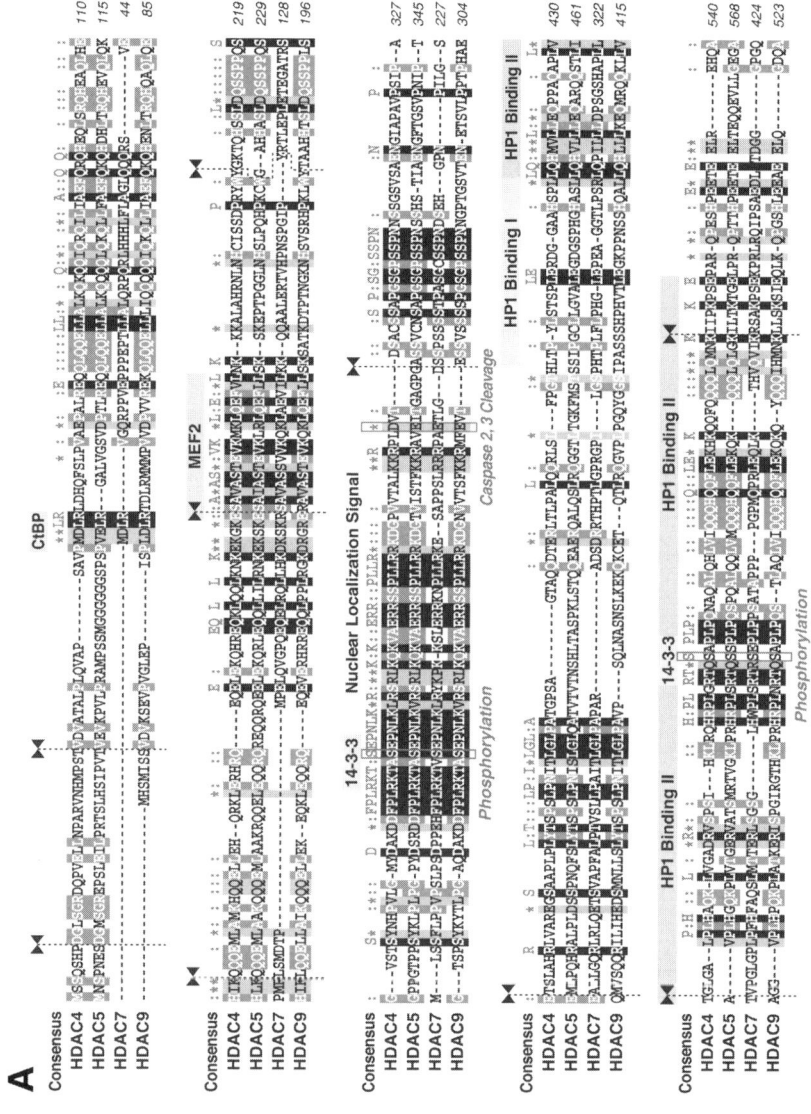

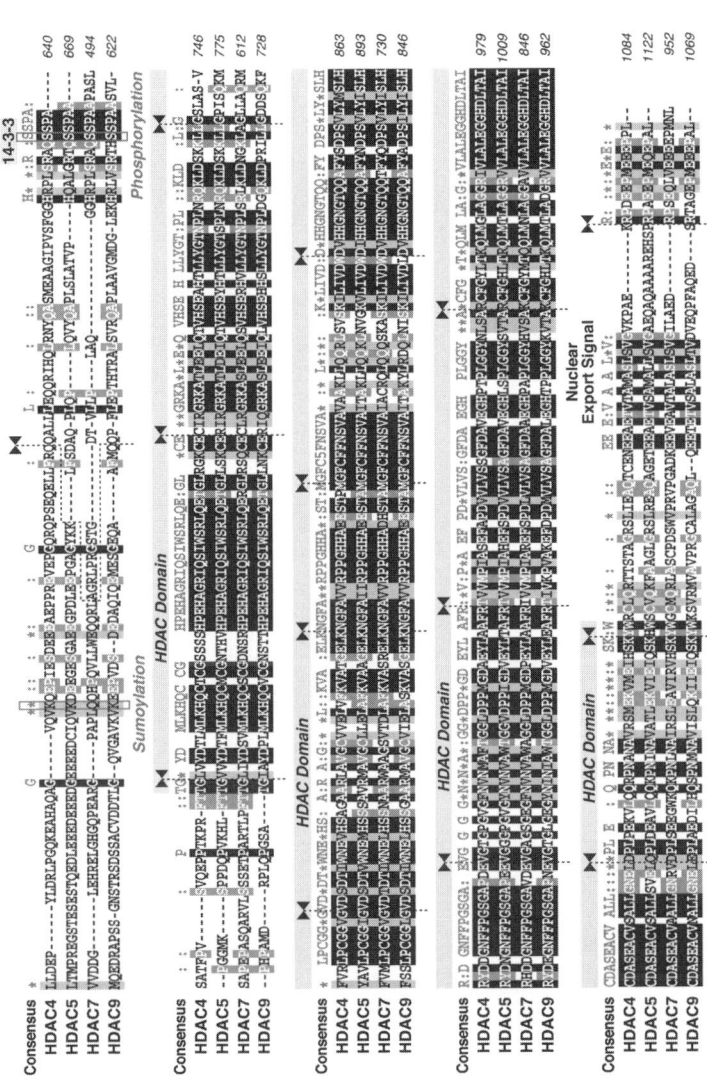

Fig. 1. Clustal alignment of human class IIa histone deacetylases (HDACs). Human HDACs were aligned using the ClustalX alignment tool and then formatted using GeneDoc. The longest isoform of each class IIa HDAC was used for the alignment. Black shading indicates identity. Gray shading indicates similarity according to the PAM 200 scoring matrix. Shaded boxes indicate regions with indicated functions. Light blue dashed boxes represent exon boundaries. Residues that are the targets of posttranslational modifications are indicated by rectangular boxes. **(A)** The four human class IIa HDACs aligned with one another. **(B,C)** The alignments between human HDAC4 and *D. melanogaster* dHDAC4 and *C. elegans* ce-HDA 7, respectively.

135

B

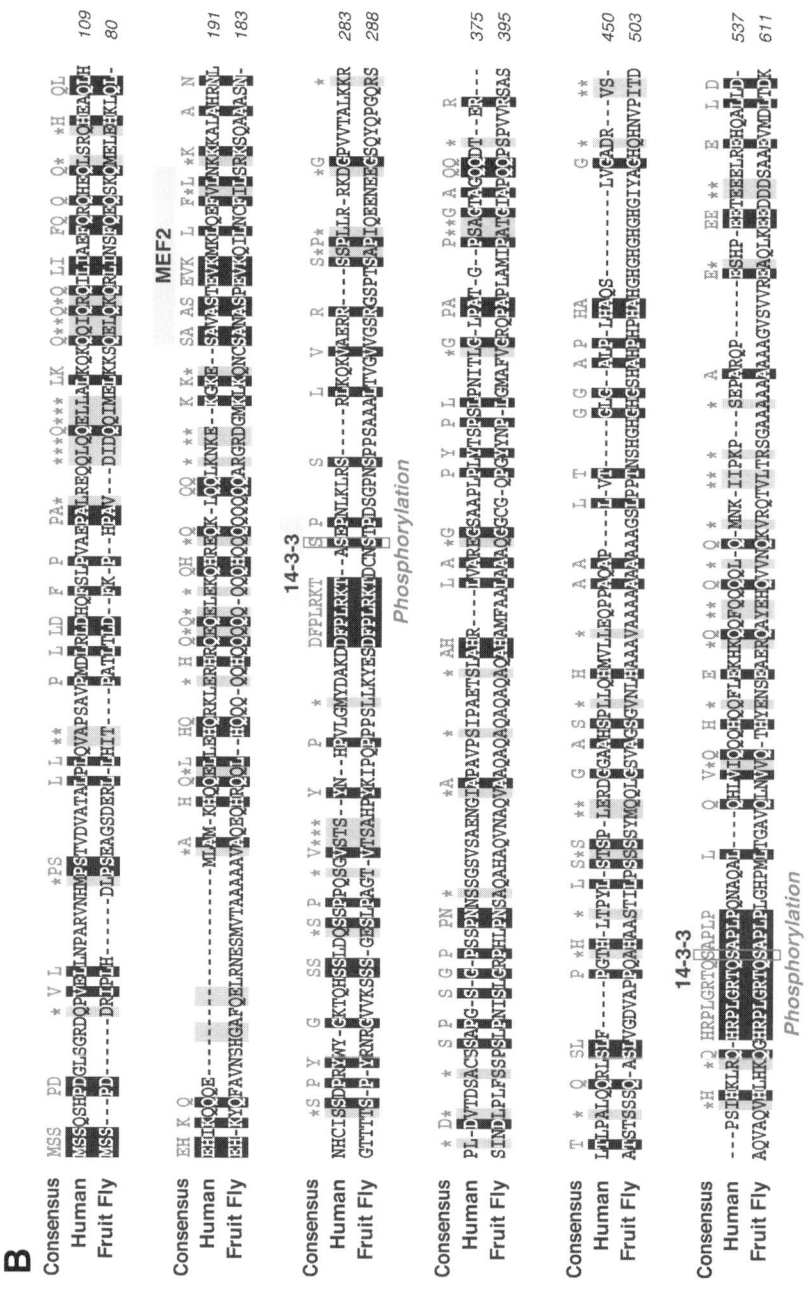

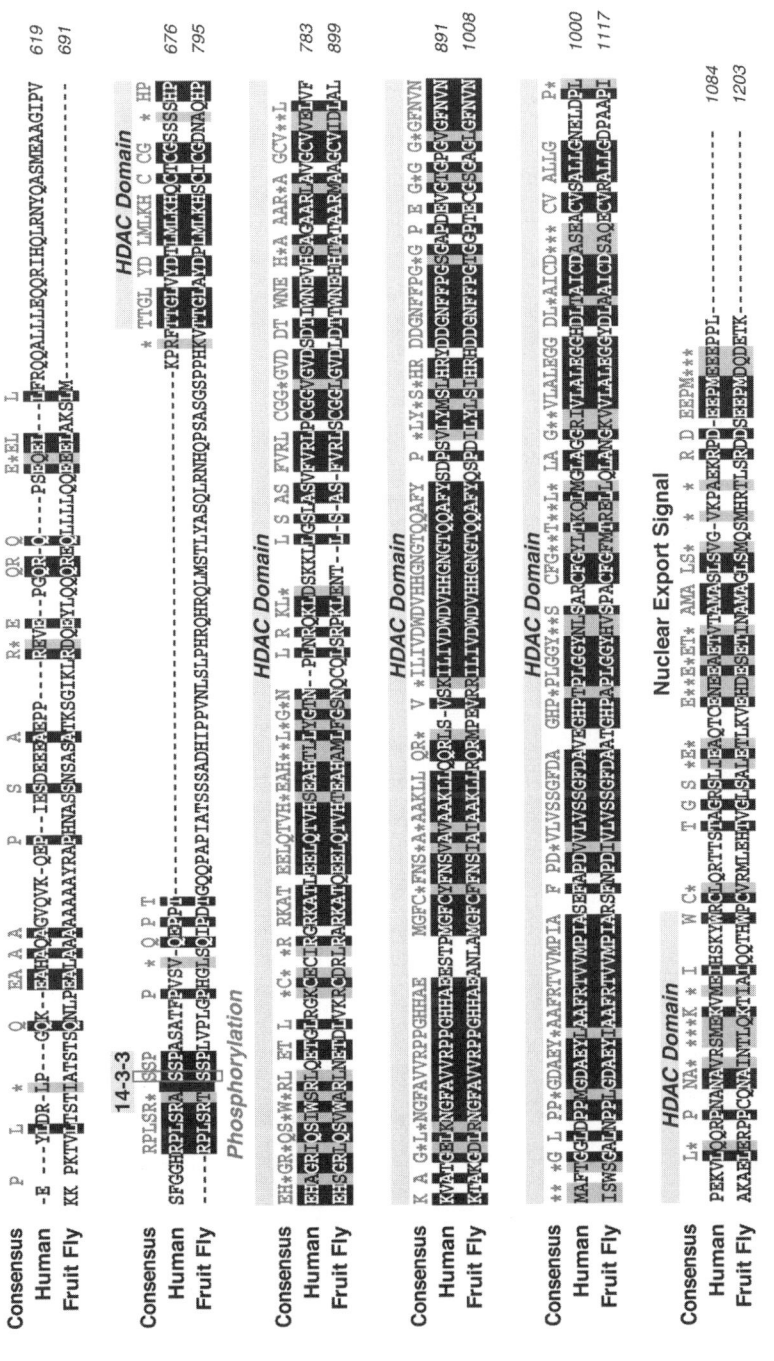

Fig. 1 (*Continued*)

137

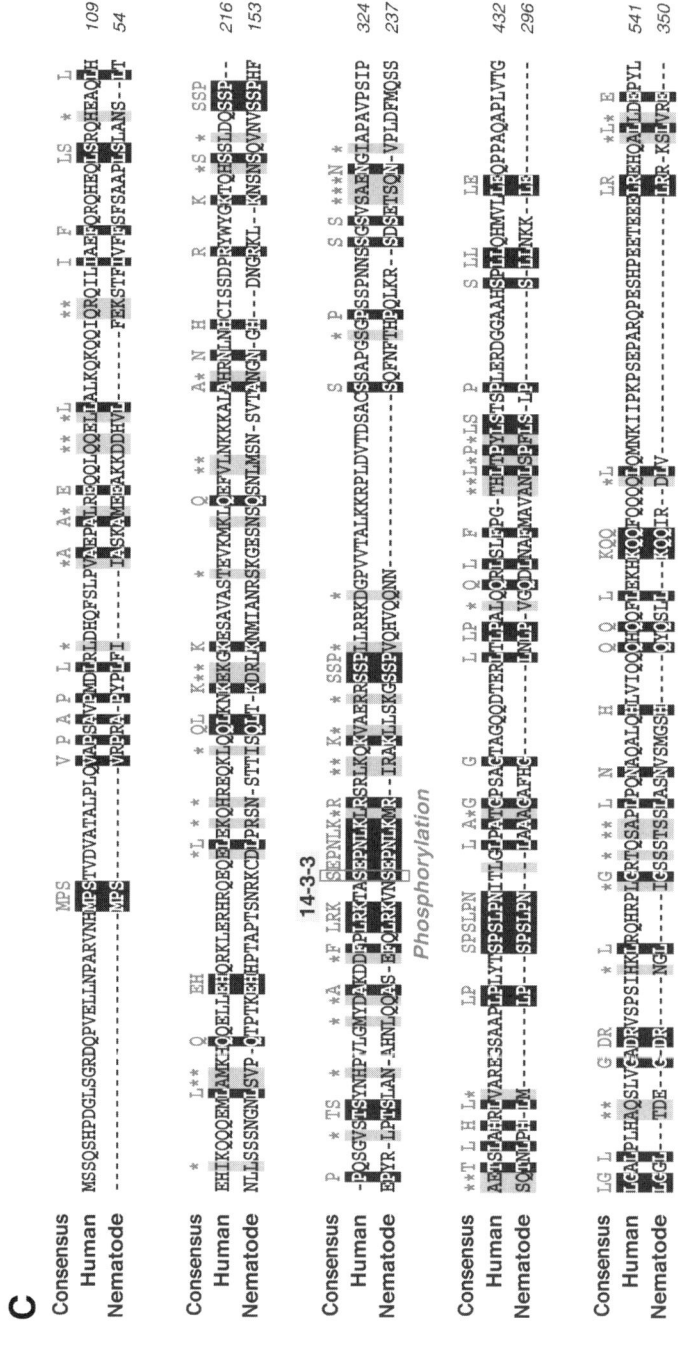

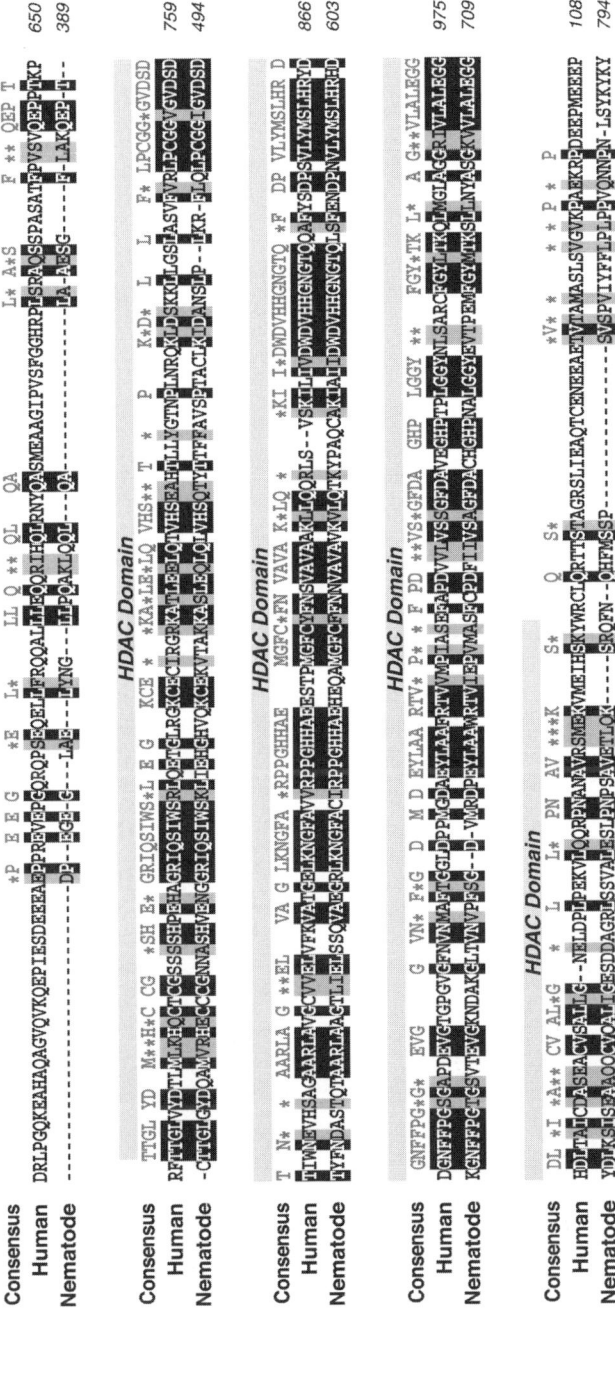

Fig. 1 (*Continued*)

139

Table 1

Genomic Structure and Known Isoforms of the Four Human Class IIa HDAC Genes[a]

Gene name	Chromosomal location	Exons	Locus size (kb)	mRNA size (bp)	Protein size (aa)	Comments
HDAC4	2q37.2	27	352	8458	1084	Sole isoform
HDAC5	17q21	25–27	47	3573	1122	Variant 1
				5041	1037	Variant 2 (cat. domain disrupted)
HDAC7	12q13.1	24	16.4	4189	952	Variant 1
				4069	912	Variant 2
				3036	1011	Variant 1 (no NES)
				2790	879	Variant 2 (cat. domain disrupted)
HDAC9	7p21.p15	12–26	500	4230	590	Variant 3 (MITR/HDRP)
				4659	1066	Variant 4
				3210	1069	Variant

Abbreviations: HDAC, histone deacetylase; HDRP, HDAC-related protein; MITR, myocyte enhancer factor 2-interacting transcription repressor; NES, nuclear export sequence.

[a]Data compiled from the Genatlas data resource at the Université René Descartes, Paris, France (http://www.dsi.univ-paris5.fr/genatlas).

beginning of exon 4 that is found in HDACs 4 and 5. Variant 1 encodes a protein of 1011 amino acids that follows the consensus sequence until exon 24 and then diverges, terminating after seven more residues. Loss of the last two coding exons does not affect the catalytic domain but does delete the C-terminal nuclear export signal, resulting in a protein that is constitutively localized to the nucleus *(5)*. Variant 3 encodes the protein that was originally cloned from the frog *Xenopus laevis* as the MITR *(6)*. It follows the consensus class IIa HDAC sequence through exon 12 and then diverges and terminates after 16 residues because of an out-of-frame splice to exon 13, resulting in a protein of 590 amino acids. Interestingly, this molecule was the first class IIa HDAC cloned but was not identified as such owing to the absence of any HDAC catalytic sequences. The same isoform of HDAC9 was cloned from human cDNA after other class IIa HDACs had been identified; it was called HDAC-related protein (HDRP) *(7)*. Even without an HDAC catalytic domain, these molecules still repress MEF2-dependent transcription (*see* the MEF2 Transcription Factors section under "Protein–Protein Interactions" following), indicating that histone deacetylation is not the only function of these molecules *(6,7)*. Variant 2 of HDAC9 goes out of frame after exon 20, resulting in a protein of 879 amino acids. This protein, like MITR, lacks a functional catalytic domain but does possess a 14-3-3 interaction and phosphorylation site that MITR lacks.

Tissue-Specific Expression

Although the conventional wisdom is that expression of the class IIa HDACs is tissue restricted—unlike the ubiquitous class I HDACs 1, 2, and 3—the reality is a bit more complex. Analysis of recovery of expressed sequence tags (ESTs) from different tissue libraries, as catalogued in the NCBI Unigene resource, suggests that all four class IIa HDACs are widely expressed. Close examination of published (and sometimes contradictory) studies using Northern blots suggests that, although the class IIa HDACs are widely expressed, they are clearly expressed much more strongly in a limited subset of cell types (Table 2). HDACs 4, 5, and 9 are particularly well expressed in brain, heart, and skeletal muscle, whereas HDAC7 is highly expressed in heart, thymus, and lung. HDAC4 also appears to be very highly expressed in ovary and intestine. Studies on the expression patterns of HDAC7 in the thymus (by fluorescence-activated cell sorting/reverse transcriptase polymerase chain reaction) and of HDAC9 in the developing mouse embryo (by *in situ* RNA hybridization) revealed that they are expressed within defined subsets of the cells within these tissues. In thymus, HDAC7 appears to be expressed predominantly in the cd4/cd8 double-positive subset of thymocytes *(8)*. In the central nervous system of the developing mouse, HDAC9 is localized to the neural tube,

Table 2
Tissue Distribution of Class IIa HDAC mRNA Expression[a]

Tissue	HDAC4	HDAC5	HDAC7	HDAC9/MITR
Brain	+++	++	–	+++
Colon	++	ND	+	+
Gall bladder	ND	ND	ND	+
Heart	++	+++	+++	+++
Kidney	+	+	–	+
Liver	+/–	++	+	+
Lung	+/–	+	++	–/+
Ovary	+++	ND	+	ND
Pancreas	+	+	+	+
PBL	+	ND	+	ND
Placenta	+/–	+	+	+
Prostate	+	ND	+	ND
Skeletal muscle	+++	++	+	++/–
Small intestine	++	ND	+	+
Spleen	+	–	–/+	+
Testis	+	+	–	ND
Thymus	++	ND	+++	ND

Abbreviations: HDAC, histone deacetylase; MITR, myocyte enhancer factor 2-interacting transcription repressor; PBL, peripheral blood lymphocytes.

[a]Expression levels were evaluated visually from Northern blots presented in the following publications: refs. 7, 8, 13, 36, 45, 46, and 93–95. +++, and ++, highly expressed; +, detectably expressed, –, not detected; ND, no data. Conflicting findings are separated by slashes (e.g., +/–).

neuroepithelium, and dorsal root ganglia (9). Transient expression in a specific cell type, as is observed in thymocytes, suggests that class IIa HDACs might play important roles in the development of tissues with low overall expression levels. Their overlapping patterns of low-level expression and their apparent functional redundancy may present significant technical challenges to studies of specific roles for class IIa HDACs with transgenic animals.

PROTEIN–PROTEIN INTERACTIONS OF THE CLASS IIa HDACs

Numerous protein–protein interactions involving class IIa HDACs have been identified (Fig. 2), as well as possible mechanisms for recruiting chromatin-modifying activities to specific DNA sequences. Clearly, both the C-terminal catalytic and N-terminal domains of the class IIa HDACs interact with a host of other proteins. Some of these interactions,

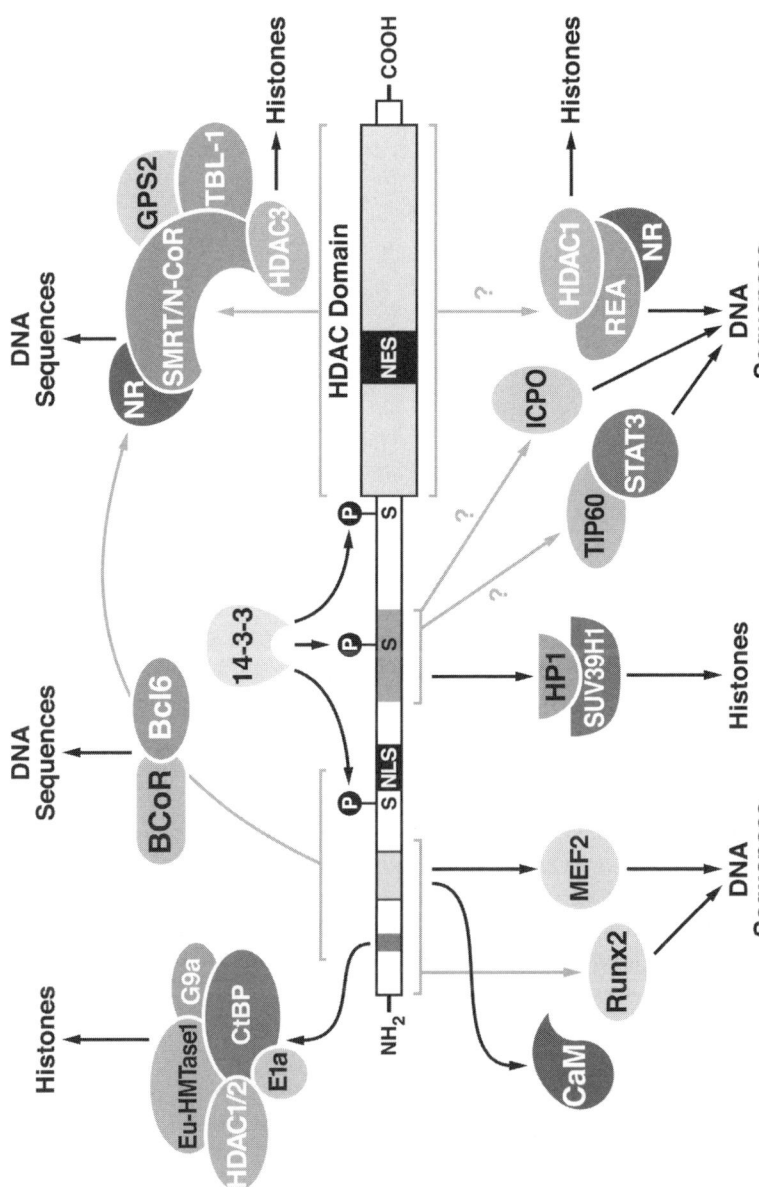

Fig. 2. Protein–protein interactions of the class IIa histone deacetylases (HDACs). Class IIa HDACs can act as adapters between many different specific DNA sequences and several sources of histone-modifying activity.

143

such as those with MEF2, BCL6, and nuclear receptor corepressor (NCoR), potentially serve to recruit the class IIa HDACs to different promoters. Other interactions, such as those with calmodulin or 14-3-3, are involved in the regulation of the association of the class IIa HDACs with promoters. Still others, such as the interactions with CtBP and heterochromatin protein 1 (HP1), are involved in the recruitment of enzymatic activities distinct from the catalytic domains of the class IIa HDACs themselves to potential target promoters. These numerous interactions allude to a bewildering array of possible roles played by the class IIa HDACs in the regulation of a large number of different genes. Although a few have been characterized, the great majority have yet to be investigated. A thorough screen for potential class IIa HDAC target genes, with DNA microarrays and class IIa HDAC molecules mutated for each of the individual interactions, will be required to determine which of these many possibilities are physiologically relevant.

The MEF2 Transcription Factors

The interaction of the class IIa HDACs with members of the MEF2 family of transcription factors is by far the best characterized in terms of biological significance. The fairly well-defined roles thought to be played by the class IIa HDACs in myogenesis, cardiac hypertrophy, and T-cell development are all mediated by MEF2 family molecules. In vertebrates, there are four MEF2 family members, MEF2A, -B, -C, and -D. In an intriguing parallel to the evolution of the class IIa HDACs, only one member of the MEF2 family occurs in *Drosophila* and *C. elegans* (reviewed in ref. *10*). They were originally isolated from skeletal muscle as factors binding to AT-rich DNA motifs in the promoter of the muscle creatine kinase (MCK) gene *(11)*. Whereas MEF2A, -B, and -C are all restricted to some degree in their expression patterns, MEF2D appears to be ubiquitously expressed (reviewed in ref. *12*). The MEF2 family members share a highly conserved MADS domain, as well as a unique MEF2 domain. These two domains together constitute the N-terminal 87 amino acids of the MEF2 transcription factors, and mediate DNA binding, dimerization, and interaction with multiple coactivators and corepressors, including the class IIa HDACs. The first class IIa HDAC to be identified, MITR/HDAC9, was recovered in a yeast two-hybrid screen for MEF2-interacting proteins *(6)*. All four class IIa HDACs interact with MEF2 proteins via a highly conserved 17-amino acid motif located near the N terminus (*see* Fig. 1A) *(6,13,14)*. Via this motif, the class IIa HDACs repress transcription at the MEF2-regulated promoters of genes, such as Nur77, myogenin, and *c-jun* *(15,16)*.

Runx2

The three members of the Runx family of transcription factors in mammals share homology throughout most of their sequences and in their N-terminal DNA binding domains to the *Drosophila* transcription factor Runt. The Runx family members transcriptionally regulate a wide variety of target genes and can function as either activators or repressors of transcription (reviewed in ref. *17*). Runx1 appears to be essential for hematopoietic development, and runx3-deficient mice have defects in limb development and the digestive system *(18–20)*. Both molecules play important roles in the developmental regulation of the CD4 and CD8 T-cell coreceptors *(21,22)*. Mice deficient in Runx 2 display a profound defect in the calcification of bone tissue owing to a block in osteoblast differentiation *(23,24)*.

Strikingly, the recently published phenotype of HDAC4-deficient mice turns out to involve a premature calcification of bone tissue, as would be expected from a Runx2 gain-of-function mutation *(25)*. Conversely, overexpression of HDAC4 in developing bone produces a phenotype similar to that of Runx2 deficiency. The authors of this study hypothesized that HDAC4 might therefore function as a corepressor of runx2. They proceed to demonstrate this, showing that the N-terminal Runt domain of runx2 interacts with the first 220 amino acids of HDAC4, which contain the MEF2 and CtBP-interacting regions. Interestingly, rather than repressing runx2 activity via the expected mechanism of histone deacetylation, HDAC4 appears instead to inhibit the DNA binding of Runx2. This model is supported by the finding that a construct of only the first 220 amino acids of HDAC4 represses runx2-mediated transcription almost as effectively as the full-length HDAC4. However, the model is weakened by the finding that a construct consisting of just the C-terminal catalytic domain of HDAC4 is also a significant repressor.

The concept that HDAC4 might act as a corepressor of Runx2 both via the novel mechanism proposed by the authors and via a mechanism involving HDAC activity and interaction with the HDAC4 catalytic domain is supported by another recent finding that runx2 interacts with HDAC3, which lacks the N-terminal domain characteristic of the class IIa HDACs *(25a)*. Clearly, this is an exciting new chapter in the biology of class IIa HDACs. It is tempting to speculate that, since the interacting domains of both class IIa HDACs and the Runx family members are conserved across their respective families, other class IIa HDAC-Runx interactions may be important in the development of other tissues, particularly in the case of HDAC7 and Runx1 or Runx3 in developing T cells.

BCL6 and BCoR

BCL6 is an oncogene involved in the pathogenesis of non-Hodgkin's B-cell lymphomas. It contains Krüppel-like zinc finger motifs and acts as a sequence-specific transcriptional repressor *(26–28)*. Microarray studies show that it has a role in regulating genes involved in B-cell activation and differentiation, inflammation, and cell-cycle regulation *(29)*. Recent experiments showed that BCL6 can recruit the class IIa HDACs *(30)* via a direct interaction between a conserved region in the N-terminal domain of class IIa HDACs (corresponding to residues 123–292 of HDAC5) and the C-terminal zinc finger region of BCL6. The N-terminal BTB/POZ domain of BCL6 can also bind either to silencing mediator for retinoid and thyroid receptors (SMRT), leading to the recruitment of class IIa HDACs via a complex, described below *(31–33)*, or to BCoR. BCoR is a corepressor that was cloned via its interaction with BCL6 and that interacts specifically with both class I and class IIa HDACs *(34)*. Thus, class IIa HDACs can be recruited by BCL6 via three separate mechanisms and may participate in a ternary complex containing both BCL6 and BCoR. Hopefully, future experiments will elucidate the role of this complex in regulating BCL6 target genes.

Nuclear Hormone Receptor Corepressors

Recently, class IIa HDACs were shown to interact directly with two closely related corepressors, SMRT and NCoR *(35–37)*. SMRT and NCoR derive their names from their interaction with nuclear receptors *(38,39)*. However, they also interact with a host of other DNA binding factors, including Rpx2, Hox, MyoD, Mad, PLZF, ETO, and B-Myb (reviewed in ref. *40*). They repress transcription of target genes via three autonomous repression domains, called RD1, -2, and -3. SMRT and NCoR interact with the C-terminal catalytic domains of class IIa HDACs via RD3. Interestingly, they also interact with the class I molecule HDAC3 through a different domain, called the SANT domain *(41–44)*, an observation that explains why class IIa HDACs coimmunoprecipitate with HDAC3 *(45–47)*. The interaction with HDAC3 was demonstrated by biochemical fractionation experiments that identified a stable complex containing SMRT/NCoR, HDAC3, transducin β-like protein 1 (TBL1) *(41,43)*, and GPS2, a protein involved in G-protein signaling *(48)*. Importantly, it appears that the class IIa HDACs are only enzymatically active when they are associated with this SMRT/ NCoR/HDAC3 complex *(45,47)*. In contrast, HDAC3 is catalytically active when bound to SMRT/NCoR alone *(44,47)*. Therefore, SMRT and NCoR may serve as critical cofactors in the function of class IIa HDACs by recruiting HDAC3, an active catalytic subunit. A similar complex, containing two different nonclass II HDAC molecules (Hos2 and Hst1) and a WD40 protein with homology to TBL1, seems to exist in the budding yeast *Saccharomyces cerevisiae (49)*.

In an interesting parallel to the complex described above, both HDAC1 and HDAC5 can interact with repressor of estrogen receptor activity (REA), a molecule that was originally identified as a transcriptional corepressor of the estrogen receptor *(50,51)*. REA-HDAC1 and REA-HDAC5 interact with distinct domains on both REA and HDAC1/5, suggesting the possible existence of a ternary complex among HDAC1, HDAC5, and REA. Although REA has no sequence homology with SMRT/NCoR, it apparently interacts with multiple nuclear hormone receptors *(50)* and might represent another adaptor between a class IIa HDAC, a catalytically active class I HDAC, and nuclear hormone receptors.

14-3-3 Proteins

Members of the widely distributed family of 14-3-3 proteins, comprising seven different molecules in humans, bind to and regulate the nucleocytoplasmic shuttling of more than 100 signaling proteins (reviewed in ref. *52*). 14-3-3 proteins bind to specific motifs in target proteins that contain phosphorylated serine or threonine residues. These motifs are of the general forms RxxS/TxP and RxxxS/TxP. Proteins thus bound by 14-3-3 proteins are anchored in the cytoplasm, where the 14-3-3 family members are localized. The N-terminal domains of all class IIa HDACs contain multiple potential 14-3-3 interacting motifs *(53)*. In HDAC5 and HDAC9, two of these motifs, 254 to 260 RKTa/vSEP and 495 to 500 RTQSxP (as numbered on HDAC5; *see* Fig. 1A), bind to 14-3-3 when phosphorylated. In HDAC4 and HDAC7, a third motif, 629 to 634 RAQSSP, is similarly phosphorylated, leading to 14-3-3 binding and consequent cytoplasmic localization *(9,16,53–55)*. This extracellular signal-dependent cytoplasmic localization of the class IIa HDACs is a critical aspect of their regulation and will be discussed more extensively in section, "Regulation and Posttranslational modifications…" following.

Calmodulin

The MEF2 binding domain of HDAC4 has similarity to calmodulin (CaM) binding domains *(56)*. HDAC4 binds to CaM in a Ca^{2+}-sensitive manner in vitro, and binding of CaM disrupts the MEF2-HDAC4 interaction. This mechanism could account for the Ca^{2+}-dependent activation of MEF2, independent of the phosphorylation of the 14-3-3 binding serine residues described in the previous paragraph *(57)*. The physiologic significance of these findings is still uncertain, however, since in all the experimental systems employed thus far, mutation of the 14-3-3-interacting residues of class IIa HDACs totally abrogates the release of their transcriptional repression of MEF2 by calcium signaling.

Heterochromatin Protein 1

The HDAC9 isoform MITR, which lacks an HDAC catalytic domain, is still capable of repressing MEF2 transcription. Similarly, the N-terminal domains of other class IIa HDACs can repress transcription independently of the C-terminal catalytic domains. In a recent study, a yeast two-hybrid screen seeking MITR-interacting proteins that might mediate this HDAC-independent repression mechanism found HP1α *(58)*. HP1 contains a chromodomain involved in the specific recognition of methylated lysine 9 of histone H3. HP1 also interacts with the histone methyltransferase SUV39H1, which coimmunoprecipitates with class IIa HDACs. The interaction is mediated by an N-terminal domain of class II HDACs, distinct from other interacting sites (Fig. 1A), and has been demonstrated for HDACs 4 and 5 as well as MITR. These observations establish an important link between histone deacetylase and histone methyltransferase activities. Since the deacetylation of histone H3 must occur as a prelude to its methylation, the class II HDAC/ HP1/SUV39H1 complex could mediate a coupled deacetylation-methylation activity that is important in the establishment and maintenance of heterochromatin *(58)*.

E1A C-Terminal Binding Protein

E1A C-terminal binding protein (CtBP1), originally identified as an adenovirus E1A-interacting protein *(59,60)*, is an important corepressor of a number of *Drosophila* DNA binding proteins, including Hairy, Snail, Krüppel, and Knirps *(61,62)*. In mammals, it interacts with the Krüppel homologs mammalian basic Krüppel-like factor 3 (BKLF/KLF3), hKLF8, and Ikaros *(63–65)*. CtBP associates with these proteins through a PXDLS motif, acting as a transcriptional corepressor. The same PXDLS motif is involved in the interaction between CtBP and several HDACs, including HDAC4, HDAC5, and MITR *(66)*. Interestingly, the CtBP binding motif is conserved in mouse HDAC7 but is missing in the human protein *(45)*. One might surmise that recruitment of class IIa HDACs and their associated NCoR/HDAC3 complex might account for the ability of CtBP to repress transcription. However, in at least some cases, CtBP can still repress transcription in the presence of HDAC inhibitors *(67,68)*. The interactions among CtBP, class IIa HDACs, and all the DNA-bound factors mentioned above via the PXDLS motif are also presumably mutually exclusive, making CtBP an unlikely adapter for the class IIa HDACs unless it can itself multimerize.

A recent study using extensive biochemical fractionation showed that CtBP is part of a stable complex that contains HDAC1, HDAC2, and two histone methyltransferases, G9a and Eu-HMTase1. Knockdown of the methyltransferases by small interfering RNA (siRNA) abrogated the

CtBP-mediated repression of the E-cadherin promoter, suggesting that these molecules play an important role in CtBP-mediated repression *(69)*. Since class IIa HDACs can associate with multiple DNA-bound factors and CtBP at the same time, a perhaps more attractive hypothesis is that the class IIa HDACs use CtBP as another means, in addition to HP1, to recruit methyltransferase activity to the promoters they target via MEF2 and other interaction partners. However, no experimental evidence yet supports this idea.

Homotypic Interactions

A number of studies have shown that class IIa HDACs are capable of participating in homotypic interactions. MITR associates with HDAC1, -3, -4, and -5 *(6)*. Similarly, HDAC7 binds to HDAC1, -2, -4, and -5, as well as itself *(15)*. A recent study presented a computational analysis, using the COILS program, of the predicted secondary structure of HDAC4 *(70)*. The analysis assigned a high probability of a coiled-coil dimerization domain to the region encompassing amino acids 90 to 179 of HDAC4, a region that is fairly well conserved between HDACs 4, 5, and 9 but is absent in HDAC7. Deletion of this region disrupted the previously observed localization of HDAC4 to discrete nuclear bodies, the ability of HDAC4 to self-associate in vitro, and its sumoylation *(37,70)*. However, this region also contains the MEF2-interacting domain of HDAC4, so whether or not the change in localization really has to do with self-aggregation rather than binding to MEF2 is an open question. Also, HDAC7, which diverges from the other family members through most of the putative dimerization region, is still found in the discrete nuclear bodies. It is nonetheless pleasing to speculate that this dimeric region of HDAC4, encompassing the MEF2 binding site, might interface in a bivalent manner with the similarly dimeric MADS/MEF2 domain. Resolution of the question must await either a solution of the MEF2-HDAC4 structures or an analysis of self-association in a more physiologic context.

Other Reported Interactions

A number of interactions between class IIa HDACs and other cellular factors have been reported, but are as yet not structurally or functionally well characterized. A brief discussion of each of these follows.

ERK1/ERK2

A study looking for kinase activity associated with HDAC4 in HEK 293T cells found that the mitogen-activated protein (MAP) kinases Erk1 and Erk2 coimmunoprecipitate with overexpressed HDAC4. The authors noted that HDAC4 is phosphorylated in their system and that transfection of constitutively activated Ras, which among other things activates Erk1/Erk2, increased the degree of nuclear localization of HDAC4 *(71)*. The authors did not, however, demonstrate that Erk1/Erk2 can phosphorylate HDAC4 in vivo, nor did they directly connect Erk1/Erk2 activity to a relocalization of HDAC4. No experiments identified the interacting regions in either molecule.

TAT-INTERACTING PROTEIN

Tat-interacting-protein (TIP60), a 60-kDa acetyltransferase of the MYST family, is thought to function both as a coactivator and as a corepressor of transcription. Published reports from two different groups place TIP60 and HDAC7 in the same protein complex. In the first study, both HDAC7 and Tip60 are purported to interact with endothelin receptor A (ETA) to modulate its activity *(72)*. The three molecules colocalized upon stimulation of ETA by its ligand. However, no further attempt to characterize the interactions or the functional significance of HDAC7 in the complex was made. In the second study, TIP60 and HDAC7 were found to interact directly, and the interacting regions in each protein were narrowed down to residues 241 to 533 of HDAC7, encompassing most of the HP1-interacting region, and residues 261 to 366 of Tip60, containing a zinc finger. They further showed that HDAC7 potentiated the repression of signal transducer and activator of infection 3 (Stat3) transcriptional activation by TIP60. This points to a possible role for HDAC7 in cytokine signaling, although the authors make no suggestion as to how the signal-dependent regulation of HDAC7 may be involved in this mechanism.

ICP0

ICP0, an immediate-early protein of the herpes simplex virus (HSV), is an activator of gene expression. HDACs 4, 5, and 7 all interact with ICP0 in transfected HeLa cells. The interaction regions were localized to residues 106 to 241 of ICP0 and residues 242 to 450 of HDAC5, corresponding to roughly the same region of HDAC7 that interacts with Tip60 *(73)*. Expression of ICP0 resulted in a relocalization of cellular class IIa HDACs to the same subnuclear structure that ICP0 occupies and in a loss of HDAC-mediated repression of MEF2 transactivation. The authors speculate that this derepression of MEF2 might keep the host cells of HSV1 in a state that would support lytic infection or, alternately, that the putative role of HDAC4 in DNA repair (*see* next section) might be affected to promote maintenance of the HSV genome in a linear form.

53BP1

A recent study implicates HDAC4 in the DNA damage repair pathway by finding that, in response to irradiation in HeLa cells, HDAC4 interacts and colocalizes with 53BP1, a p53-interacting DNA damage-response protein *(74)*. 53BP1 and HDAC4 were found together in transient nuclear foci after irradiation. These foci failed to resolve in cells that were deficient in DNA repair because of the loss of DNA-PK. Furthermore, siRNA knockdown of HDAC4 affected the level of 53BP1, abrogated G2 cell-cycle arrest in response to irradiation, and radiosensitized the cells. No tests were proposed or conducted to discover how HDAC4 might carry out this role in DNA repair. However, the finding does appear to be worthy of further investigation, preferably in the context of untransformed cells.

REGULATION AND POSTTRANSLATIONAL MODIFICATIONS OF CLASS IIA HDAC ACTIVITY

The most important feature of the class IIa HDACs is their extensive non-catalytic domains that comprise multiple distinct targeting and regulatory modules. These modules allow extracellular signals to regulate the association with and repression of specific promoters by class IIa HDACs (Fig. 3). By far the best understood instance of this regulatory function is the activation of MEF2 target genes through signal-dependent dissociation of class IIa HDACs. These genes include molecules involved in multiple signal-dependent pathways of cellular differentiation. Genes regulating muscle differentiation (e.g., myogenin, muscle creatine kinase, and MRF4), genes involved in thymic selection of T cells (e.g., Nur77), and genes involved in the regulation of Epstein-Barr virus (EBV) latency (e.g., ZEBRA), are all regulated through MEF2-binding sites in their promoters (reviewed in ref. *10*). Although the biological contexts and significance of the regulation of each of these target genes are different (as will be discussed in depth in Chapter 5), the basic mechanism underlying their regulation is the same. Conserved serine residues in the N-terminal domains of the class IIa HDACs are phosphorylated in response to extracellular signals, resulting in the dissociation of the class IIa HDACs from MEF2 and the resulting derepression of the MEF2 target genes. Although a great deal is known about the functioning of this mechanism, very little is known about the significance of other posttranslational modifications of class IIa HDACs (i.e., sumoylation and caspase cleavage). Similarly, although many clear possibilities exist, little is known about how signal-dependent modifications of class IIa HDACs might regulate putative target genes to which class IIa HDACs might be recruited via factors other than MEF2. Future studies will hopefully soon shed some light on this large, unexplored territory.

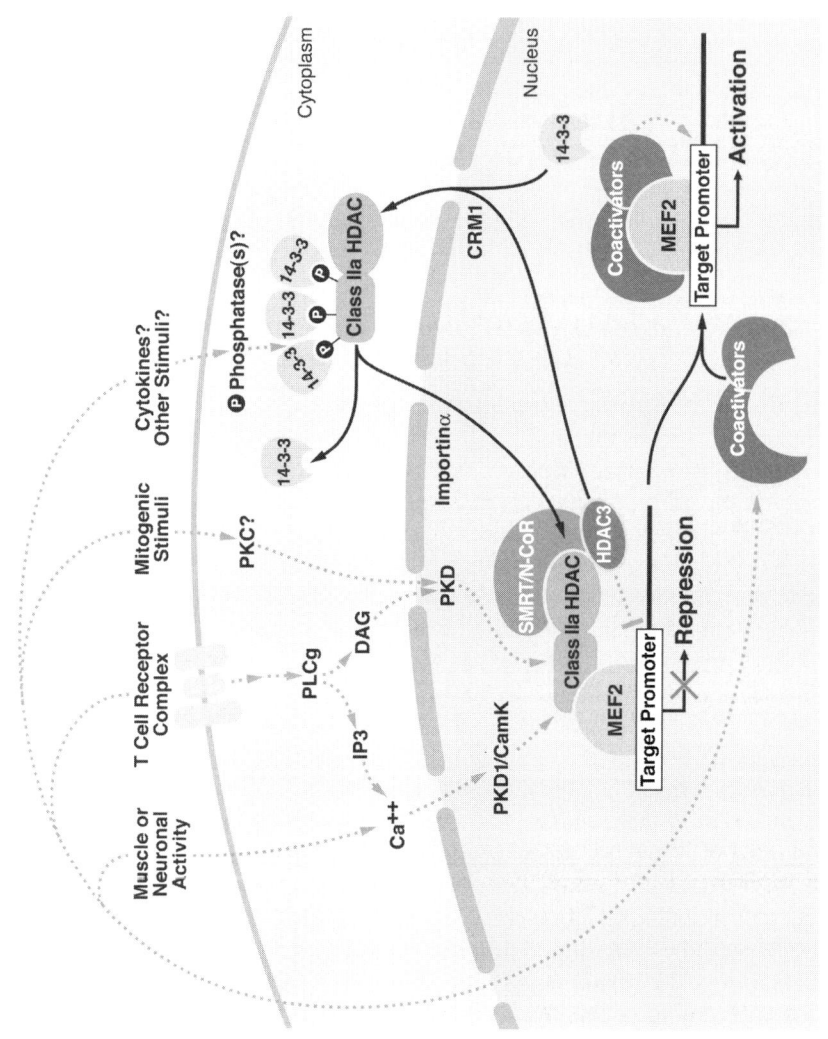

Regulation of Nucleocytoplasmic Shuttling

Signal-dependent nucleocytoplasmic shuttling is a hallmark of the class IIa HDACs. All the full-length isoforms of the class IIa HDACs *(15,16,53,54)* can move between the cytoplasm and the nucleus and localize exclusively to the nucleus upon treatment with inhibitors of nuclear export *(53,57,75–77)*. As discussed above, the subcellular distribution of class IIa HDACs can be regulated by binding to 14-3-3 proteins, and the binding of these proteins to the class IIa HDACs is phosphorylation dependent *(16,53,54)*. Mutations of the conserved 14-3-3-interacting phosphorylation sites in the class IIa HDACs (Fig. 1A) prevent class IIa HDACs from being exported to the cytoplasm in response to extracellular signals *(9,16,53–55,71,77)*.

The 14-3-3 proteins are thought to modify the subcellular localization of targets by modulating the activity of nuclear localization (NLS) and nuclear export signals (NES). An NLS containing an arginine/lysine-rich motif is present in the N-terminal domains of all four class IIa HDACs, just to the C-terminal side of the first 14-3-3 binding site (Fig. 1A) *(57,78)*. Phosphorylation-dependent binding of 14-3-3 proteins to the amino-termini of class II HDACs masks this NLS and prevents nuclear import. Conversely, a chromosome region maintenance 1 (CRM1)-dependent nuclear export signal is present at the extreme C termini of HDACs 4, 5, and 7 and the full-length isoforms of HDAC9 (Fig. 1A) *(5,78)*. The truncated isoforms of HDAC9, variants 1, 2, and 3, lack the C-terminal NES and are constitutively nuclear. This NES, in those class IIa HDACs that have it, becomes active upon binding of 14-3-3 proteins to the N terminus of class II HDACs and drives their relocalization to the cytoplasm.

Phosphorylation of Class IIa HDACs

Several lines of evidence suggest that signal-dependent phosphorylation of 14-3-3 binding sites is the critical mechanism regulating the nucleocytoplasmic shuttling of the class IIa HDACs and the signal-dependent repression of target genes. As mentioned in the previous section, mutation of these conserved serine residues results in constitutive nuclear localization of the class IIa HDACs and signal-refractory repression of their target genes *(8,9,77,79)*. Treatment of cells with staurosporine, a protein kinase

---

Fig. 3. Regulation of class IIa HDACs by signal-dependent phosphorylation. Phosphorylation of 14-3-3 binding sites in the N termini of class IIa HDACs by either PKD or Cam kinase in response to extracellular signals results in the export of class IIa HDACs to the cytoplasm and derepression of target genes. As yet unknown phosphatases, possibly also regulated by extracellular signals, may mediate reimportation of class IIa HDACs to the nucleus and consequent rerepression of target genes.

inhibitor, leads to the nuclear localization of HDAC4 *(54)*. Conversely, treatment of cells with calyculin A, a phosphatase inhibitor, increases the cytoplasmic retention of HDAC4.

Initial examination of sequences of the phosphorylation sites in class IIa HDACs determined that they were closely related to consensus phosphorylation sites for the calcium/calmodulin-dependent protein kinases (CaMKs) *(79)*. These kinases represent attractive candidates for the regulators of class IIa HDACs, since the activity of MEF2 is regulated by calcium flux *(80)* and since calcium signaling is an important mechanism in the muscle, immune, and neural cells where class IIa HDACs are abundant. Subsequent studies showed that CaMKI and CaMKIV could phosphorylate all four class IIa HDACs, promote their association with 14-3-3 proteins, and stimulate their export to the cytoplasm *(5,9,16,53,55)*. Overexpression of constitutively active CaMKs or signal-dependent activation of CaMKs in cell culture models induced relocalization of class IIa HDACs to the cytoplasm, derepressed class IIa HDAC target genes, and induced both the myogenic conversion program and cardiac hypertrophy *(55,81–83)*.

However, recent studies have revealed that phosphorylation of class IIa HDACs by CaMKs is not the whole story. In the cardiomyocytes of HDAC9-deficient mice, an HDAC kinase activity stimulated by cardiac pressure overload was resistant to CaMK inhibitors *(84)*. Since then, another study from the same group has revealed that protein kinase D (PKD), a recently described protein kinase related to both protein kinase C (PCK) and CaMK, is activated by hypertrophic stimuli and phosphorylates HDAC5. Phosphorylation of HDAC5 by a constitutively active PKD mutant stimulated nuclear export of HDAC5 *(85)*. Similarly, work done in our laboratory showed that PKD is activated by antigen receptor signaling in thymocytes.

We also found that PKD can phosphorylate HDAC7 in a T-cell hybridoma, and that expression of constitutively active PKD leads to nuclear export of HDAC7 and derepression of the Nur77 promoter. Interestingly, in at least one model of T-cell apoptosis and Nur77 regulation, the PKC-PKD pathway, and not calcium signaling, appeared to be the key regulator of HDAC7. Treatment of antigen receptor-stimulated DO11.10 T-cell hybridoma cells with PKC/PKD inhibitors, but not CaMK inhibitors, was able to block the expression of Nur77. Also, the cytoplasmic relocalization of transfected HDAC7 was driven by phorbol myristate acetate treatment, which activates PKD, but not by treatment with ionomycin, which activates CaMK *(86)*.

The recent discovery of a new kinase that is responsive to distinct extracellular signals and can mediate the nuclear export of class IIa HDACs raises some intriguing possibilities. In some circumstances, the two kinases might function redundantly, as in T-cell antigen receptor signaling, which results in both PKC activation and calcium flux. However, in other cases, such as muscle, the activation of these two kinases may arise from different signals entirely. A dynamic equilibrium between the activities of the two kinases and the activities of the cognate phosphatases, all in response to different or overlapping extracellular signals, might thus determine the localization of class IIa HDACs as the result of a complex integration of the extracellular environment.

Such a complex integration of different signals might play an important role in regulating cell-fate decisions in processes of differentiation in which class IIa HDACs might play a role, such as early T-cell development or the formation of structures in the developing heart or nervous system. Indeed, a recent study showed that PKD appears to play a role during β-selection in the early development of T cells, a process that involves numerous cell-fate decisions (87). This finding, as well as the elucidation of other differentiation processes involving PKD and CaMK, will provide new clues as to the possible functions of the class IIa HDACs. How effective each kinase is at phosphorylating each potential substrate is also still an open question. Currently, there are only data on PKD for HDAC5 and HDAC7, so it is still formally possible that HDAC4 and HDAC9 are not substrates.

Finally, there is still nothing known about what cellular phosphatases are responsible for the dephosphorylation of the class IIa HDACs, either constitutively or in response to extracellular signals. Modulation of the activity of HDAC phosphatases may be important in adding a combinatorial element to the regulation of class IIa HDAC subcellular localization. Finding and characterizing these phosphatases is an active area of research in our laboratory and undoubtedly in others as well.

Other Posttranslational Modifications

Although phosphorylation of 14-3-3 binding sites is an important and well-characterized posttranslational modification of the class IIa HDACs, it is not the only one. HDACs 4, -9, 1, and 6 are conjugated to the small ubiquitin-like modifier-1 (SUMO-1) through the SUMO E3 ligase RanBP2 (70). This modification occurs at K559 of HDAC4, a residue that is conserved in HDACs 4, 5, and 9, but not HDAC7 (Fig. 1A). A mutant version of HDAC4 that cannot be sumoylated, K559R, was found to have diminished repressive activity and markedly diminished enzymatic activity. The effect may be owing to a structural problem in the mutant protein. One hypothetical function of SUMO is the proper targeting of sumoylated proteins to the nuclear pore complex and to nuclear bodies. However, there was no difference between the subnuclear localizations of HDAC4 K559R and wild-type HDAC4. Mutation of the sumoylation site of HDAC4 did not affect binding to any known interaction partners, but SUMO might mediate interaction of HDAC4 with an as-yet unknown cofactor.

Finally, two reports have come out this year that HDAC4 can be cleaved by caspases 2 and 3 in response to proapoptotic stimuli (88,89). Cleavage occurs at D289 of HDAC4, a residue that is not conserved in any of the other class IIa HDACs. Interestingly, the cleaved N-terminal fragment of HDAC4 promotes apoptosis by itself, through the mitochondrial pathway, and was also found to be a more potent repressor of MEF2-mediated transcription than the full-length HDAC4. Unfortunately, the authors did not determine the effect of a caspase-resistant mutant of HDAC4 on the susceptibility of cells to various apoptotic stimuli, so it is impossible to assess how important this mechanism is to the regulation of apoptosis.

SUMMARY AND FUTURE QUESTIONS

Much has been learned about the class IIa HDACs in the short time since they were discovered. A host of interaction partners have been identified, mediating targeting to specific promoters, recruitment of different enzymatic activities such as histone methylation, and regulation of subcellular localization. Many of these interactions have been tied to the signal-dependent regulation of specific target genes that play important roles in differentiation processes in heart, skeletal muscle, and the immune system and in the regulation of viral latency. Other biological roles are being defined in the context of knockout animals. However, many questions remain to be answered.

The host of protein–protein interactions in which the class IIa HDACs participate offers a vast array of possible transcriptional targets for these regulators; however, to date, only one systematic study looking for targets of the class IIa HDACs has been undertaken (90). In Saccharomyces cerevisiae, a technically impressive study (91) defined the histone deacetylation targets genome-wide of five HDAC molecules: reduced potassium dependency 3 (RPD3; the class I prototype), histone decetylase1 (HDA1; the class II prototype), silent information regulator 2 (Sir2), Hos1/3, and Hos2. The authors used a chromatin immunoprecipitation/DNA microarray strategy to analyze the effects of deletion of each of these molecules on the acetylation state of approx 6700 distinct intergenic regions (IGRs).

There was a clear division of labor between the yeast molecules. For example, of the 815 IGRs hyperacetylated in the RPD3-deleted mutant and the 647 IGRs hyperacetylated as a result of HDA1 deletion, only 139, or about 10% of the total, were affected by both mutations. Although deletion of HDA1 affected acetylation near a broad range of genes, there was a preference for genes involved in responses to metabolic stress. Interestingly, these genes were concentrated in regions around 10 to 25 kb from the telomeres, which are repressed under normal growth conditions. The authors termed these regions HAST domains. They also found a good correlation between genes hyperacetylated by HDA1 deletion and genes derepressed by deletion of the sequence-specific factor tup1, which recruits HDA1 to promoters *(92)*. However, only about 31% of the genes affected by HDA1 deletion are differentially regulated by tup1 deletion, suggesting that as yet undefined mechanisms are responsible for the recruitment of HDA1 to the remaining loci. Unfortunately, the lack of the N-terminal domain characteristic of the vertebrate class IIa HDACs in HDA1 clearly limits the degree to which this study can shed light on the potential targets of the human class IIa HDACs.

Although recent work implies strongly that a number of targets of runx2 are regulated by HDAC4, the great majority of known class IIa HDAC targets are recruited via interaction with MEF2 family transcription factors. In part, this dearth of other modes of class IIa HDAC recruitment may have to do with the tendency of the field thus far to start with a MEF2-regulated gene and work backward toward the class IIa HDACs. DNA microarray technology should make it fairly straightforward to undertake studies that start with the class IIa HDACs and proceed forward from there. The one such study published so far failed to identify any genes that were regulated by HDAC5 in a MEF2-independent manner. Microarray comparisons were made between murine cardiomyocytes that were expressing a signal-resistant mutant of HDAC5 vs wild-type cardiomyocytes. The one differentially regulated gene that was not already known to be a MEF2 target that was investigated was peroxisome proliferator-activated receptor γ coactivator 1α, an important regulator of mitochondrial biogenesis *(90)*. As it turns out, this gene also has MEF2 binding sites in its promoter. Hopefully, future microarray studies will have better luck in identifying MEF2-independent targets of the class IIa HDACs.

In our own laboratory, we are currently undertaking microarray studies aimed at identifying targets of HDAC7 in T-cell development. Although the results are still too preliminary to discuss in detail, we appear to have identified at least a few genes that are regulated by a mechanism unrelated to MEF2, but further confirmation will be required before we can assert this with confidence. Hopefully, as several laboratories undertake similar studies in different physiologic contexts, a clearer picture of the doubtlessly highly complex role of the class IIa HDACs in developmental gene regulation will begin to emerge.

REFERENCES

1. Gregoretti IV, Lee YM, Goodson HV. Molecular evolution of the histone deacety-lase family: functional implications of phylogenetic analysis. J Mol Biol 2004; 338:17–31.
2. Zeremski M, Stricker JR, Fischer D, Zusman SB, Cohen D. Histone deacetylase dHDAC4 is involved in segmentation of the *Drosophila* embryo and is regulated by gap and pair-rule genes. Genesis 2003;35:31–38.
3. Dichoso D, Brodigan T, Chwoe KY, et al. The MADS-Box factor CeMEF2 is not essential for *Caenorhabditis elegans* myogenesis and development. Dev Biol 2000;223:431–440.
4. Choi KY, Ji YJ, Jee C, Kim do H, Ahnn J. Characterization of CeHDA-7, a class II histone deacetylase interacting with MEF-2 in *Caenorhabditis elegans*. Biochem Biophys Res Commun 2002;293:1295–1300.
5. McKinsey TA, Zhang CL, Olson EN. Identification of a signal-responsive nuclear export sequence in class II histone deacetylases. Mol Cell Biol 2001;21: 6312–6321.
6. Sparrow DB, Miska EA, Langley E, et al. MEF-2 function is modified by a novel co-repressor, MITR. EMBO J 1999;18:5085–5098.
7. Zhou X, Richon VM, Rifkind RA, Marks PA. Identification of a transcriptional repressor related to the noncatalytic domain of histone deacetylases 4 and 5. Proc Natl Acad Sci U S A 2000;97:1056–1061.
8. Dequiedt F, Kasler H, Fischle W, et al. HDAC7, a thymus-specific class II his-tone deacetylase, regulates Nur77 transcription and TCR-mediated apoptosis. Immunity 2003;18:687–698.
9. Zhang CL, McKinsey TA, Olson EN. The transcriptional corepressor MITR is a signal-responsive inhibitor of myogenesis. Proc Natl Acad Sci U S A 2001;98: 7354–7359.
10. Black BL, Olson EN. Transcriptional control of muscle development by myocyte enhancer factor-2 (MEF2) proteins. Annu Rev Cell Dev Biol 1998;14: 167–196.
11. Gossett LA, Kelvin DJ, Sternberg EA, Olson EN. A new myocyte-specific enhancer-binding factor that recognizes a conserved element associated with multiple muscle-specific genes. Mol Cell Biol 1989;9:5022–5033.
12. McKinsey TA, Zhang CL, Olson EN. MEF2: a calcium-dependent regulator of cell division, differentiation and death. Trends Biochem Sci 2002,27.40–47.
13. Wang AH, Bertos NR, Vezmar M, et al. HDAC4, a human histone deacetylase related to yeast HDA1, is a transcriptional corepressor. Mol Cell Biol 1999; 19:7816–7827.
14. Lemercier C, Verdel A, Galloo B, Curtet S, Brocard MP, Khochbin S. mHDA1/HDAC5 histone deacetylase interacts with and represses MEF2A tran-scriptional activity. J Biol Chem 2000;275:15,594–15,599.
15. Dressel U, Bailey PJ, Wang SC, Downes M, Evans RM, Muscat GE. A dynamic role for HDAC7 in MEF2-mediated muscle differentiation. J Biol Chem 2001;276:17,007–17,013.
16. Kao HY, Verdel A, Tsai CC, Simon C, Juguilon H, Khochbin S. Mechanism for nucleocytoplasmic shuttling of histone deacetylase 7. J Biol Chem 2001;276: 47,496–47,507.
17. Otto F, Lubbert M, Stock M. Upstream and downstream targets of RUNX pro-teins. J Cell Biochem 2003;89:9–18.

18. Okuda T, van Deursen J, Hiebert SW, Grosveld G, Downing JR. AML1, the target of multiple chromosomal translocations in human leukemia, is essential for normal fetal liver hematopoiesis. Cell 1996;84:321–330.

19. Li QL, Ito K, Sakakura C, et al. Causal relationship between the loss of RUNX3 expression and gastric cancer. Cell 2002;109:113–124.

20. Levanon D, Bettoun D, Harris-Cerruti C, et al. The Runx3 transcription factor regulates development and survival of TrkC dorsal root ganglia neurons. EMBO J 2002;21:3454–3463.

21. Taniuchi I, Osato M, Egawa T, et al. Differential requirements for Runx proteins in CD4 repression and epigenetic silencing during T lymphocyte development. Cell 2002;111:621–633.

22. Ehlers M, Laule-Kilian K, Petter M, et al. Morpholino antisense oligonucleotide-mediated gene knockdown during thymocyte development reveals role for Runx3 transcription factor in CD4 silencing during development of CD4–/CD8+ thymocytes. J Immunol 2003;171:3594–3604.

23. Komori T, Yagi H, Nomura S, et al. Targeted disruption of Cbfa1 results in a complete lack of bone formation owing to maturational arrest of osteoblasts. Cell 1997;89:755–764.

24. Otto F, Thornell AP, Crompton T, et al. Cbfa1, a candidate gene for cleidocranial dysplasia syndrome, is essential for osteoblast differentiation and bone development. Cell 1997;89:765–771.

25. Vega RB, Matsuda K, Oh J, et al. Histone deacetylase 4 controls chondrocyte hypertrophy during skeletogenesis. Cell 2004;119:555–566.

25a. Schroeder TM, Kahler RA, Li X, Westendorf JJ. Histone deacetylase 3 interacts with runx2 to repress the osteocalcin promoter and regulate osteoblast differentiation. J Biol Chem 2004;279:41,998–42,007. Epub 2004 Aug 2.

26. Kerckaert JP, Deweindt C, Tilly H, Quief S, Lecocq G, Bastard C. LAZ3, a novel zinc-finger encoding gene, is disrupted by recurring chromosome 3q27 translocations in human lymphomas. Nat Genet 1993;5:66–70.

27. Ye BH, Lista F, Lo Coco F, et al. Alterations of a zinc finger-encoding gene, BCL-6, in diffuse large-cell lymphoma. Science 1993;262:747–750.

28. Deweindt C, Albagli O, Bernardin F, et al. The LAZ3/BCL6 oncogene encodes a sequence-specific transcriptional inhibitor: a novel function for the BTB/POZ domain as an autonomous repressing domain. Cell Growth Differ 1995;6:1495–1503.

29. Shaffer AL, Yu X, He Y, Boldrick J, Chan EP, Staudt LM. BCL-6 represses genes that function in lymphocyte differentiation, inflammation, and cell cycle control. Immunity 2000;13:199–212.

30. Lemercier C, Brocard MP, Puvion-Dutilleul F, Kao HY, Albagli O, Khochbin S. Class II histone deacetylases are directly recruited by BCL6 transcriptional repressor. J Biol Chem 2002;277:22,045–22,052.

31. Dhordain P, Albagli O, Lin RJ, et al. Corepressor SMRT binds the BTB/POZ repressing domain of the LAZ3/BCL6 oncoprotein. Proc Natl Acad Sci U S A 1997;94:10,762–10,767.

32. Wong CW, Privalsky ML. Components of the SMRT corepressor complex exhibit distinctive interactions with the POZ domain oncoproteins PLZF, PLZF-RARalpha, and BCL-6. J Biol Chem 1998;273:27,695–27,702.

33. Huynh KD, Bardwell VJ. The BCL-6 POZ domain and other POZ domains interact with the co-repressors N-CoR and SMRT. Oncogene 1998;17:2473–2484.

34. Huynh KD, Fischle W, Verdin E, Bardwell VJ. BCoR, a novel corepressor involved in BCL-6 repression. Genes Dev 2000;14:1810–1823.

35. Huang EY, Zhang J, Miska EA, Guenther MG, Kouzarides T, Lazar MA. Nuclear receptor corepressors partner with class II histone deacetylases in a Sin3-independent repression pathway. Genes Dev 2000;14:45–54.

36. Kao HY, Downes M, Ordentlich P, Evans RM. Isolation of a novel histone deacetylase reveals that class I and class II deacetylases promote SMRT-mediated repression. Genes Dev 2000;14:55–66.

37. Downes M, Ordentlich P, Kao HY, Alvarez JG, Evans RM. Identification of a nuclear domain with deacetylase activity. Proc Natl Acad Sci U S A 2000;97: 10,330–10,335.

38. Chen JD, Evans RM. A transcriptional co-repressor that interacts with nuclear hormone receptors. Nature 1995;377:454–457.

39. Horlein AJ, Naar AM, Heinzel T, et al. Ligand-independent repression by the thyroid hormone receptor mediated by a nuclear receptor co-repressor. Nature 1995;377:397–404.

40. Aranda A, Pascual A. Nuclear hormone receptors and gene expression. Physiol Rev 2001;81:1269–1304.

41. Li J, Wang J, Wang J, et al. Both corepressor proteins SMRT and N-CoR exist in large protein complexes containing HDAC3. EMBO J 2000;19:4342–4350.

42. Wen YD, Perissi V, Staszewski LM, et al. The histone deacetylase-3 complex contains nuclear receptor corepressors. Proc Natl Acad Sci U S A 2000;97: 7202–7207.

43. Guenther MG, Lane WS, Fischle W, Verdin E, Lazar MA, Shiekhattar R. A core SMRT corepressor complex containing HDAC3 and TBL1, a WD40- repeat protein linked to deafness. Genes Dev 2000;14:1048–1057.

44. Guenther MG, Barak O, Lazar MA. The SMRT and N-CoR corepressors are activating cofactors for histone deacetylase 3. Mol Cell Biol 2001;21: 6091–6101.

45. Fischle W, Dequiedt F, Fillion M, Hendzel MJ, Voelter W, Verdin E. Human HDAC7 histone deacetylase activity is associated with HDAC3 in vivo. J Biol Chem 2001;276:35,826–35,835.

46. Grozinger CM, Hassig CA, Schreiber SL. Three proteins define a class of human histone deacetylases related to yeast Hda1p. Proc Natl Acad Sci U S A 1999; 96:4868–4873.

47. Fischle W, Dequiedt F, Hendzel MJ, et al. Enzymatic activity associated with class II HDACs is dependent on a multiprotein complex containing HDAC3 and SMRT/N-CoR. Mol Cell 2002;9:45–57.

48. Zhang J, Kalkum M, Chait BT, Roeder RG. The N-CoR-HDAC3 nuclear receptor corepressor complex inhibits the JNK pathway through the integral subunit GPS2. Mol Cell 2002;9:611–623.

49. Pijnappel WW, Schaft D, Roguev A, et al. The *S. cerevisiae* SET3 complex includes two histone deacetylases, Hos2 and Hst1, and is a meiotic-specific repressor of the sporulation gene program. Genes Dev 2001;15:2991–3004.

50. Kurtev V, Margueron R, Kroboth K, Ogris E, Cavailles V, Seiser C. Transcriptional regulation by the repressor of estrogen receptor activity via recruitment of histone deacetylases. J Biol Chem 2004;279:24,834–24,843.

51. Montano MM, Ekena K, Delage-Mourroux R, Chang W, Martini P, Katzenellenbogen BS. An estrogen receptor-selective coregulator that potentiates the effectiveness of antiestrogens and represses the activity of estrogens. Proc Natl Acad Sci U S A 1999;96:6947–6952.

52. Fu H, Subramanian RR, Masters SC. 14-3-3 proteins: structure, function, and regulation. Annu Rev Pharmacol Toxicol 2000;40:617–647.

53. Wang AH, Kruhlak MJ, Wu J, et al. Regulation of histone deacetylase 4 by binding of 14-3-3 proteins. Mol Cell Biol 2000;20:6904–6912.

54. Grozinger CM, Schreiber SL. Regulation of histone deacetylase 4 and 5 and transcriptional activity by 14-3-3-dependent cellular localization. Proc Natl Acad Sci U S A 2000;97:7835–7840.

55. McKinsey TA, Zhang CL, Olson EN. Activation of the myocyte enhancer factor-2 transcription factor by calcium/calmodulin-dependent protein kinase-stimulated binding of 14-3-3 to histone deacetylase 5. Proc Natl Acad Sci U S A 2000; 97:14,400–14,405.

56. Youn H-D, Grozinger CM, Liu JO. Calcium regulates transcriptional repression of myocyte enhancer factor 2 by histone deacetylase 4. J Biol Chem 2000;275: 22,563–22,567.

57. McKinsey TA, Zhang CL, Lu J, Olson EN. Signal-dependent nuclear export of a histone deacetylase regulates muscle differentiation. Nature 2000;408: 106–111.

58. Zhang CL, McKinsey TA, Olson EN. Association of class II histone deacetylases with heterochromatin protein 1: potential role for histone methylation in control of muscle differentiation. Mol Cell Biol 2002;22:7302–7312.

59. Boyd JM, Subramanian T, Schaeper U, La Regina M, Bayley S, Chinnadurai G. A region in the C-terminus of adenovirus 2/5 E1a protein is required for association with a cellular phosphoprotein and important for the negative modulation of T24-ras mediated transformation, tumorigenesis and metastasis. EMBO J 1993;12:469–478.

60. Schaeper U, Boyd JM, Verma S, Uhlmann E, Subramanian T, Chinnadurai G. Molecular cloning and characterization of a cellular phosphoprotein that interacts with a conserved C-terminal domain of adenovirus E1A involved in negative modulation of oncogenic transformation. Proc Natl Acad Sci U S A 1995;92: 10,467–10,471.

61. Poortinga G, Watanabe M, Parkhurst SM. *Drosophila* CtBP: a Hairy-interacting protein required for embryonic segmentation and hairy-mediated transcriptional repression. EMBO J 1998;17:2067–2078.

62. Nibu Y, Zhang H, Levine M. Interaction of short-range repressors with *Drosophila* CtBP in the embryo. Science 1998;280:101–104.

63. Turner J, Crossley M. Cloning and characterization of mCtBP2, a co-repressor that associates with basic Kruppel-like factor and other mammalian transcriptional regulators. EMBO J 1998;17:5129–5140.

64. Koipally J, Georgopoulos K. Ikaros interactions with CtBP reveal a repression mechanism that is independent of histone deacetylase activity. J Biol Chem 2000;275:19,594–19,602.

65. van Vliet J, Turner J, Crossley M. Human Kruppel-like factor 8: a CACCC-box binding protein that associates with CtBP and represses transcription. Nucleic Acids Res 2000;28:1955–1962.

66. Zhang CL, McKinsey TA, Lu J-R, Olson EN. Association of COOH-terminal-binding protein (CtBP) and MEF2-interacting transcription repressor (MITR) contributes to transcriptional repression of the MEF2 transcription factor. J Biol Chem 2001;276:35–39.

67. Turner J, Crossley M. The CtBP family: enigmatic and enzymatic transcriptional co-repressors. Bioessays 2001;23:683–690.

68. Chinnadurai G. CtBP, an unconventional transcriptional corepressor in development and oncogenesis. Mol Cell 2002;9:213–224.

69. Shi Y, Sawada J, Sui G, et al. Coordinated histone modifications mediated by a CtBP co-repressor complex. Nature 2003;422:735–738.

70. Kirsh O, Seeler J-S, Pichler A, et al. The SUMO E3 ligase RanBP2 promotes modification of the HDAC4 deacetylase. EMBO J 2002;21:2682–2691.

71. Zhou X, Richon VM, Wang AH, Yang XJ, Rifkind RA, Marks PA. Histone deacetylase 4 associates with extracellular signal-regulated kinases 1 and 2, and its cellular localization is regulated by oncogenic Ras. Proc Natl Acad Sci U S A 2000;97:14,329–14,333.

72. Lee HJ, Chun M, Kandror KV. Tip60 and HDAC7 interact with the endothelin receptor a and may be involved in downstream signaling. J Biol Chem 2001;276:16,597–16,600.

73. Lomonte P, Thomas J, Texier P, Caron C, Khochbin S, Epstein AL. Functional interaction between class II histone deacetylases and ICP0 of herpes simplex virus type 1. J Virol 2004;78:6744–6757.

74. Kao GD, McKenna WG, Guenther MG, Muschel RJ, Lazar MA, Yen TJ. Histone deacetylase 4 interacts with 53BP1 to mediate the DNA damage response. J Cell Biol 2003;160:1017–1027.

75. Miska EA, Karlsson C, Langley E, Nielsen SJ, Pines J, Kouzarides T. HDAC4 deacetylase associates with and represses the MEF2 transcription factor. EMBO J 1999;18:5099–5107.

76. Zhao X, Ito A, Kane CD, et al. The modular nature of histone deacetylase HDAC4 confers phosphorylation-dependent intracellular trafficking. J Biol Chem 2001;276:35,042–35,048.

77. Miska EA, Langley E, Wolf D, Karlsson C, Pines J, Kouzarides T. Differential localization of HDAC4 orchestrates muscle differentiation. Nucleic Acids Res 2001;29:3439–3447.

78. Wang AH, Yang XJ. Histone deacetylase 4 possesses intrinsic nuclear import and export signals. Mol Cell Biol 2001;21:5992–6005.

79. McKinsey TA, Zhang C-L, Lu J, Olson EN. Signal-dependent nuclear export of a histone deacetylase regulates muscle diferentiation. Nature 2000;408:106–111.

80. Woronicz JD, Lina A, Calnan BJ, Szychowski S, Cheng L, Winoto A. Regulation of the Nur77 orphan steroid receptor in activation-induced apoptosis. Mol Cell Biol 1995;15:6364–6376.

81. Lu J, McKinsey TA, Zhang CL, Olson EN. Regulation of skeletal myogenesis by association of the MEF2 transcription factor with class II histone deacetylases. Mol Cell 2000;6:233–244.

82. Lu J, McKinsey TA, Nicol RL, Olson EN. Signal-dependent activation of the MEF2 transcription factor by dissociation from histone deacetylases. Proc Natl Acad Sci U S A 2000;97:4070–4075.

83. Passier R, Zeng H, Frey N, et al. CaM kinase signaling induces cardiac hypertrophy and activates the MEF2 transcription factor in vivo. J Clin Invest 2000;105:1395–1406.

84. Zhang CL, McKinsey TA, Chang S, Antos CL, Hill JA, Olson EN. Class II histone deacetylases act as signal-responsive repressors of cardiac hypertrophy. Cell 2002;110:479–488.

85. Vega RB, Harrison BC, Meadows E, et al. Protein kinases C and D mediate agonist-dependent cardiac hypertrophy through nuclear export of histone deacetylase 5. Mol Cell Biol 2004;24:8374–8385.

86. Parra M, Kasler H, McKinsey TA, Olson EN, Verdin E. Protein kinase D1 phosphorylates HDAC7 and induces its nuclear export after TCR activation. J Biol Chem 2005;280:13,762–13,770; epub Dec., 2004.

87. Marklund U, Lightfoot K, Cantrell D. Intracellular location and cell context-dependent function of protein kinase D. Immunity 2003;19:491–501.

88. Paroni G, Mizzau M, Henderson C, Del Sal G, Schneider C, Brancolini C. Caspase-dependent regulation of histone deacetylase 4 nuclear-cytoplasmic shuttling promotes apoptosis. Mol Biol Cell 2004;15:2804–2818.

89. Liu F, Dowling M, Yang XJ, Kao GD. Caspase-mediated specific cleavage of human histone deacetylase 4. J Biol Chem 2004;279:34,537–34,546.

90. Czubryt MP, McAnally J, Fishman GI, Olson EN. Regulation of peroxisome proliferator-activated receptor gamma coactivator 1 alpha (PGC-1 alpha) and mitochondrial function by MEF2 and HDAC5. Proc Natl Acad Sci U S A 2003; 100:1711–1716.

91. Robyr D, Suka Y, Xenarios I, et al. Microarray deacetylation maps determine genome-wide functions for yeast histone deacetylases. Cell 2002;109:437–446.

92. Wu J, Suka N, Carlson M, Grunstein M. TUP1 utilizes histone H3/H2B-specific HDA1 deacetylase to repress gene activity in yeast. Mol Cell 2001;7:117–126.

93. Fischle W, Emiliani S, Hendzel MJ, et al. A new family of human histone deacetylases related to *Saccharomyces cerevisiae* HDA1p. J Biol Chem 1999; 274:11,713–11,720.

94. Verdel A, Khochbin S. Identification of a new family of higher eukaryotic histone deacetylases. Coordinate expression of differentiation-dependent chromatin modifiers. J Biol Chem 1999;274:2440–2445.

95. Zhou X, Marks PA, Rifkind RA, Richon VM. Cloning and characterization of a histone deacetylase, HDAC9. Proc Natl Acad Sci U S A 2001;98: 10,572–10,577.

7 Histone Deacetylases in the Response to Misfolded Proteins

J. Andrew McKee, MD
and Tso-Pang Yao, PhD

CONTENTS

From: *Cancer Drug Discovery and Development*
Histone Deacetylases: Transcriptional Regulation and Other Cellular Functions
Edited by: E. Verdin © Humana Press Inc., Totowa, NJ

SUMMARY

Until recently, reversible acetylation was thought to occur exclusively in the nucleus. Now it is known that several cytoplasmic processes require reversible acetylation. The first identified cytoplasmic deacetylase was HDAC6, a member of the histone deacetylase (HDAC) family. HDAC6 modulates α-tubulin acetylation and thus can regulate cytoskeletal dynamics and cell motility. HDAC6 has also been shown recently to play an essential role in the cell's response to misfolded proteins. Using the characterization of HDAC6 as a starting point, in this chapter we review the role of HDACs in the cellular response to misfolded proteins. Specifically, we address how HDACs regulate the formation of aggresomes. We also discuss the relevance of these findings to neurodegenerative disease.

Key Words: HDAC, deacetylation, aggresome, misfolded protein, inclusion body, ubiquitin, proteasome, polyglutamine, Huntington, neurodegenerative disease.

INTRODUCTION

In 1966, reversible protein acetylation was discovered by virtue of its correlation with gene transcription (reviewed in ref. *1*). Because this pioneering research concerned gene transcription, subsequent work has focused exclusively on the role of acetylation in histone modification and downstream events. These studies have led to a molecular understanding of gene transcription and chromatin remodeling, as well as the identification of enzymes that regulate reversible histone acetylation (reviewed in refs. *2* and *3*). Because of the intense focus on histone acetylation, it is commonly thought that reversible acetylation, and therefore enzymes that regulate acetylation, are mostly dedicated to chromatin-related processes. Recent studies, however, have begun to challenge this simplistic paradigm and implicate reversible protein acetylation in a surprising array of cellular processes including cell motility *(4)* immune synapse formation *(5)*, and misfolded protein trafficking *(6)*. These new studies suggest that reversible acetylation might have many nongenomic functions that are just now being discovered. In this chapter, we discuss recent findings that have identified novel and essential roles for members of the histone deacetylase (HDAC) gene family in the cellular response to misfolded proteins. We will also touch on the significance of these findings for neurodegenerative disease.

HDAC6 IS A CYTOPLASMIC DEACETYLASE

The first evidence of nonnuclear and nonhistone-associated activity for a HDAC member came from the characterization of HDAC6 *(7)*. Among the 11 identified HDAC family members, HDAC6 is uniquely localized to the cytoplasm under most conditions *(8–10)*. In the cytoplasm, HDAC6 concentrates distinctly at the perinuclear region and at the leading edge. Interestingly, this pattern is also shared by p150^{Glued}, which is a component of the dynein motor complex. Dynein is a large protein complex that hydrolyzes ATP to move cargo such as organelles and proteins from the plus (+) to the minus (–) ends of microtubules (reviewed in ref. *11*).

The similarities between the subcellular distribution of HDAC6 and p150^{Glued} suggest a functional link among HDAC6, microtubules, and the dynein motor. Indeed, it was discovered that HDAC6 dynamically associates with microtubules *(4,12)*. One key function of this microtubule connection might be linked to microtubule acetylation *(13)*, a modification that was known to be associated with microtubule stability *(14)*. Through cell biological, biochemical, and genetic approaches, it was discovered that HDAC6 is the α-tubulin deacetylase that had long eluded researchers *(4,12,15)*. Although the exact function of tubulin acetylation remains unknown, the demonstration of HDAC6 as a tubulin deacetylase provides the first experimental evidence that HDAC family members have functions outside the nucleus.

HDAC6 HAS AN INTRINSIC UBIQUITIN-BINDING ACTIVITY

In characterizing the protein structure of HDAC6, additional nongenomic functions of HDAC6 have been discovered. In addition to its tandem catalytic domains *(7)*, HDAC6 also contains a zinc finger motif that is absent in other members of the HDAC family. Intriguingly, such a motif (known as a binding-of-ubiquitin zinc [BUZ] finger and also as the PAZ domain *[16]* or the HUB domain *[9,10]*) is also found almost exclusively in deubiquitinating enzymes *(17)*, suggesting that HDAC6 might be functionally connected to protein ubiquitination (Fig. 1). Indeed, biochemical studies demonstrate that this zinc finger motif (BUZ finger) has ubiquitin-binding activity *(16–18)*. Remarkably, the BUZ finger also mediates HDAC6 monoubiquitination *(17)*. Thus, HDAC6 can bind ubiquitinated proteins and be a target of monoubiquitination.

This unusual ubiquitin connection is characteristic of proteins involved in vesicular transport and protein trafficking. Such proteins often contain specific domains such as the ubiquitin interactive motif (UIM) and CUE domains. Similar to the BUZ finger, the UIM and CUE domains can also bind ubiquitin and mediate monoubiquitination *(19)*. These similarities suggest that HDAC6 might be involved with protein trafficking. This idea, albeit completely unexpected for a HDAC, is consistent with the fact that HDAC6 associates with the microtubule network and dynein motor

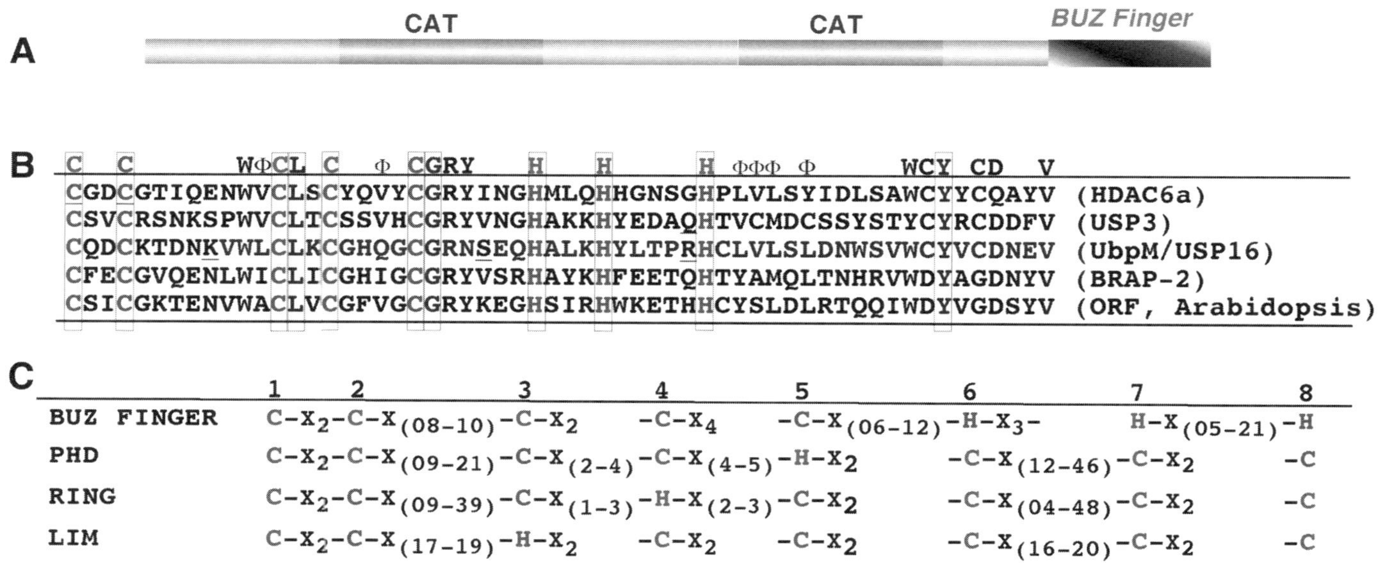

A

CAT   CAT   *BUZ Finger*

B

```
      C  C  WDΦCL C  φ CGRY  H       H    H  φφφ φ    WCY CD  V
CGDCGTIQENWVCLSCYQVYCGRYINGHMLQHHGNSGHPLVLSYIDLSAWCYYCQAYV  (HDAC6a)
CSVCRSNKSPWVCLTCSSVHCGRYVNGHAKKHYEDAQHTVCMDCSSYSTYCYRCDDFV  (USP3)
CQDCKTDNKVWLCLKCGHQGCGRNSEQHALKHYLTPRHCLVLSLDNWSVWCYVCDNEV  (UbpM/USP16)
CFECGVQENLWICLICGHIGCGRYVSRHAYKHFEETQHTYAMQLTNHRVWDYAGDNYV  (BRAP-2)
CSICGKTENVWACLVCGFVGCGRYKEGHSIRHWKETHHCYSLDLRTQQIWDYVGDSYV  (ORF, Arabidopsis)
```

C

	1	2	3	4	5	6	7	8
BUZ FINGER	C-X$_2$-C-X$_{(08-10)}$-C-X$_2$			-C-X$_4$	-C-X$_{(06-12)}$-	H-X$_3$-	H-X$_{(05-21)}$-	H
PHD	C-X$_2$-C-X$_{(09-21)}$-C-X$_{(2-4)}$			-C-X$_{(4-5)}$-	H-X$_2$	-C-X$_{(12-46)}$-	C-X$_2$	-C
RING	C-X$_2$-C-X$_{(09-39)}$-C-X$_{(1-3)}$			-H-X$_{(2-3)}$-	C-X$_2$	-C-X$_{(04-48)}$-	C-X$_2$	-C
LIM	C-X$_2$-C-X$_{(17-19)}$-H-X$_2$			-C-X$_2$	-C-X$_2$	-C-X$_{(16-20)}$-	C-X$_2$	-C

Fig. 1. The protein structure of HDAC6. (**A**) HDAC6 possesses two catalytic deacetylase domains and a binding-of-ubiquitin zinc (BUZ) finger (also referred to as a PAZ domain or a HUB domain). (**B**) Homology alignment of the HDAC6 BUZ finger with putative zinc fingers in several deubiquitinating enzymes. The genes, their species of origin, and accession numbers include: HDAC6 (*Homo sapiens*), Q9UBN7; USP3 (*H. sapiens*), AF073344; UbpM (*H. sapiens*), BC030777; BRAP-2 (*H. sapiens*), AF035620; ORF (*Arabidopsis thaliana*), NM_129779. Key conserved cysteine and histidine residues are boxed. Note that spacing and the number of key residues is conserved throughout the different species, as shown in the top consensus sequence line. (**C**) The HDAC6 BUZ finger is compared with the plant homeodomain (PHD), RING, and LIM zinc finger domains.

168

complex *(4)*. Thus the initial characterization of HDAC6 as a microtubule-associated ubiquitin-binding deacetylase provided exciting clues to the cellular processes that HDAC6 regulates.

AGGRESOMES AND THE PROCESSING OF MISFOLDED PROTEINS

One critical process known to involve both dynein motors and protein ubiquitination is the management of misfolded protein aggregates. Protein misfolding and aggregation are unavoidable consequences of protein production in the cell. Under normal conditions, the production of misfolded proteins is kept in check by quality control processes *(20,21)*, which use molecular chaperones to maintain the proper tertiary structure of newly synthesized or unfolded proteins. If a protein fails to fold properly, it is targeted for degradation by the proteasome. However, stress and pathological conditions, including temperature, oxidative stress, and genetic alterations, can cause an accumulation of misfolded proteins that exceeds the capacity of proteasomal degradation. The misfolded proteins that escape proteasomal degradation can be toxic if they are not sequestered or otherwise degraded *(21,22)*. Failure to degrade misfolded proteins is a dominant factor contributing to the cell death observed in many human disorders *(21,23)*.

Specific cellular processes have evolved to eliminate misfolded proteins. One important response to the accumulation of misfolded proteins is the cellular formation of an aggresome *(21,24–26)*. Aggresomes are perinuclear inclusion bodies that are major repositories and processing centers for misfolded protein aggregates. The formation of aggresomes requires an intact microtubule network and microtubule-associated dynein motors *(24)*. It was proposed that misfolded proteins in the cytoplasm were collected by dynein motors and transported along the microtubule network to the microtubule-organizing center (MTOC), forming an aggresome *(24)*. As dynein is a minus-end-directed motor that moves cargo toward the MTOC, this model elegantly explains the invariant perinuclear and MTOC-centered localization of aggresomes. Once misfolded proteins arrive at the MTOC, they are probably processed by local concentrations of proteasomes and by autophagy machinery (reviewed in ref. *21*).

The formation of aggresomes probably reflects two important functions: (1) to sequester misfolded proteins that would otherwise cause widespread cellular toxicity, and (2) to permit efficient degradation of misfolded proteins by MTOC-localized machinery, such as proteasomes or autophagy. This model predicts that aggresomes have a critical role in managing the cellular stress induced by misfolded proteins.

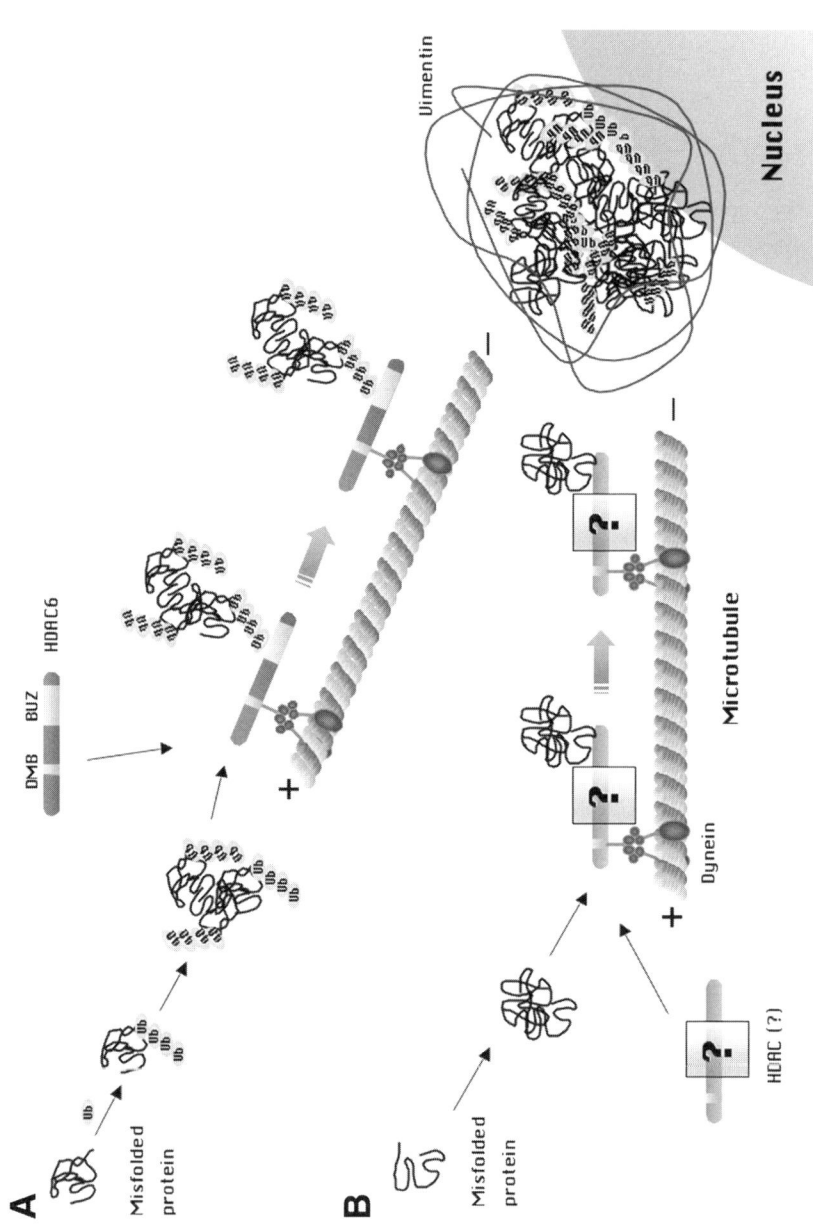

170

HDAC6 and Aggresome Formation

For misfolded proteins to be transported to the MTOC, the dynein motor must first bind them. However, it was not known how dynein could recognize and bind misfolded proteins. A clue for this fundamental question came from characterizing the subcellular localization of HDAC6 *(6)*. It was discovered that HDAC6 underwent a dramatic relocalization and became concentrated in the aggresome under conditions that induce misfolded protein accumulation. The significance of this observation was revealed when it was found that cells deficient in HDAC6 cannot form aggresomes. HDAC6 is required for aggresomes induced by inhibition of proteasome activity or by the expression of ubiquitinated misfolded proteins, such as a mutant form of the cystic fibrosis transmembrane conducting regulator (CFTR)-ΔF508 *(6)*. In HDAC6-deficient cells, many small clusters of misfolded protein are observed instead of a single prominent aggresome. These observations show that HDAC6 is required for aggresome formation and implicate HDAC6 in the microtubule-based shuttling of misfolded protein cargo to the MTOC.

By what mechanism is HDAC6 essential for aggresome formation? Investigations revealed that HDAC6 mediates aggresome formation by associating simultaneously with the dynein motor complex and with ubiquitinated proteins (Fig. 2A) *(6)*. HDAC6 interacts with dynein motors through sequences at the N terminus, whereas it binds ubiquitinated misfolded CFTRΔF508 via the BUZ finger. Thus, HDAC6 may represent a "missing link" between misfolded protein cargo and dynein, since HDAC6 allows for the efficient transport of misfolded proteins along the microtubule network to the MTOC and aggresome formation *(6)*. In support of this model, it was shown that the ubiquitin-binding BUZ finger is essential for HDAC6 to regulate aggresome formation. An HDAC6 mutant that

---

Fig. 2. The role of cytoplasmic HDACs in transporting misfolded proteins to the aggresome. **(A)** Misfolded proteins are polyubiquitinated to target them for proteasomal degradation. When the proteasomes are overwhelmed, however, misfolded ubiquitinated proteins form small aggregates in the cytoplasm. HDAC6, with its dynein motor-binding domain (DMB) and binding-of-ubiquitin zinc (BUZ) finger, functions to bind this misfolded cargo and the dynein motor complex. This enables shuttling of misfolded proteins to the aggresome via (–)-ended movement along microtubules (shown at right). **(B)** Some cytoplasmic misfolded proteins are not ubiquitinated. Examples include the chimera protein GFP250 and mutant superoxide dismutase (SOD-1). As with ubiquitinated proteins, these can form small aggregates that are recognized and transported via dynein and microtubules to the aggresome. Recent evidence implicates an as-yet unidentified non-HDAC6 histone deacetylase ("HDAC?") in mediating the formation of non-ubiquitinated aggresomes.

lacks the BUZ finger does not bind ubiquitinated misfolded CFTR and hence does not support aggresome formation. This model would explain why, in HDAC6-deficient cells, misfolded ubiquitinated proteins are not transported to the MTOC (Fig. 2A).

Reversible Protein Acetylation and Aggresome Formation

HDAC6 possesses a unique ability to link misfolded protein cargo with the dynein motor complex. Is HDAC6 merely a bridging protein, or does it have additional functions that are conferred by its deacetylase activity? Two lines of evidence suggest that HDAC6 functions as more than just an adaptor for misfolded protein cargo and dynein motors. First, a catalytically inactive HDAC6 mutant cannot support aggresome formation *(6)*. Second, HDAC inhibitors can suppress aggresome formation induced by misfolded mutant superoxide dismutase (SOD-1) *(27)*. These results argue that specific protein deacetylation is probably important for aggresome formation. What might be the target(s) of HDAC6 deacetylation during aggresome formation? The obvious candidates are proteins in the dynein motor complex including α-tubulin, molecular chaperone machinery, proteasomes, and autophagy components. The deacetylation of these factors by HDAC6 might be necessary for the initial aggresome-delivery complex to form and/or to allow efficient transport for aggresome maturation. Because the deacetylase activity of HDAC6 is required for aggresome formation, yet no targets for HDAC6 deacetylation have been identified in the aggresomal response, several important and exciting unanswered questions remain concerning the misfolded protein response and reversible acetylation.

WHAT INITIATES AGGRESOME FORMATION?

The aggresome is only one of several cellular responses to misfolded proteins. The first line of defense involves chaperone proteins that direct proper protein folding in the endoplasmic reticulum (ER) and cytoplasm (reviewed in ref. *28*). When this fails, a second defense mechanism uses ubiquitin-conjugating enzymes to target misfolded proteins for degradation. One prominent example of such machinery is ER-associated degradation (ERAD) *(28)*. Finally, aggresomal response is activated when other mechanisms, such as the proteasome and ERAD, have been overwhelmed.

How do cells sense the presence of aggregated proteins and activate the aggresomal response? Do ubiquitinated misfolded proteins, HDAC6, and dynein form a complex merely by chance or through a regulated mechanism? Evidence indicates that the association between HDAC6 and dynein motors is indeed regulated. Under normal conditions, the interaction between HDAC6 and dynein is weak. However, when the proteasome is inhibited, and ubiquitinated misfolded proteins accumulate in the cell, the HDAC6-dynein motor complexes are significantly induced (6). One interpretation is that the accumulation of ubiquitinated, misfolded proteins can stimulate or stabilize the interaction between HDAC6 and dynein motors. This could then promote the efficient transport of misfolded proteins to the MTOC and the aggresome. Misfolded proteins might induce this response by binding to HDAC6 via the BUZ finger. One can speculate that this would then induce a conformational change in HDAC6, thereby allowing more favorable binding to the dynein motor complex. Subsequently, the shuttling of misfolded proteins via HDAC6 could proceed to the aggresome. In this case, the BUZ finger would function as a sensor for the accumulation of misfolded proteins.

Another possibility is that the machinery involved in degrading the misfolded proteins, such as ERAD, can somehow communicate with the machinery that regulates the formation of aggresomes. Given that both ERAD and the aggresome are responses to the accumulation of misfolded proteins, this suggestion is plausible. Furthermore, if ERAD and the aggresome represent a response to moderate and severe levels of misfolded proteins, respectively, then it makes sense that if the moderate response (ERAD) became overwhelmed, it would activate a more severe response (aggresome). Interestingly, HDAC6 has been reported to interact with cdc48/p97 (18), a key component of the ERAD machinery. One can speculate that the association of HDAC6 and cdc48/p97 could form the connection between ER and cytoplasmic misfolded protein responses, permitting a cell overwhelmed by misfolded ER proteins to signal and initiate the formation of the aggresome.

THE NONUBIQUITINATED MISFOLDED PROTEIN CARGO DILEMMA

Thus far, we have discussed reversible acetylation in the context of aggresomes that are composed of ubiquitinated proteins. However, aggresomes can also form with ubiquitin-negative misfolded proteins. One example is aggresomes formed by overexpression of GFP250, a chimeric protein between green fluorescent protein (GFP) and part of p115 (26). Interestingly, HDAC6 does not bind nonubiquitinated misfolded model protein GFP250 and is not required for GFP250-induced aggresome formation (6). This specificity of HDAC6 toward ubiquitinated proteins, however, poses a potential problem for cells.

The concept has been proposed that nonubiquitinated proteins can be degraded by proteasomes (reviewed in ref. 29). It is likely that some misfolded proteins might not be subject to polyubiquitination. In addition to GFP250, another example of an aggresome-forming, nonubiquitinated protein is mutant SOD-1. The mutant form of this enzyme causes neuro-degenerative familial amyotrophic lateral sclerosis (ALS) *(30)*. These nonubiquitinated misfolded proteins, however, are still toxic to cells and need to be cleared *(31)*. Importantly, aggresomes induced by SOD-1 and GFP250 share many other features of aggresomes formed by ubiquitinated proteins. For instance, aggresomes from both ubiquitinated and nonubiquitinated proteins localize to the MTOC and require transport via micro-tubules and the dynein motor complex *(25,26)*. Therefore, it is apparent that ubiquitination is not essential for misfolded proteins to be recognized by the dynein motor for transport to the MTOC.

How, then, does the dynein motor complex recognize nonubiquitinated misfolded proteins? As a related question, are other members of the HDAC family involved in the processing of nonubiquitinated misfolded proteins? In a screen for molecules that suppress SOD-1 aggresome formation, a general HDAC inhibitor, Scriptaid, was identified *(27)*. Although it remains possible that Scriptaid inhibits SOD-1 aggresome formation through a transcription-dependent mechanism, the most likely interpretation is that one or more HDAC family members is involved in the transport of SOD-1 misfolded proteins. As with Scriptaid, another HDAC inhibitor, Trapoxin-B, was also able to inhibit SOD-1 aggresome formation *(27)*. Trapoxin-B, however, inhibits all HDACs except HDAC6 *(32)*. Thus, in the presence of a drug that blocks all HDACs but HDAC6, aggresomes of nonubiquitinated proteins could not form *(27)*. This is consistent with the finding of Kawaguchi et al. *(6)* that HDAC6 is not required to form aggresomes of the nonubiquitinated protein GFP250. Taken together, these data suggest that one or more HDAC family members, other than HDAC6, are impor-tant for forming aggresomes with nonubiquitinated proteins (Fig. 2B). Identifying a putative HDAC that is important for SOD-1 aggresome formation would be of great significance and would suggest that HDAC family members might play a more general role in regulating misfolded proteins. Elucidating how nonubiquitinated misfolded proteins are recog-nized and processed will be critical for our understanding of how cells manage misfolded protein stress. This would be especially relevant to diseases that involve the aggregation of nonubiquitinated proteins, such as SOD-1-induced ALS.

HDACs AND THE EXPANDED POLYGLUTAMINE-ASSOCIATED INCLUSION BODY

As discussed, aggresomes share many similarities with inclusion bodies found in many diseases. Proteins that contain expanded glutamine tracts form another type of protein aggregate. These poly-glutamine (polyQ) aggregates are thought to be toxic and are involved in the pathogenesis of many diseases, including Huntington's disease and several forms of spinocerebellar ataxia (SCA; reviewed in ref. *33*). PolyQ aggregates, like aggresomes, are enriched in ubiquitin and molecular chaperones *(33)*. It remains unclear, however, whether the formation of the polyQ inclusion body is mediated by an active mechanism, as with aggresomes, or whether polyQ aggregates form by a passive mechanism of self-assembly.

Similar to aggresomes, however, polyQ-associated inclusion body has been linked to HDAC family members. For example, HDAC3 was reported to be present in the disease-inducing mutant Ataxin-1-associated nuclear inclusion bodies *(34)*. Furthermore, in a model of neurodegeneration in *Drosophila*, in which a polyQ-expanded ataxin-1 gene is expressed, a mutation of the dRpd3 gene leads to enhanced neurotoxicity *(35)*. dRpd3 is a homolog of mammalian HDAC1 and HDAC3 *(10)*. These results suggest a functional connection between members of the HDAC families and polyQ inclusion bodies. Interestingly, the well-characterized acetyltransferase cyclic AMP-responsive binding protein (CREB) binding protein (CBP) is also present in the polyQ inclusion body *(36)*, further suggesting a role for enzymes that regulate protein acetylation in the pathogenesis of polyQ inclusion bodies.

In contrast to the active role proposed for HDAC6 in regulating aggresome formation, it is thought that CBP and HDACs are trapped in polyQ inclusion bodies by a passive mechanism. The sequestration of these enzymes in polyQ aggregates causes CBP and HDACs deficiency, subsequent alteration in gene transcription, and ultimate cell death. Although a large body of experimental data supports this model, several interesting observations suggest that other mechanisms might be in operation. For example, CBP was found to move in and out of the polyQ inclusion body dynamically instead of simply being physically trapped in the inclusion body *(37)*. Furthermore, in a *Drosophila* model of polyQ-expanded aggregates of the Huntingtin gene, elevated expression of CBP prevented the formation of polyQ aggregates *(31)*. Given the importance of HDAC6 in regulating aggresome formation, it would be of great interest and significance to consider whether HDAC members and the CBP acetyltransferase might play a similar active role in regulating the formation of polyQ inclusion bodies.

INCLUSION BODIES, HDAC, AND GENE TRANSCRIPTION

In cell culture models of aggresomes, substantial evidence has accrued to argue that the cytoplasmic behavior of HDAC6 is involved with misfolded proteins. It remains possible, however, that HDAC6 could directly or indirectly regulate transcriptional activities that are important for the processing of misfolded proteins. For example, HDAC6 may shuttle into the nucleus and alter gene transcription, which may then in turn affect key components of the aggresomal response. Although a minor nuclear pool of HDAC6 has been reported under specific conditions *(8,9)*, there is no evidence that such a nuclear translocation occurs in response to misfolded protein's stress *(6)*. On the other hand, it is worth noting that the effect of Scriptaid in preventing SOD1-induced aggresome formation can be reversed when transcription is inhibited by actinomycin D *(27)*. However, considering that many heat shock proteins are induced transcriptionally in response to misfolded protein stress *(38)*, actinomycin D treatment could prevent the induction of heat shock proteins and increase misfolded protein levels, thereby promoting aggresome formation. Further studies would be required to determine whether HDAC6 and possibly other members of the HDAC family regulate aggresome formation independently of transcriptional events.

In contrast to the aggresome, the toxicity associated with polyQ inclusion bodies has been linked to transcriptional perturbation in many studies. It was initially reported that a mutant fragment of the Huntingtin gene with an expanded polyQ tract can interact with CBP, affect its acetyltransferase activity, cause a decrease in histone acetylation, and induce neuronal cell death *(36,39)*. Importantly, these phenotypes can be ameliorated by treatment with either of two HDAC inhibitors, sodium butyrate and suberoylanilide hydroxamic acid (SAHA) *(39)*. In this case, however, whether the nature of the cytoplasmic aggregates was altered by HDAC inhibition was not known. In another *Drosophila* model discussed previously, it was found that elevated expression of CBP returned acetylated H3 and H4 to baseline levels, rescued the neurodegenerative phenotype, and, most importantly, prevented the formation of intraneuronal inclusions caused by mutant Huntingtin fragments *(31)*. The latter observation is of great interest. If mutant Huntingtin induces cell death by trapping CBP in the inclusion bodies, as was proposed *(36)*, it is not clear how elevated levels of CBP could lead to clearance of the inclusion bodies. An interesting possibility is that CBP might not be simply trapped in the polyQ inclusion bodies, rather, CBP could also actively regulate the formation of inclusion bodies, possibly by enhancing the clearance of misfolded proteins. Whether CBP and HDAC members regulate polyQ-associated protein aggregates through a genomic-dependent or -independent mechanism is a critical issue. It is possible that CBP and HDACs regulate proteins that are critical for polyQ inclusion body formation via reversible acetylation. Such a scenario would suggest that protein acetylation machinery could have a general role in the regulation of various inclusion bodies induced by misfolded proteins.

HDACs AND NEURODEGENERATIVE DISEASE

Many human diseases are characterized by the presence of intracellular protein aggregates that usually correlate with regions of increased cell death. In such diseases, aggregates are termed inclusion bodies. In Parkinson's disease and dementia with Lewy bodies, for instance, inclusion bodies appear in neurons of involved regions of the brain (reviewed in ref. *40*). There are many striking similarities, biochemically and morphologically, between inclusion bodies and aggresomes. These similarities include the presence of a restructured intermediate filament network, microtubule organizational machinery (γ-tubulin, pericentrin), ubiquitinated proteins and ubiquitin-conjugating enzymes, and molecular chaperones *(21,41)*. These observations suggest that aggresomes are fundamentally important in both misfolded protein-induced stress response and the pathogenesis of neurodegenerative and other diseases.

However, whether the formation of inclusion bodies is the cause of cellular toxicity or part of a beneficial stress response is still heatedly debated. The study of HDAC6 and aggresome formation provides a tentative clue to this important question. It was observed that in HDAC6-deficient cells, failure to form aggresomes in response to misfolded protein accumulation is accompanied by dramatic apoptosis *(6)*. The hypersensitivity of HDAC6-deficient cells to misfolded proteins strongly supports the idea that HDAC6-dependent aggresome formation is an important cytoprotective response to misfolded protein stress. Accordingly, inclusion bodies are probably part of the stress response that is important to protect neurons from toxicity caused by misfolded proteins.

However, the function of HDAC members in managing misfolded protein induced-stress and neurodegenerative disease could be a complex one. For example, as was already discussed, the loss of *Drosophila* Rpd3 (a HDAC homolog) aggravates cell death that is caused by aggregated polyQ-expanded Ataxin-1 *(34)*. A conflicting story is told by results from studies in fly and mouse models of protein aggregation. In these reports, the toxicity of polyQ-expanded, aggregated proteins can be ameliorated by treatment with HDAC inhibitors *(35,39,42)*. These apparently contradictory observations underscore the importance of fully characterizing the roles of different HDAC members and CBP acetyltransferase in various types of misfolded protein inclusion body formation. Expanding our knowledge of these issues will be essential for exploring the protein acetylation machinery as a therapeutic target in treating neurodegenerative disease.

CONCLUSIONS

Although they were initially considered as enzymes dedicated to histone deacetylation, the finding that HDAC6 is critical for aggresome formation has revealed unexpected nongenomic functions for a HDAC family member. It is probable that there will be additional HDAC members involved in aggresome or other types of inclusion body formation. Delineating the roles and the mechanisms by which HDAC family members, and possibly acetyltransferases, regulate misfolded protein responses could have an important impact on our understanding of protein acetylation in the pathogenesis of diseases caused by misfolded proteins. Such knowledge could also expose new opportunities for treatment of these devastating diseases. Future studies of the nongenomic functions of HDACs and acetyltransferases may further reveal that reversible protein acetylation is a highly versatile signaling system whose role extends far beyond histones and chromatin.

ACKNOWLEDGMENTS

The authors are grateful to Todd Cohen, Charlotte Hubbert, and Dr. Yoshi Kawaguchi for their critical reading of the manuscript.

REFERENCES

1. Allfrey VG. Chromatin and chromatin structure. In: Li HJ, Eckhardt R, eds. New York: Academic, 1977:167–191.
2. Strahl BD, Allis CD. The language of covalent histone modifications. Nature 2000;403:41–45.
3. Roth SY, Denu JM, Allis CD. Histone acetyltransferases. Annu Rev Biochem 2001;70:81–120.
4. Hubbert C, Guardiola A, Shao R, et al. HDAC6 is a microtubule-associated deacetylase. Nature 2002;417:455–458.
5. Serrador JM, Cabrero JR, Sancho D, Mittelbrunn M, Urzainqui A, Sanchez-Madrid F. HDAC6 deacetylase activity links the tubulin cytoskeleton with immune synapse organization. Immunity 2004;20:417–428.
6. Kawaguchi Y, Kovacs JJ, McLaurin A, Vance JM, Ito A, Yao TP. The deacetylase HDAC6 regulates aggresome formation and cell viability in response to misfolded protein stress. Cell 2003;115:727–738.
7. Grozinger CM, Hassig CA, Schreiber SL. Three proteins define a class of human histone deacetylases related to yeast Hda1p. Proc Natl Acad Sci U S A 1999;96:4868–4873.
8. Westendorf JJ, Zaidi SK, Cascino JE, et al. Runx2 (Cbfa1, AML-3) interacts with histone deacetylase 6 and represses the p21(CIP1/WAF1) promoter. Mol Cell Biol 2002;22:7982–7992.
9. Verdel A, Curtet S, Brocard MP, et al. Active maintenance of mHDA2/mHDAC6 histone-deacetylase in the cytoplasm. Curr Biol 2000;10:747–749.
10. de Ruijter AJ, van Gennip AH, Caron HN, Kemp S, van Kuilenburg AB. Histone deacetylases (HDACs): characterization of the classical HDAC family. Biochem J 2003;370:737–749.
11. Vale RD. The molecular motor toolbox for intracellular transport. Cell 2003;112:467–480.
12. Zhang Y, Li N, Caron C, et al. HDAC-6 interacts with and deacetylates tubulin and microtubules in vivo. EMBO J 2003;22:1168–1179.

13. L'Hernault SW, Rosenbaum JL. Chlamydomonas alpha-tubulin is posttranslationally modified by acetylation on the epsilon-amino group of a lysine. Biochemistry 1985;24:473–478.

14. Piperno G, LeDizet M, Chang XJ. Microtubules containing acetylated alpha-tubulin in mammalian cells in culture. J Cell Biol 1987;104:289–302.

15. Matsuyama A, Shimazu T, Sumida Y, et al. In vivo destabilization of dynamic microtubules by HDAC6-mediated deacetylation. EMBO J 2002;21:6820–6831.

16. Hook SS, Orian A, Cowley SM, Eisenman RN. Histone deacetylase 6 binds polyubiquitin through its zinc finger (PAZ domain) and copurifies with deubiquitinating enzymes. Proc Natl Acad Sci U S A 2002;99:13,425–13,430.

17. Kovacs JJ, Murphy PJM, Zhao X, et al. The deacetylase HDAC6 regulates molecular chaperone Hsp90 acetylation and function. Cell 2003;115:727–738.

18. Seigneurin-Berny D, Verdel A, Curtet S, et al. Identification of components of the murine histone deacetylase 6 complex: link between acetylation and ubiquitination signaling pathways. Mol Cell Biol 2001;21:8035–8044.

19. Hicke L, Dunn R. Regulation of membrane protein transport by ubiquitin and ubiquitin-binding proteins. Annu Rev Cell Dev Biol 2003;19:141–172.

20. Goldberg AL. Protein degradation and protection against misfolded or damaged proteins. Nature 2003;426:895–899.

21. Kopito RR. Aggresomes, inclusion bodies and protein aggregation. Trends Cell Biol 2000;10:524–530.

22. Ellis RJ, Pinheiro TJ. Medicine: danger—misfolding proteins. Nature 2002;416: 483, 484.

23. Garcia-Mata R, Gao YS, Sztul E. Hassles with taking out the garbage: aggravating aggresomes. Traffic 2002;3:388–396.

24. Johnston JA, Ward CL, Kopito RR. Aggresomes: a cellular response to misfolded proteins. J Cell Biol 1998;143:1883–1898.

25. Johnston JA, Illing ME, Kopito RR. Cytoplasmic dynein/dynactin mediates the assembly of aggresomes. Cell Motil Cytoskelet 2002;53:26–38.

26. Garcia-Mata R, Bebok Z, Sorscher EJ, Sztul ES. Characterization and dynamics of aggresome formation by a cytosolic GFP-chimera. J Cell Biol 1999;146: 1239–1254.

27. Corcoran LJ, Mitchison TJ, Liu Q. A novel action of histone deacetylase inhibitors in a protein aggresome disease model. Curr Biol 2004;14:488–492.

28. Sitia R, Braakman I. Quality control in the endoplasmic reticulum protein factory. Nature 2003;426:891–894.

29. Verma R, Deshaies RJ. A proteasome howdunit: the case of the missing signal. Cell 2000;101:341–344.

30. Rosen DR, Siddique T, Patterson D, et al. Mutations in Cu/Zn superoxide dismutase gene are associated with familial amyotrophic lateral sclerosis. Nature 1993;362:59–62.

31. Taylor JP, Taye AA, Campbell C, Kazemi-Esfarjani P, Fischbeck KH, Min KT. Aberrant histone acetylation, altered transcription, and retinal degeneration in a *Drosophila* model of polyglutamine disease are rescued by CREB-binding protein. Genes Dev 2003;17:1463–1468.

32. Furumai R, Komatsu Y, Nishino N, Khochbin S, Yoshida M, Horinouchi S. Potent histone deacetylase inhibitors built from trichostatin A and cyclic tetrapeptide antibiotics including trapoxin. Proc Natl Acad Sci U S A 2001;98:87–92.

33. Michalik A, Van Broeckhoven C. Pathogenesis of polyglutamine disorders: aggregation revisited. Hum Mol Genet 2003;12:R173–R186.

34. Tsai CC, Kao HY, Mitzutani A, et al. Ataxin 1, a SCA1 neurodegenerative disorder protein, is functionally linked to the silencing mediator of retinoid and thyroid hormone receptors. Proc Natl Acad Sci U S A 2004;101:4047–4052.

35. Fernandez-Funez P, Nino-Rosales ML, de Gouyon B, et al. Identification of genes that modify ataxin-1-induced neurodegeneration. Nature 2000;408:101–106.

36. Nucifora FC Jr, Sasaki M, Peters MF, et al. Interference by Huntingtin and atrophin-1 with CBP-mediated transcription leading to cellular toxicity. Science 2001;291:2423–2428.

37. Stenoien DL, Mielke M, Mancini MA. Intranuclear ataxin1 inclusions contain both fast- and slow-exchanging components. Nat Cell Biol 2002;4:806–810.

38. Morimoto RI. Dynamic remodeling of transcription complexes by molecular chaperones. Cell 2002;110:281–284.

39. Steffan JS, Bodai L, Pallos J, et al. Histone deacetylase inhibitors arrest polyglutamine-dependent neurodegeneration in *Drosophila*. Nature 2001;413:739–743.

40. Taylor JP, Hardy J, Fischbeck KH. Toxic proteins in neurodegenerative disease. Science 2002;296:1991–1995.

41. McNaught KS, Shashidharan P, Perl DP, Jenner P, Olanow CW. Aggresome-related biogenesis of Lewy bodies. Eur J Neurosci 2002;16:2136–2148.

42. Hockly E, Richon VM, Woodman B, et al. Suberoylanilide hydroxamic acid, a histone deacetylase inhibitor, ameliorates motor deficits in a mouse model of Huntington's disease. Proc Natl Acad Sci U S A 2003;100:2041–2046.

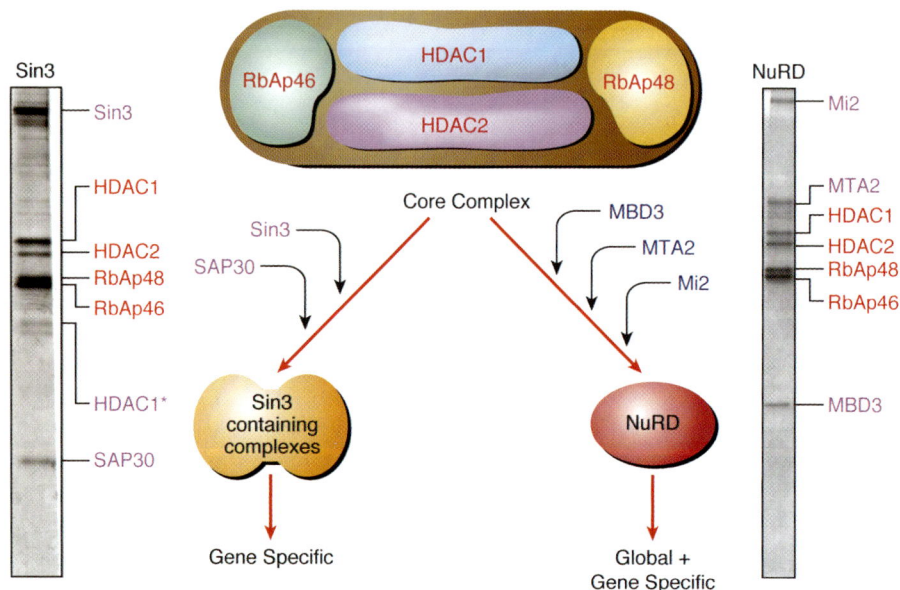

Color Plate 1, Fig. 1. Polypeptides composing the Sin3 and NuRD corepressor complexes. (Ch. 2; *see* full caption and discussion on p. 29.)

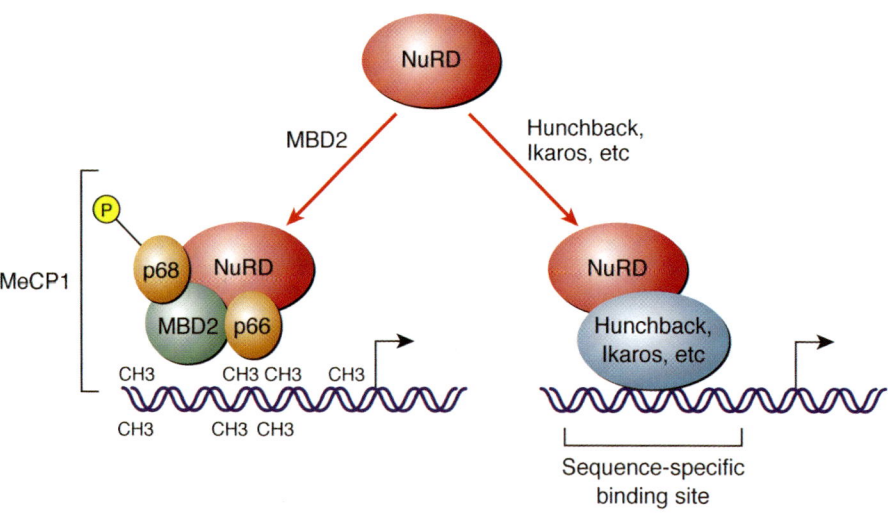

Color Plate 2, Fig. 2. The NuRD complex. (Ch. 2; *see* full caption on p. 33 and discussion on p. 32.)

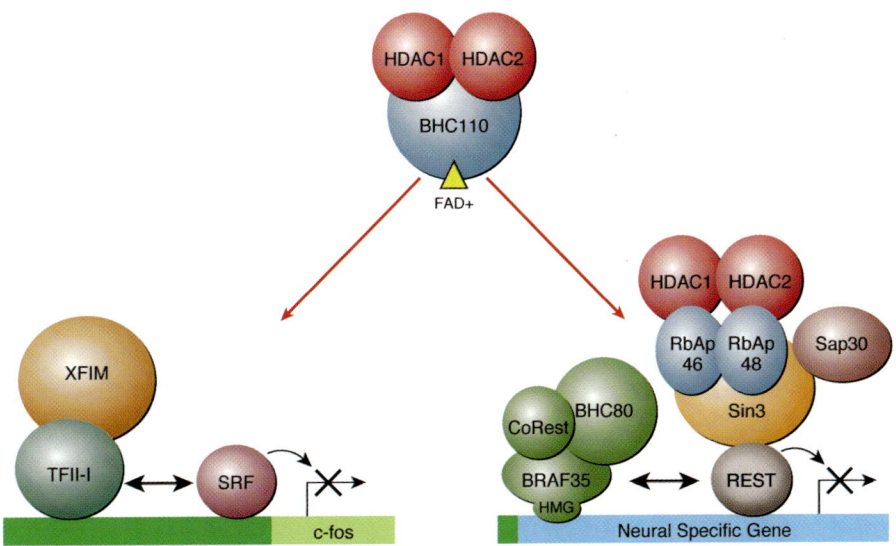

Color Plate 3, Fig. 3. BCH10-containing complexes. (Ch. 2; *see* full caption and discussion on p. 37.)

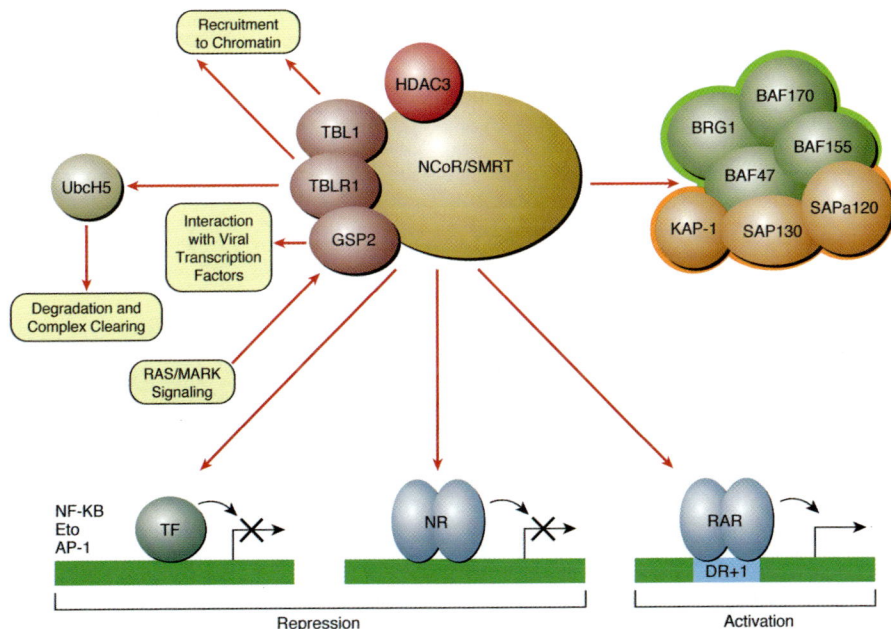

Color Plate 4, Fig. 4. *HDAC3* complex. (Ch. 2; *see* full caption and discussion on p. 39.)

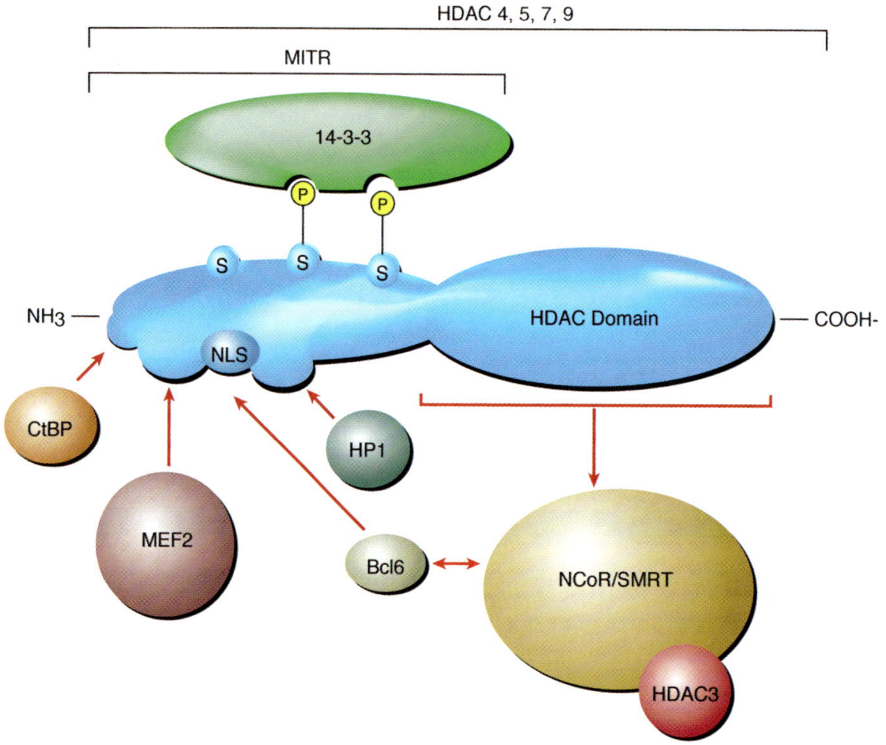

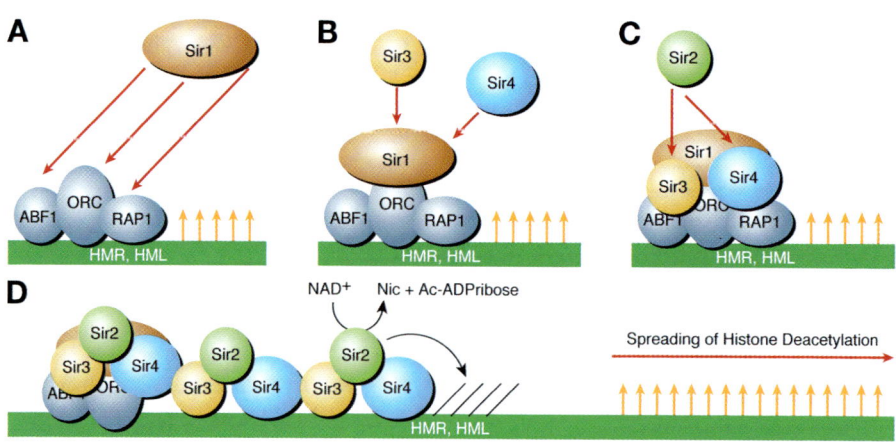

Color Plate 5, Fig. 5. HDACIIa interactions. (Ch. 2; *see* full caption on p. 43 and discussion on p. 42.)

Color Plate 6, Fig. 6. Sequential model of *Sir2p* action at the mating-type loci. (Ch. 2; *see* full caption and discussion on p. 45.)

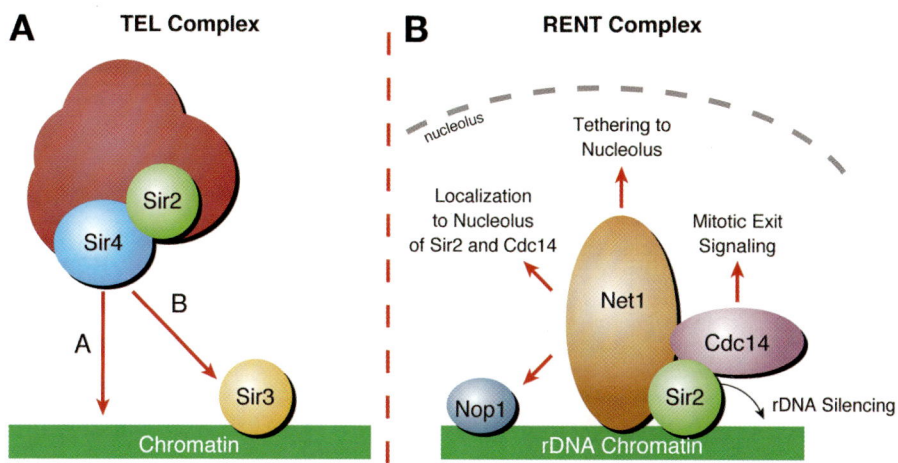

Color Plate 7, Fig. 7. *Sir2p*-containing complexes. (Ch. 2; *see* full caption and discussion on p. 46.)

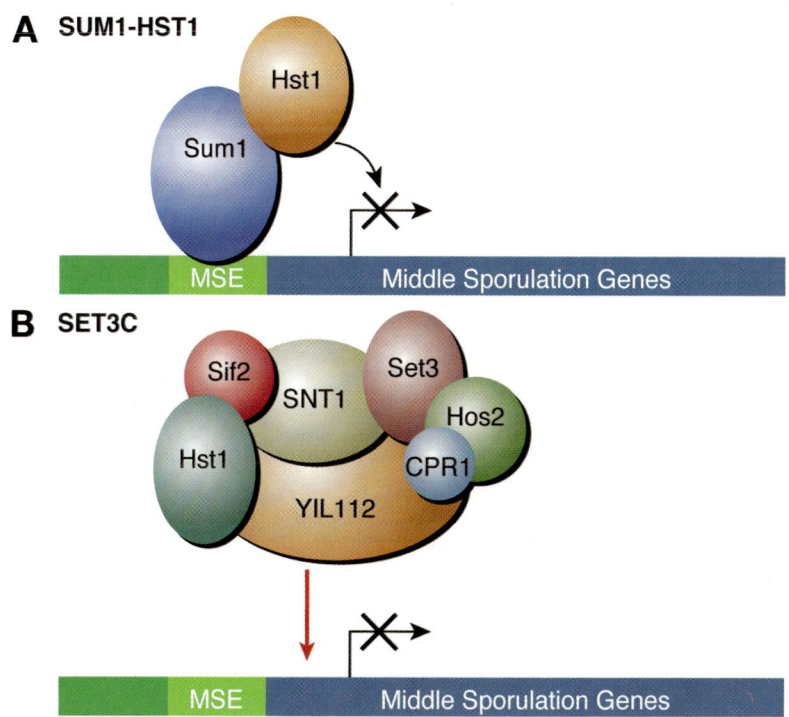

Color Plate 8, Fig. 8. *Hst1p* complexes. (Ch. 2; *see* full caption on p. 48 and discussion on p. 47.)

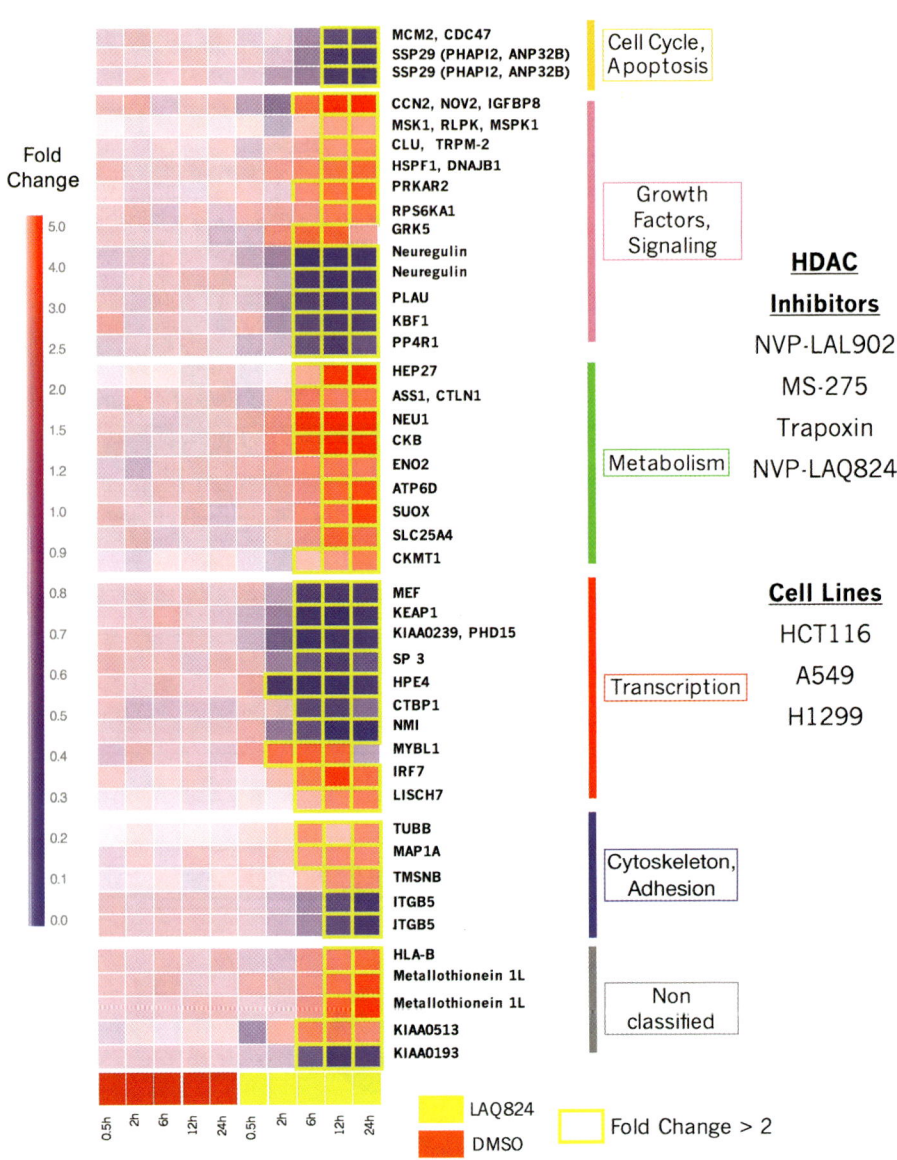

Color Plate 9, Fig. 2. Genes and pathways modified by HDAC inhibitors. (Ch. 14; *see* discussion on p. 321.)

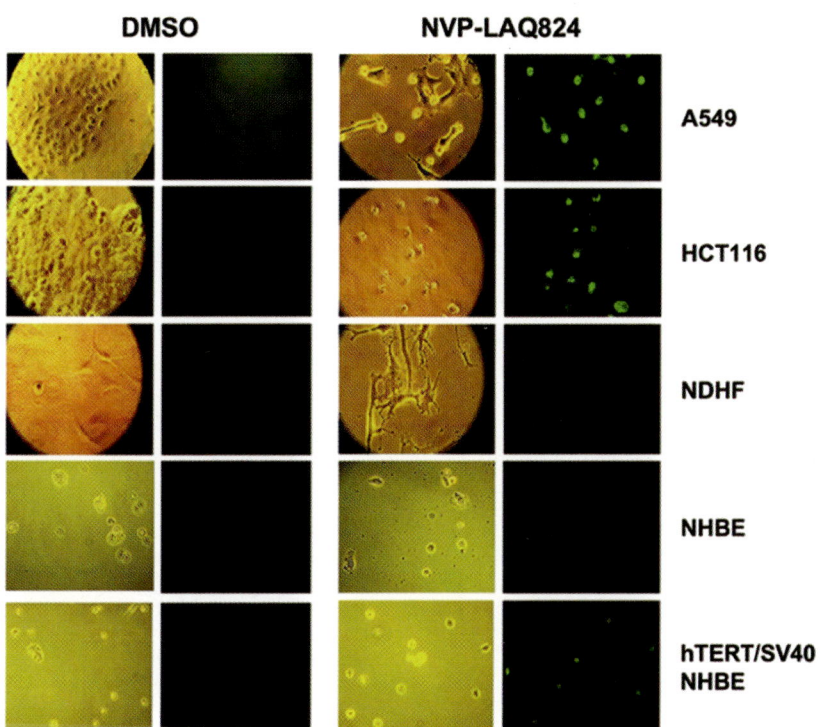

Color Plate 10, Fig. 3. NVP-LAQ824 induces apoptosis in transformed but not in normal cells. (Ch. 14; *see* discussion on p. 324).

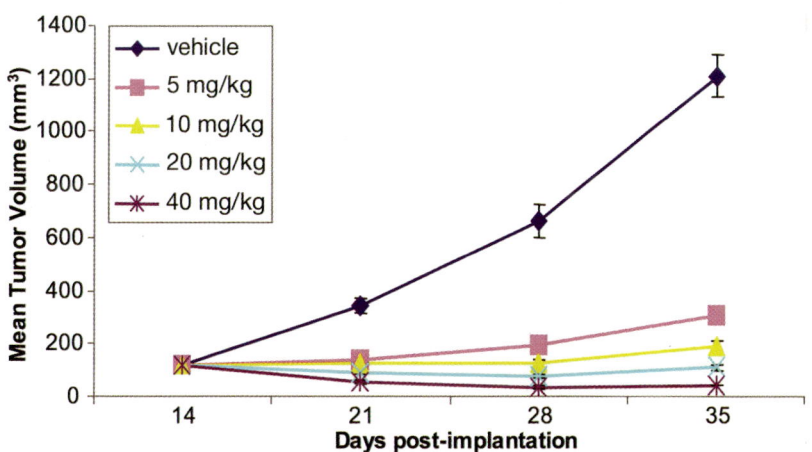

Color Plate 11, Fig. 4. NVP-LBH589 causes regression in HCT116 xenografts. (Ch. 14; *see* discussion on p. 326).

III CLASS III HISTONE DEACETYLASES

8 Evolution of Sirtuins From Archaea to Vertebrates

Roy A. Frye, MD, PhD

CONTENTS

SUMMARY

Most eukaryotic sirtuins (sir2-like proteins) can be grouped into four classes. In deuterostomes such as vertebrates, the urochordate sea squirt *Ciona*, and the echinoderm sea urchin *Strongylocentrotus*, there are seven sirtuins. Class I includes SIRT1, SIRT2, and SIRT3. SIRT4 is in class II and SIRT5 is in class III. Class IV includes SIRT6 and SIRT7. Fish have two SIRT5 orthologs while most other vertebrates have only one version of each of the seven sirtuins. Arthropods lack SIRT3, and some arthropods (e.g., *Drosophila*) lack SIRT5, but other arthropods have SIRT1, SIRT2,

From: *Cancer Drug Discovery and Development*
Histone Deacetylases: Transcriptional Regulation and Other Cellular Functions
Edited by: E. Verdin © Humana Press Inc., Totowa, NJ

SIRT4, SIRT5, SIRT6, and SIRT7. Most prokaryotic sirtuins can be grouped into three categories: the same class II and class III categories as seen in eukaryotes, and a class U, which could be the precursor of the eukaryotic class I and class IV sirtuins. A model is proposed in which the first eukaryote (which resulted from the engulfment of an α-proteobacterium by an archaean) received a class III sirtuin from the archaean parent, while the class II sirtuin and a class U sirtuin came from the α-proteobacterium parent. While most eukaryotic class III sirtuins appear to be derived from an archaeal class III sirtuin, the Kinetoplastida (*Leishmania* and *Trypanosoma*) have a class III sirtuin gene that appears to be of γ-proteobacterial origin, possibly an example of lateral gene transfer. The seven mammalian sirtuins are aligned and contrasted with sirtuins from diverse eukaryotic and prokaryotic organisms.

Key Words: sir2, sirtuin, evolution, homology, phylogeny, SIRT1, SIRT2, SIRT3, SIRT4, SIRT5, SIRT6, SIRT7.

INTRODUCTION

The sirtuins are a family of regulatory proteins that are of ancient evolutionary origin since they are found in most prokaryotes and in all eukaryotes *(1,2)*. Sirtuins are NAD-dependent acetyllysine deacetylases; the prototype of the sirtuins is the *Saccharomyces cerevisiae* protein silent information regulator 2 (sir2), which regulates epigenetic gene silencing, stability of the nucleolar rDNA, and yeast aging *(3,4)*. Studies have shown that caloric restriction causes activation of sir2, which then inhibits the yeast aging process *(5)*. In the nematode worm *Caenorhabditis elegans*, a sirtuin that is an ortholog of sir2 has been implicated in the regulation of an aging pathway related to caloric restriction that involves a FOXO protein called daf-16 *(6)*. Recent work has indicated that aspects of the sir2/caloric restriction/FOXO/aging paradigm may be germane to mammalian systems *(7–11)*. In mammals the ortholog of yeast sir2 is called SIRT1.

Mammals have seven sirtuins *(1)*. In addition to the intranuclear SIRT1, there is the cytoplasmic SIRT2, three mitochondrial sirtuins (SIRT3, SIRT4, and SIRT5), and also within the nucleus are the heterochromatin-associated SIRT6 and the nucleolar SIRT7 *(12–16)*. Most eukaryotic sirtuins can be grouped into four classes *(1)*. The SIRT1, SIRT2, and SIRT3 sequences are rather similar, and they comprise the class I sirtuins. SIRT4 is in class II, and SIRT5 is in class III. SIRT6 and its paralog SIRT7 are class IV sirtuins. Mammals and other vertebrates are in the subphylum Craniata within the phylum Chordata. Other chordates include the subphyla Cephalochordata and Urochordata. Recently there has been extensive sequencing of the urochordate sea squirts *Ciona intestinalis* and

Table 1
Presence of Sirtuins in Various Eukaryotes[a]

Organism	Class I			Class II	Class III	Class IV	
	SIRT1-like	SIRT2-like	SIRT3-like	SIRT4-like	SIRT5-like	SIRT6-like	SIRT7-like
Vertebrata	+	+	+	+	+	+	+
Urochordata	+	+	+	+	+	+	+
Echinodermata	+	+	+	+	+	+	+
Arthropoda	+	+	−	+	+/−	+	+
Nematoda	+	−	−	+	−	+	−
Trematoda (Schistosoma)	+	+	−	−	+	+	−
Fungi (Filamentous)	+	+	−	+/−	+	+/−	−
Fungi (yeasts)	+	+	−	+/−	+/−	−	−
Giardia lamblia	+	+	−	−	+	−	−
Dictyostelium	+	+	−	−	−	−	−
Plasmodium (malaria)	−	−	−	−	+	+	−
Kinetoplastida (Trypanosoma)	−	+	−	+	+	−	−
Viridiplantae	−	−	−	+	+/−	+	−
Rhodophyta (red algae)	+	+	−	−	−	+	−

[a] +, present; −, absent; +/−, present in some but not all species within the category.

185

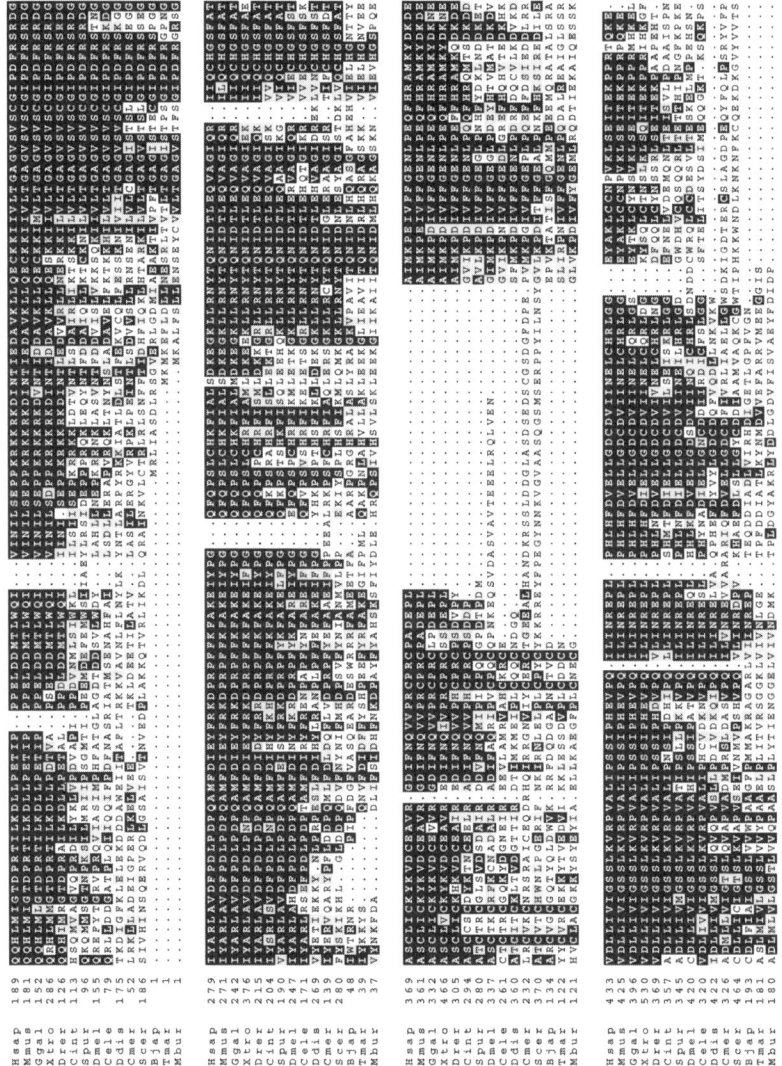

Fig. 1. SIRT1 orthologs (enzymatic domain region) from human, mouse, chicken, frog, zebrafish, sea squirt, fruitfly, nematode, *Dictyostelium*, red algae, budding yeast, and are compared with class U sirtuins from three prokaryotes: *Bradyrhizobium japonicum*, *Thermotoga maritima*, and *Methanococcoides burtonii*. Shading indicates similarity to the human sequence. For abbreviations, *see* Table 2.

Ciona savignyi. All seven sirtuins appear to be present in all vertebrates, and furthermore they are all represented in the urochordate *Ciona* and the echinoderm *Strongylocentrotus* (Table 1, Figs. 1–7). Thus

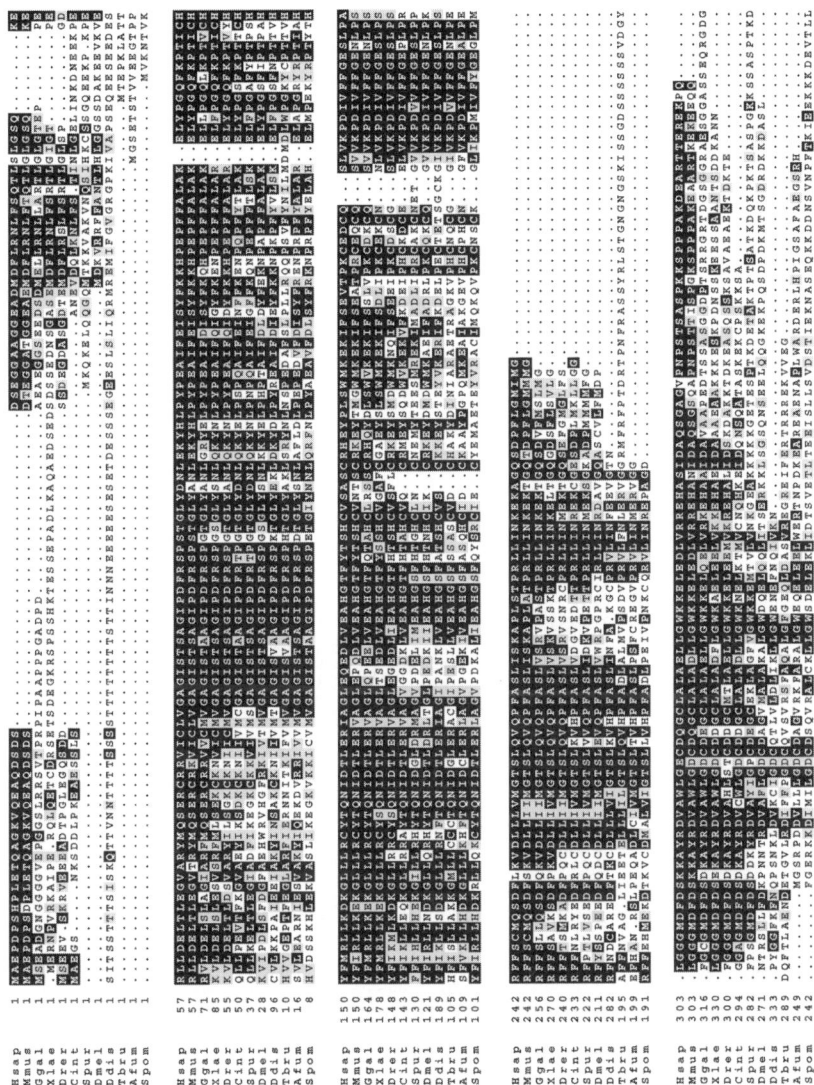

Fig. 2. SIRT2 orthologs from human, mouse, chicken, frog, sea squirt, sea urchin, fruitfly, *Dictyostelium*, trypanosome, filamentous fungus, and fission yeast are compared. (The first amino acid of the *Dictyostelium* sequence portrayed here is actually the 135th amino acid.) Shading indicates similarity to the human sequence. For abbreviations, *see* Table 2.

Deuterostomia (which includes chordates and echinoderms) appear to possess all seven types of SIRTs.

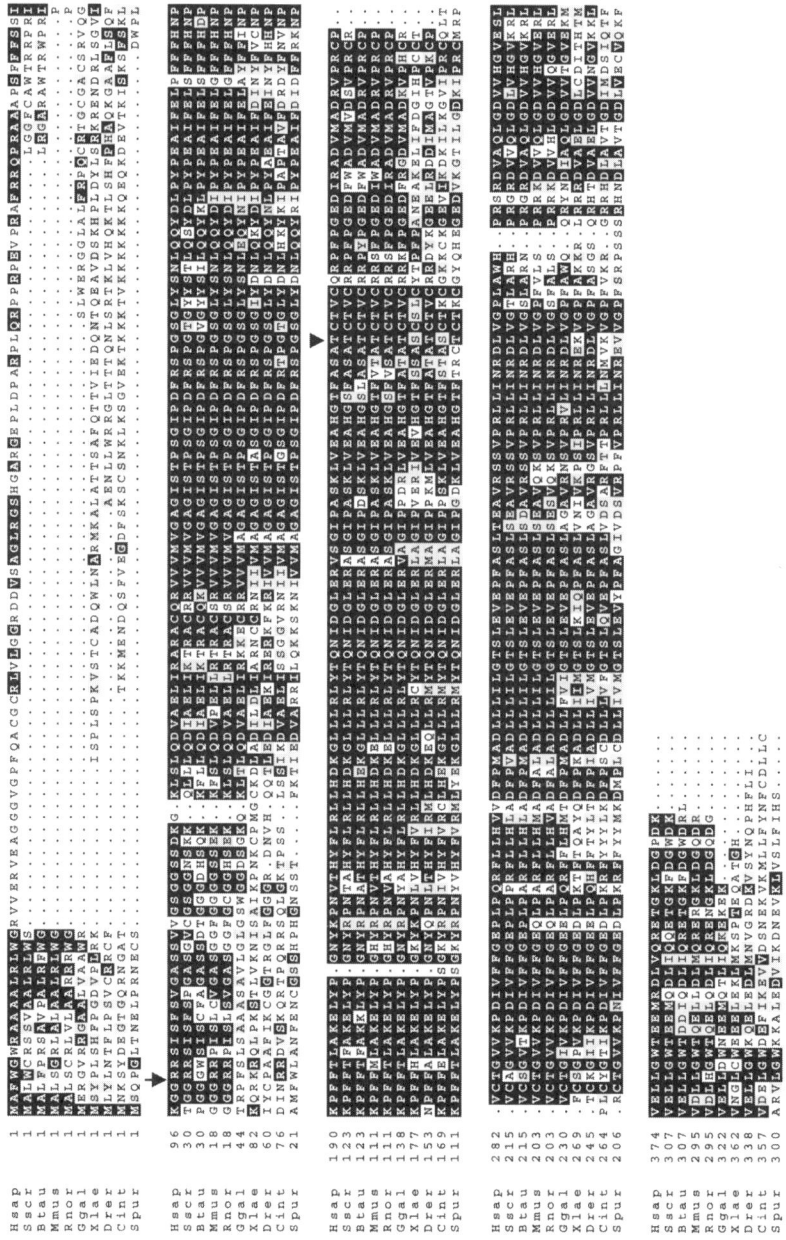

Fig. 3. SIRT3 orthologs from human, pig, cow, mouse, rat, chicken, frog, zebrafish, sea squirt, and sea urchin are compared. The arrow indicates the cleavage site for the mitochondrial matrix protease. The arrowhead indicates the T159N nonsynonymous SNP site. Shading indicates similarity to the human sequence. For abbreviations, *see* Table 2.

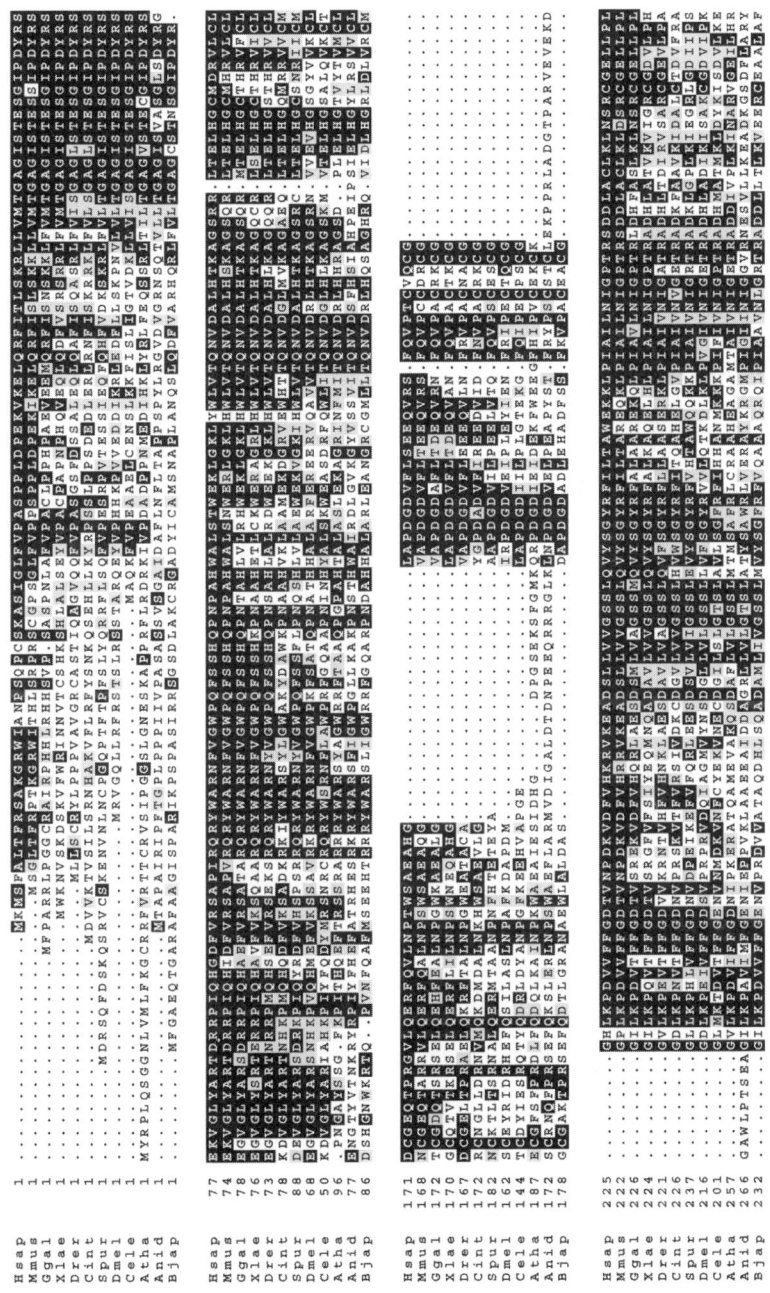

Fig. 4. SIRT4 ortologs from human, mouse, chicken, frog, zebrafish, sea squirt, sea urchin, fruitfly, nematode, green plant, and filamentous fungus are compared with the class II sirtuin from *Bradyrhizobium japonicum*. Shading indicates similarity to the human sequence. For abbreviations, *see* Table 2.

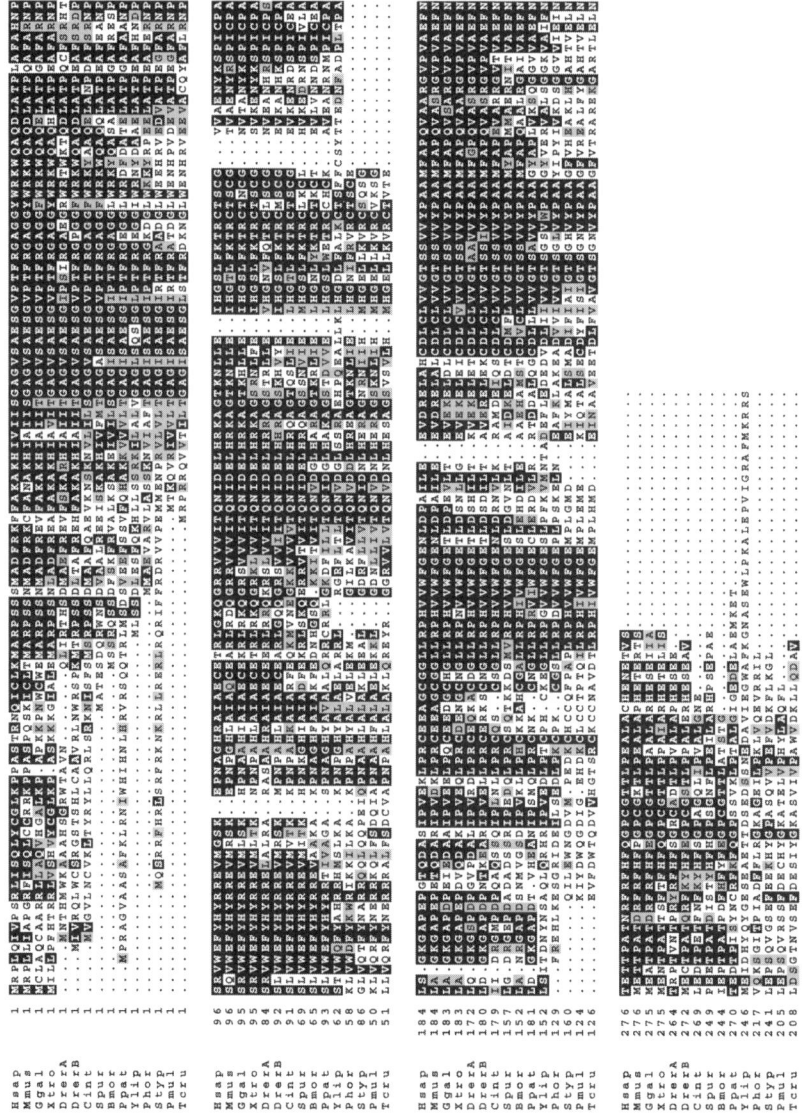

Fig. 5. SIRT5 orthologs from human, mouse, chicken, frog, zebrafish, sea squirt, sea urchin (incomplete sequence), silk moth, green plant (moss), and a yeast are compared with prokaryotic class III sequences from the archaean, *Pyrococcus horikoshii*, two γ-proteobacteria, *Salmonella typhimurium* and *Pasteurella multocida,* and *Trypanosoma cruzi*. Shading indicates similarity to the human sequence. For abbreviations, *see* Table 2.

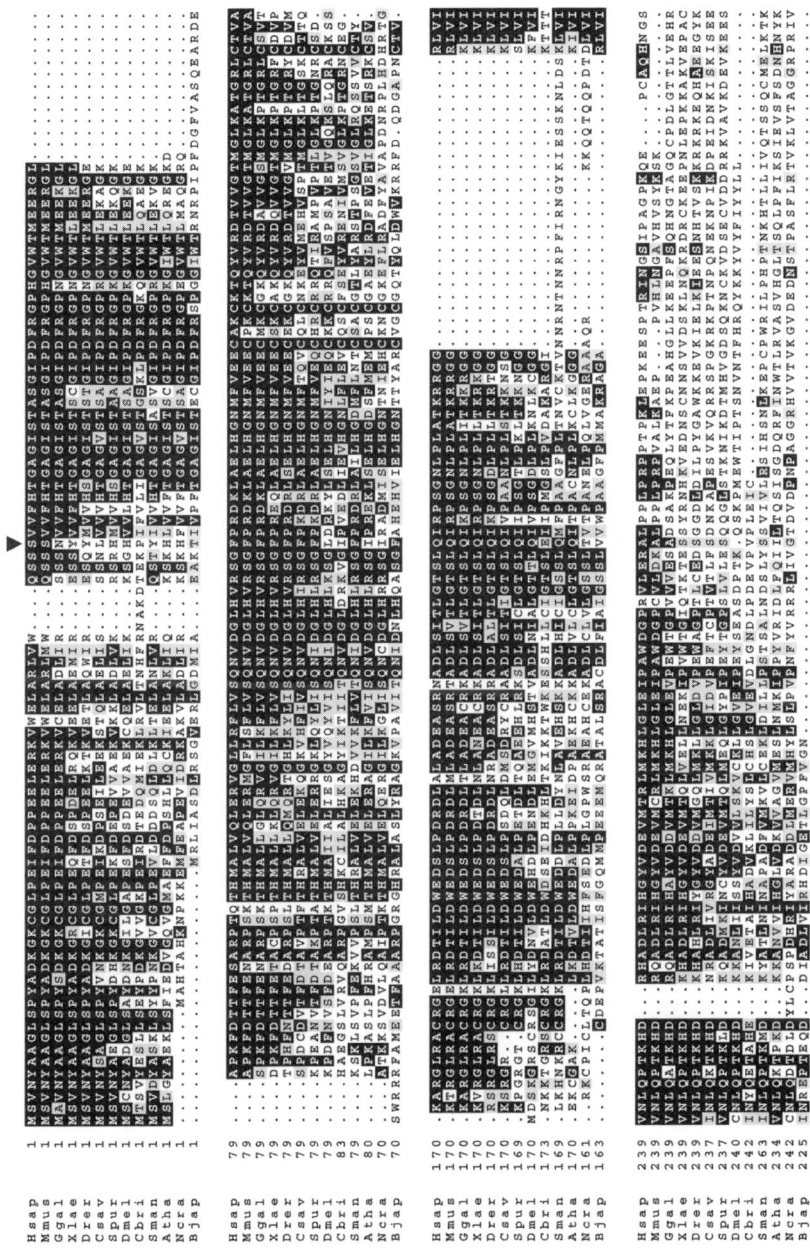

Fig. 6. SIRT6 orthologs from human, cow, mouse, chicken, frog, zebrafish, sea squirt, sea urchin, fruitfly, nematode, trematode, green plant, and filamentous fungus are compared with the class U sirtuin from *Bradyrhizobium japonicum*. The arrowhead indicates the S46N nonsynonymous SNP site. For abbreviations, *see* Table 2.

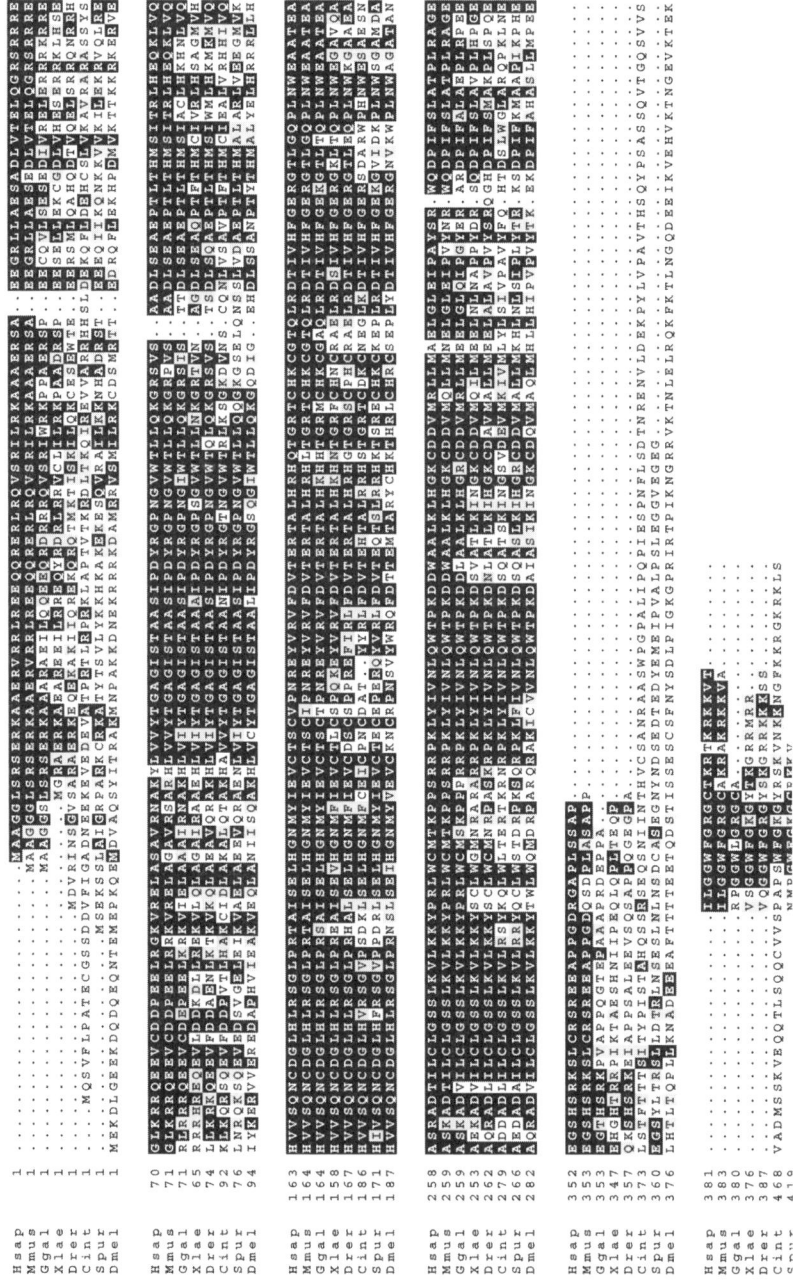

Coelomata is a broader category that encompasses (in addition to Deuterostomia) the Protostomia, which include the mollusck and arthropod phyla. Arthropods possess orthologs of all seven SIRTs except for SIRT3. The Bilateria division of metazoans includes in addition to Coelomata: the Pseudocoelomata (includes nematode roundworms) and the Acoelomata (includes trematode flatworms). The nematode *Caenorhabditis elegans* has orthologs of SIRT1, SIRT4, and SIRT6, but it lacks orthologs of SIRT2, SIRT3, SIRT5, and SIRT7. In regard to the lower forms of eukaryotes, it is notable that fungi are associated with the major branch called Opisthokonts, which includes metazoans *(17,18)*; and some fungi have orthologs of SIRT1, SIRT2, SIRT4, SIRT5, and SIRT6 (Table 1, Figs. 1, 2, 4, and 6). Thus, although the SIRT3 and SIRT7 genes (paralog genes to SIRT2 and SIRT6, respectively) appear to be more recent Deuterostomia- and Coelomata-specific developments, the other five sirtuins (SIRT1, SIRT2, SIRT4, SIRT5, and SIRT6) are all quite ancient and were present in very early forms of eukaryotes.

Because sirtuins are present in prokaryotes, this then raises the question of what types of sirtuin genes were present in the first eukaryotic cell. Current theory indicates that the first eukaryotic cell was formed when an archaean engulfed an α-proteobacterium, which then subsequently evolved into the eukaryotic mitochondria *(19–21)*. Many archaeans possess class III sirtuins that are highly similar to SIRT5. An α-proteobacterium called *Bradyrhizobium japonicum* contains a class II sirtuin that is highly similar to SIRT4 and a class U sirtuin that is intermediate between SIRT1 and SIRT6 (Figs. 1, 4, and 6). Thus the first eukaryotic cell may have received its class III (SIRT5 ortholog) sirtuin from its archaean parent and its class II (SIRT4 ortholog) sirtuin from its α-proteobacterium parent (Fig. 8). The third sirtuin gene, a class U sirtuin with sequence similarity to both SIRT1 and SIRT6, probably evolved into the SIRT1 and SIRT2 genes (and subsequently, with deuterostomes, SIRT3 evolved as a paralog of SIRT2), thus producing the class I sirtuins. In a similar fashion, class IV genes may have resulted from this same α-proteobacterium-derived class U gene evolving first into the SIRT6 sequence; then subsequently with Coelomata, a duplicated copy of the SIRT6 gene evolved into the SIRT7 gene, thus producing a paralog of the SIRT6 gene.

SIRTUIN SEQUENCE SURVEY
AND ALIGNMENT METHODS

Blast searches of the sequence databases (Expressed Sequence Tag, cDNA, and genomic sequences) offered through the NCBI web portal

Fig. 7. SIRT7 orthologs from human, mouse, chicken, frog, zebrafish, sea squirt, sea urchin, and fruitfly are compared. Shading indicates similarity to the human sequence. For abbreviations, *see* Table 2.

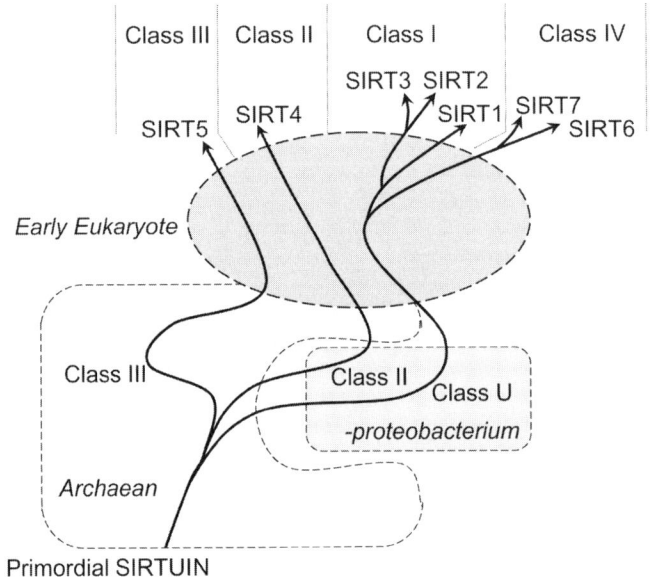

Fig. 8. Model for the evolution of the class I, class II, class III, and class IV sirtuins. Previously it has been postulated that an α-proteobacterium became engulfed by an archaean cell to produce the first eukaryotic cell. Here it is proposed that the engulfed α-proteobacterium (similar to *Bradyrhizobium japonicum*) contributed a class II sirtuin and a class U sirtuin and that the archaean parent contributed the class III sirtuin.

(National Center for Biotechnology Information of the National Institutes of Health/National Library of Medicine) yielded numerous sirtuin sequences from hundreds of prokaryotes and numerous protozoan and metazoan eukaryotes. Some of the eukaryotic genomic sequences were processed into predicted cDNA and protein sequences using the software available at the Softberry website. Initial protein sequence alignments were produced by the ClustalW 1.8 program at the Baylor College of Medicine website, and they were further adjusted manually using the SeqPup program. The alignments were transformed into figures using the BOXSHADE program. For each of the seven SIRTs, sequences from mammals, chicken, frog, fish, urochordate (sea squirt), and echinoderm (sea urchin) are included in the figures. In these figures the organism names are abbreviated (e.g., *Homo sapiens* to Hsap); the key to the abbreviations is in Table 2.

SIRT1 ORTHOLOGS

Over the past few years much more attention has been directed toward SIRT1 than any other mammalian sirtuin, probably because of the

Table 2
Abbreviations

Abbreviation	Scientific name	Comment
Afum	*Aspergillus fumigatus*	Filamentous fungus
Anid	*Aspergillus nidulans*	Filamentous fungus
Atha	*Arabidopsis thaliana*	Green plant
Bjap	*Bradyrhizobium japonicum*	α-Proteobacterium
Bmor	*Bombyx mori*	Silk moth
Btau	*Bos taurus*	Cow
Cbri	*Caenorhabditis briggsae*	Nematode worm
Cele	*Caenorhabditis elegans*	Nematode worm
Cint	*Ciona intestinalis*	Sea squirt (urochordate)
Cmer	*Cyanidioschyzon merolae*	Red algae
Csav	*Ciona savignyi*	Sea squirt (urochordate)
Ddis	*Dictyostelium discoideum*	"Slime mold"
Dmel	*Drosophila melanogaster*	Fruitfly
Drer	*Danio rerio*	Zebrafish
Ggal	*Gallus gallus*	Chicken
Hsap	*Homo sapiens*	Human
Mbur	*Methanococcoides burtonii*	Archaean
Mmus	*Mus musculus*	Mouse
Phor	*Pyrococcus horikoshii*	Archaean
Pmul	*Pasteurella multocida*	γ-Proteobacterium
Ppat	*Physcomitrella patens*	Green plant (moss)
Rnor	*Rattus norvegicus*	Rat
Scer	*Saccharomyces cerevisiae*	Fungus (brewer's yeast)
Sman	*Schistosoma mansoni*	Trematode worm
Spom	*Schizosaccharomyces pombe*	Fungus (fission yeast)
Spur	*Strongylocentrotus purpuratus*	Sea urchin (echinoderm)
Sscr	*Sus scrofa*	Pig
Styp	*Salmonella typhimurium*	γ-Proteobacterium
Tcru	*Trypanosoma cruzi*	Trypanosome
Tmar	*Thermotoga maritima*	Early eubacterium
Ylip	*Yarrowia lipolytica*	Fungus (yeast)
Xlae	*Xenopus laevis*	Frog (tetraploid genome)
Xtro	*Xenopus tropicalis*	Frog (diploid genome)

widespread speculation that SIRT1 may regulate mammalian aging. SIRT1 modulates cell survival, muscle differentiation, and fat cell metabolism; these pleotrophic effects probably reflect the ability of SIRT1 to regulate several important proteins including p53, CTIP2, PCAF, MyoD, FOXO proteins, Ku70, PPAR-γ, and NF-κB *(7–9,12,22–28)*. Recently caloric restriction, a regimen that has well proven antiaging effects in many animals including mammals, was found to upregulate SIRT1 expression in rats *(11)*.

SIRT1 ortholog sequences are present in most eukaryotes including vertebrates, the urochordate *Ciona*, the echinoderm *Strongylocentrotus* arthropods, nematodes, fungi, *Dictyostelium discoideum*, and the red algae *Cyanidioschyzon merolae* (Table 1 and Fig. 1); however, SIRT1 orthologs appear to be absent in the Viridiplantae (green plants). SIRT1 ortholog sequences are also absent in the protozoan organisms of malaria (the completely sequenced *Plasmodium falciparum* and *Plasmodium yoelii yoelii*) and are absent in the completely sequenced *Leishmania major* genome.

Regarding the origin of the SIRT1-like gene, it may have arisen from a prokaryotic class U precursor. Although most prokaryotic sirtuins are class III (SIRT5-like) or class II (SIRT4-like), some prokaryotic sirtuins show stronger homology to class I and class IV sirtuins; these somewhat undifferentiated prokaryotic sirtuins have been grouped as class U *(1)*. Characteristically, Class U sirtuins contain the sequence motif GAGIS-TASGIPDFR, while Class III sirtuins contain GAGISAESGIPTFR, and Class II sirtuins contain GAGISTESGIPDYR. Class U sequences are present in several Archaea (*Sulfolobus* species, *Haloarcula marismortui, Pyrobaculum aerophilum,* and *Methanococcoides burtonii*). Class U sirtuins are present in many Firmicutes (gram-positive bacteria) such as *Bacillus* and *Staphylococcus* species. One of the most ancient of the Eubacteria is *Thermotoga maritime (29)*; it has a class U gene (Fig. 1). Class U sirtuins are present in some α-proteobacteria (*Bradyrhizobium japonicum, Rhodopseudomonas palustris*, and *Hyphomonas neptunium*). The model outlined in Fig. 8 proposes that the early eukaryotic cell contained at least three sirtuin genes, a class III sirtuin from its archaean parent (*see Pyrococcus horikoshii* SIRT5-like sequence in Fig. 5), a class II sirtuin from its α-proteobacterium parent (*see Bradyrhizobium japonicum* SIRT4-like sequence in Fig. 4), and also a class U sequence probably also from its α-proteobacterium parent (*see Bradyrhizobium japonicum* class U sequence in Figs. 1 and 6). Alternative possibilities are that the class U sirtuin was obtained from its archaean parent (*see Methanococcoides burtonii* class U sequence in Fig. 1) or that the class II and class U sequences were gained by the primitive eukaryotic cell via lateral gene transfer from other eubacterial species.

SIRT2 ORTHOLOGS

The SIRT2 protein is cytoplasmic and has been shown to deacetylate α-tubulin *(13)*. SIRT2 has also been implicated in control of exit from the M phase of the cell cycle in studies that found that SIRT2 becomes phosphorylated at the G2/M transition and is stabilized by the phosphory-lation *(30)*. The protein phosphatase CDC14B dephosphorylates SIRT2, which is then degraded, allowing the cell cycle exit to proceed *(30)*. It is unknown whether the effect of SIRT2 on cell cycle exit is mediated by its ability to deacetylate tubulin, but, given the importance of tubulin in the mitotic spindle apparatus, it seems this is a likely possibility. The degree of acetylation of tubulin appears to affect its stability, and this may have effects on cell motility *(31)*.

SIRT2 genes are found in many lower eukaryotes including fission yeast (*Schizosaccharomyces pombe*), filamentous fungi such as *Aspergillus fumigatus*, and members of the Kinetoplastida group such as *Leishmania* and *Trypanosoma* species (Table 1 and Fig. 2). The development of acetylation as a posttranslational modification of tubulin was an early event in eukaryotic evolution *(32,33)*; thus this may correlate tempo-rally with the early development of the SIRT2 gene. The widely studied "slime mold" organism (actually a type of soil amoeba) *Dictyostelium dis-coideum* also has a SIRT2 gene (Fig. 2). *Dictyostelium* is a model system for the study of tubulin-dependent events associated with cell motility and cell polarity, so it would be interesting to investigate the role of the SIRT2 ortholog in this system.

SIRT3 ORTHOLOGS

The SIRT3 sequence is highly similar to the SIRT2 sequence, and it is likely that during the development of the Deuterostomia a gene duplication event involving the SIRT2 gene resulted in the formation of the SIRT2-like SIRT3 gene. Coelomata are divided into Deuterostomia (includes Chordata and Echinodermata) and Protostomia (includes Mollusca and Arthropoda). Although the SIRT3 gene is not found in arthropods, it is present in the echinoderm *Strongylocentrotus*, and chrodates, including the urochordate *Ciona* and in all vertebrates (Fig. 3). The mammalian SIRT3 protein is tar-geted to the mitochondria where a mitochondrial matrix protease cleaves off the N-terminal mitochondrial targeting peptide *(14)*. The intramito-chondrial acetylated protein substrates of SIRT3 are still unknown.

One study has reported that a synonymous (silent mutation) single-nucleotide polymorphism (SNP rs12364050) located at base 477 in the 159th codon of the SIRT3 coding sequence is associated with modest vari-ations in human longevity *(34)*. The current SNP database shows that a nonsynonymous SNP (rs1734491) is present with a heterozyogosity fre-quency of 0.269; this SNP alters codon 255 from threonine to asparagine (location is marked in Fig. 3). It would be of interest to determine whether this nonsynonymous SNP is in haplotype linkage with the synonymous SNP that was linked to variation in longevity.

SIRT4 ORTHOLOGS

In prokaryotes, class II (SIRT4-like) sirtuins are absent in Archaea but they are found in some categories of the Eubacteria, especially in the Actinobacteria and in the various proteobacteria, including some β-proteobacteria (Bordetella and Burkholderiaceae) and γ-proteobacteria (Pseudomonadaceae and Xanthomonadaceae) divisions. Current sequence evidence suggests that most species of α-proteobacteria lack a Class II sirtuin gene, however a SIRT4-like gene is present in the α-proteobacterium *Bradyrhizobium japonicum* (Fig. 4). SIRT4 genes are present in all vertebrates, the urochordate sea squirt *Ciona*, the echinoderm *Strongylocentrotus* arthropods, nematodes, fungi, green plants, *Giardia*, trypanosomes, and *Leishmania* species (Table 1 and Fig. 4). The biological functions of SIRT4-like proteins are undetermined. The human SIRT4 protein has been localized to the mitochondria *(16)*.

SIRT5 ORTHOLOGS

The class III sirtuins, with their origin in Archaea, are probably the most ancient form of sirtuins. The prokaryotic sirtuins that are most similar to eukaryotic SIRT5 sequences are the class III sirtuins found in archaean organisms (e.g., the sirtuin from *Pyrococcus horikoshii*). Many of the Eubacteria, especially the γ-proteobacteria (gram-negative bacteria), also have SIRT5-like class III sirtuins, but they are significantly less similar to most eukaryotic SIRT5-like sirtuins (Fig. 5). SIRT5-like sequences are found in some arthropods (e.g., silk moth, lobster, mosquito) but absent in others (e.g., fruitfly). Similarly, most green plants lack SIRT5-like genes, but some plants such as spruce, loblolly pine, and the moss *Physcomitrella patens*, do contain class III sirtuin genes. In many eukaryotes (but not in Kinetoplastida), a sequence segment is present in the midregion of the class III sirtuin sequence that contains the conserved amino acid sequence motif "SPICPAL"; this feature is absent from prokaryotic class III sirtuins.

A Class III sirtuin gene sequence is present in Kinetoplastida organisms (Leishmania and Trypanosoma) but it is significantly different from other eukaryotic Class III sirtuins and in fact strongly resembles Class III sirtuin genes from γ-proteobacteria (e.g., *Pasteurella multocida* and *Salmonella typhimurium*; *see* sequences aligned in Fig. 5); perhaps this Class III gene in Kinetoplastida organisms was obtained via lateral gene transfer from a γ-proteobacterium.

Although generally chordates have only one version of each of the seven SIRT genes, fish have two SIRT5 genes (*see* A and B sequences from *Danio rerio* in Fig. 5). Human DNA contains a SIRT5-like pseudogene (genBank XM_372781, located at 1p31.2); perhaps this is a degenerated version of the extra SIRT5 gene that was once active in the fish ancestors of mammals.

An important function of SIRT5-like prokaryotic class III genes is to regulate the short-chain acyl CoA synthetase enzymes by deacetylating a lysine residue that functions in the active site of the enzyme. This was first shown in the *Salmonella* organism, in which the class III sirtuin called CobB was shown to activate the acetyl CoA synthetase enzyme *(35)*. These findings were subsequently extended to the yeast system, in which in a similar fashion the hst3 and hst4 sirtuins (distantly related to class I sirtuins) of *Saccharomyces cerevisiae* were found to affect ability of the yeast cells to metabolize the short-chain fatty acids acetate and proprionate *(36)*. The short-chain acyl CoA synthetase enzymes are members of the AMP-forming family of enzymes, which include in mammals over 20 different enzymes most of which are involved in acyl CoA synthetase reactions for various types of fatty acids. It was speculated that all members of this enzyme class may be modulated by sirtuins *(35)*. On the basis of homology, in vertebrates it would be predicted that SIRT5, and possibly other sirtuins, probably regulate various members of the AMP-forming enzyme family. The human SIRT5 protein has been localized to the mitochondria *(16)*.

SIRT6 ORTHOLOGS

SIRT6 is a class IV sirtuin. Class IV sirtuins are not found in prokaryotes but are present in a wide spectrum of eukaryotes including chordates, echinoderms, arthropods, nematodes, trematodes, Apicomplexa (includes malaria), and Viridiplantae (Table 1 and Fig. 6). Yeast-type fungi and Kinetoplastida (*Leishmania* and *Trypanosoma*) lack class IV sirtuins. The precursor gene for class IV sirtuins was probably derived from a prokaryotic class U sirtuin; of all prokaryotic sirtuins, the class U sirtuin from the α-proteobacterium *Bradyrhizobium japonicum* is the most similar to class IV sirtuins of eukaryotes.

A nonsynonymous SNP (rs352493) with a heterozygosity frequency of 0.21 has been found in the human SIRT6 gene at codon 46 involving a change from serine to asparagine (location is marked in Fig. 6). Mouse SIRT6 was found to be intranuclear and to catalyze an intramolecular ADP-ribosyltransferase reaction *(37)*. The human SIRT6 protein showed localization to heterochromatin regions *(16)*.

SIRT7 ORTHOLOGS

SIRT7 is a class IV sirtuin that appears to have been derived from a gene duplication of SIRT6 that occurred during evolution at the level of the Coelomata; thus both arthropods and chordates have SIRT7 genes. Other more primitive eukaryotes including protozoans, Pseudocoelomata, and Acoelomata lack SIRT7 genes.

A SIRT7 cDNA clone was isolated in a screen for genes that were over-expressed in human papillary thyroid carcinoma cells *(38,39)*. The SIRT7 protein is localized to the nucleolus *(16)*. The biological functions of the SIRT7 protein are undetermined.

CONCLUSIONS

It is evident that specific forms of sirtuin genes have been highly con-served throughout evolution in a wide spectrum of organisms ranging from prokaryotes to mammals. This conservation of different forms of sirtuins probably relates to preserving binding interactions with other proteins that are associated with sirtuins in multiprotein complexes and binding interactions with specific acetylated protein substrates. Therefore studies that reveal the function of sirtuins in both prokaryotic and primi-tive eukaryotic systems are likely to be very helpful in elucidating the function of mammalian sirtuins and vice versa. Remarkable evidence of this sort of conservation of function across a wide evolutionary time span was found recently in regard to similarities between SIRT1-containing chromatin-modifying complexes discovered in *Drosophila* and human cells. The *Drosophila* larval complex contained several proteins including SIRT1 and Enhancer of Zeste *(40)*. The corresponding human chromatin-modifying complex called PRC4 (polycomb repressive complex 4) con-tained several proteins including SIRT1 and Ezh2 (a human homolog of Enhancer of Zeste) and was found to be present in undifferentiated embryonic cells and in a variety of malignant tumor cells including prostate cancers, but—as was found in *Drosophila*—the complex was absent in normal adult cells *(41)*. As sirtuins continue to be studied in many diverse prokaryotic and eukaryotic model systems, further widely relevant insights into the functions of these highly conserved proteins can be anticipated.

REFERENCES

1. Frye RA. Phylogenetic classification of prokaryotic and eukaryotic Sir2-like pro-teins. Biochem Biophys Res Commun 2000;273:793–798.
2. Frye RA. Characterization of five human cDNAs with homology to the yeast SIR2 gene: Sir2-like proteins (sirtuins) metabolize NAD and may have protein ADP-ribosyltransferase activity. Biochem Biophys Res Commun 1999;260: 273–279.
3. Imai S, Armstrong CM, Kaeberlein M, Guarente L. Transcriptional silencing and longevity protein Sir2 is an NAD-dependent histone deacetylase. Nature 2000; 403:795–800.

4. Guarente L. Sir2 links chromatin silencing, metabolism, and aging. Genes Dev 2000;14:1021–1026.

5. Lin SJ, Defossez PA, Guarente L. Requirement of NAD and SIR2 for life-span extension by calorie restriction in *Saccharomyces cerevisiae*. Science 2000; 289:2126–2128.

6. Tissenbaum HA, Guarente L. Increased dosage of a sir-2 gene extends lifespan in *Caenorhabditis elegans*. Nature 2001;410:227–230.

7. Brunet A, Sweeney LB, Sturgill JF, et al. Stress-dependent regulation of FOXO transcription factors by the SIRT1 deacetylase. Science 2004;303:2011–2015.

8. Motta MC, Divecha N, Lemieux M, et al. Mammalian SIRT1 represses forkhead transcription factors. Cell 2004;116:551–563.

9. Van Der Horst A, Tertoolen LG, De Vries-Smits LM, Frye RA, Medema RH, Burgering BM. FOXO4 is acetylated upon peroxide stress and deacetylated by the longevity protein hSir2SIRT1. J Biol Chem 2004.

10. Daitoku H, Hatta M, Matsuzaki H, et al. Silent information regulator 2 potentiates Foxo1-mediated transcription through its deacetylase activity. Proc Natl Acad Sci U S A 2004.

11. Cohen HY, Miller C, Bitterman KJ, et al. Calorie restriction promotes mammalian cell survival by inducing the SIRT1 deacetylase. Science 2004.

12. Langley E, Pearson M, Faretta M, et al. Human SIR2 deacetylates p53 and antagonizes PML/p53-induced cellular senescence. EMBO J 2002;21:2383–2396.

13. North BJ, Marshall BL, Borra MT, Denu JM, Verdin E. The human Sir2 ortholog, SIRT2, is an NAD+-dependent tubulin deacetylase. Mol Cell 2003;11:437–444.

14. Schwer B, North BJ, Frye RA, Ott M, Verdin E. The human silent information regulator (Sir)2 homologue hSIRT3 is a mitochondrial nicotinamide adenine dinucleotide-dependent deacetylase. J Cell Biol 2002;158:647–657.

15. Onyango P, Celic I, McCaffery JM, Boeke JD, Feinberg AP. SIRT3, a human SIR2 homologue, is an NAD-dependent deacetylase localized to mitochondria. Proc Natl Acad Sci U S A 2002;99:13,653–13,658.

16. Michishita E, Park JY, Burneskis JM, Barrett JC, Horikawa I. Evolutionarily Conserved and Nonconserved Cellular Localizations and Functions of Human SIRT Proteins. Mol Biol Cell 2005;16:4623–4635.

17. Baldauf SL, Roger AJ, Wenk-Siefert I, Doolittle WF. A kingdom-level phylogeny of eukaryotes based on combined protein data. Science 2000;290:972–977.

18. Baldauf SL. The deep roots of eukaryotes. Science 2003;300:1703–1706.

19. Keeling PJ, Doolittle WF. Evidence that eukaryotic triosephosphate isomerase is of alpha-proteobacterial origin. Proc Natl Acad Sci U S A 1997;94:1270–1275.

20. Martin W, Muller M. The hydrogen hypothesis for the first eukaryote. Nature 1998;392:37–41.

21. Rotte C, Henze K, Muller M, Martin W. Origins of hydrogenosomes and mitochondria. Curr Opin Microbiol 2000;3:481–486.

22. Luo J, Nikolaev AY, Imai S, et al. Negative control of p53 by Sir2alpha promotes cell survival under stress. Cell 2001;107:137–148.

23. Vaziri H, Dessain SK, Ng Eaton E, et al. hSIR2(SIRT1) functions as an NAD-dependent p53 deacetylase. Cell 2001;107:149–159.

24. Senawong T, Peterson VJ, Avram D, et al. Involvement of the histone deacetylase SIRT1 in chicken ovalbumin upstream promoter transcription factor (COUP-TF)-interacting protein 2-mediated transcriptional repression. J Biol Chem 2003; 278:43,041–43,050.

25. Fulco M, Schiltz RL, Iezzi S, et al. Sir2 regulates skeletal muscle differentiation as a potential sensor of the redox state. Mol Cell 2003;12:51–62.

26. Cohen HY, Lavu S, Bitterman KJ, et al. Acetylation of the C terminus of Ku70 by CBP and PCAF controls Bax-mediated apoptosis. Mol Cell 2004;13:627–638.

27. Picard F, Kurtev M, Chung N, et al. Sirt1 promotes fat mobilization in white adipocytes by repressing PPAR-gamma. Nature 2004;429:771–776.

28. Yeung F, Hoberg JE, Ramsey CS, et al. Modulation of NF-kappaB-dependent transcription and cell survival by the SIRT1 deacetylase. EMBO J 2004;23: 2369–2380.

29. Achenbach-Richter L, Gupta R, Stetter KO, Woese CR. Were the original eubacteria thermophiles? Syst Appl Microbiol 1987;9:34–39.

30. Dryden SC, Nahhas FA, Nowak JE, Goustin AS, Tainsky MA. Role for human SIRT2 NAD-dependent deacetylase activity in control of mitotic exit in the cell cycle. Mol Cell Biol 2003;23:3173–3185.

31. Palazzo A, Ackerman B, Gundersen GG. Cell biology: tubulin acetylation and cell motility. Nature 2003;421:230.

32. Schneider A, Plessmann U, Felleisen R, Weber K. Posttranslational modifications of trichomonad tubulins; identification of multiple glutamylation sites. FEBS Lett 1998;429:399–402.

33. Noel C, Gerbod D, Fast NM, et al. Tubulins in *Trichomonas vaginalis*: molecular characterization of alpha-tubulin genes, posttranslational modifications, and homology modeling of the tubulin dimer. J Eukaryot Microbiol 2001;48: 647–654.

34. Rose G, Dato S, Altomare K, et al. Variability of the SIRT3 gene, human silent information regulator Sir2 homologue, and survivorship in the elderly. Exp Gerontol 2003;38:1065–1070.

35. Starai VJ, Celic I, Cole RN, Boeke JD, Escalante-Semerena JC. Sir2-dependent activation of acetyl-CoA synthetase by deacetylation of active lysine. Science 2002;298:2390–2392.

36. Starai VJ, Takahashi H, Boeke JD, Escalante-Semerena JC. Short-chain fatty acid activation by acyl-coenzyme A synthetases requires SIR2 protein function in *Salmonella enterica* and *Saccharomyces cerevisiae*. Genetics 2003;163:545–555.

37. Liszt G, Ford E, Kurtev M, Guarente L. Mouse Sir2 homolog SIRT6 is a nuclear ADP-ribosyltransferase. J Biol Chem 2005;280:21,313–21,320.

38. de Nigris F, Cerutti J, Morelli C, et al. Isolation of a SIR-like gene, SIR-T8, that is overexpressed in thyroid carcinoma cell lines and tissues. Br J Cancer 2002;86:917–923.

39. Frye R. "SIRT8" expressed in thyroid cancer is actually SIRT7. Br J Cancer 2002;87:1479.

40. Furuyama T, Banerjee R, Breen TR, Harte PJ. SIR2 is required for polycomb silencing and is associated with an E(Z) histone methyltransferase complex. Curr Biol 2004;14:1812–1821.

41. Kuzmichev A, Margueron R, Vaquero A, et al. Composition and histone substrates of polycomb repressive group complexes change during cellular differentiation. Proc Natl Acad Sci U S A 2005;102:1859–1864.

9 Structure of the Sir2 Family of NAD⁺-Dependent Histone/Protein Deacetylases

Kehao Zhao, PhD
and Ronen Marmorstein, PhD

CONTENTS

SUMMARY

Sir2 enzymes are broadly conserved from bacteria to humans, and eukaryotic organisms typically contain multiple Sir2 enzymes that target different protein substrates to mediate diverse biological processes including gene silencing, DNA repair, genome stability, longevity, metabolism,

From: *Cancer Drug Discovery and Development*
Histone Deacetylases: Transcriptional Regulation and Other Cellular Functions
Edited by: E. Verdin © Humana Press Inc., Totowa, NJ

adipogenesis, and cell physiology. These enzymes use a conserved catalytic core domain to bind NAD$^+$ and acetyl-lysine-bearing protein targets. They generate lysine, 2′-O-acetyl-ADP-ribose, and nicotinamide products and contain more variable N- and C-terminal domains that may contribute protein-specific functions. Structural and related biochemical studies on the Sir2 enzymes from several laboratories have provided important insights into their conserved mode of NAD$^+$ and acetyl-lysine binding, recognition, and catalysis, as well as the distinguishing features that allow different members of the family to target their respective cognate substrates. This chapter summarizes the results of the structural analysis of the Sir2 enzymes as well as the implications of these studies for structure-based design of Sir2-specific small-molecule compounds that might modulate Sir2 functions for therapeutic application.

Key Words: Chromatin regulation, histone deacetylase, protein deacetylase, Sir2, NAD$^+$, longevity, metabolism, gene silencing, structure.

INTRODUCTION

The yeast silent information regulator-2 (ySir2) protein is the prototype of the class III family of histone deactylase (HDAC) enzymes that deacetylate the $N\zeta$-nitrogen of acetyl-lysine residues within histones H3 and H4 to silence gene expression from the mating-type locus, telomeres, and rDNA $(1,2)$. Unlike the class I and II HDAC enzymes, which do not require a cofactor for catalysis, the Sir2 proteins require the cofactor NAD$^+$ for catalytic activity (3), which generates the products 2′-O-acetyl-ADP-ribose, nicotinamide, and deacetylated histone $(4,5)$. Interestingly, nicotinamide has also been shown to be a noncompetitive inhibitor of Sir2 proteins, thereby also implicating nicotinamide as an important physiological regulator of these proteins (6).

It is now appreciated that Sir2 proteins are conserved in the three domains of bacteria, archaea, and eukaryotes; bacteria and archaea typically contain one or two Sir2 proteins, and eukaryotic organisms contain multiple members. For example, budding yeast and human contain five (Sir2 and Hst1–4) and seven (SirT1–SirT7) Sir2 homologs, respectively. Analysis of Sir2 proteins from various species indicates that their protein targets extend beyond histones and that they mediate diverse biological functions (7). For example, of the seven known human Sir2 proteins, nuclear SIRT1 targets the p53 tumor suppressor protein for deacetylation to suppress the apoptotic program in response to DNA damage $(8,9)$. It also targets forkhead transcription factors to regulate transcriptional activity in response to insulin signaling $(10–12)$ and binds to peroxisome proliferator-activated receptor-γ (PPAR-γ) to activate the genes associated with fat mobilization in white adipocytes (13). In addition, the cytoplasmic SIRT2 homolog targets α-tubulin for deacetylation for the maintenance of cell integrity (14).

In yeast and worms, an increased dosage of Sir2 extends life span, and in yeast, both Sir2 and NAD^+ are required for the long-established link between calorie-restricted diets and longevity in many organisms *(15,16)*. In addition, since it is well documented that as cells age they are more prone to genomic instability, (a hallmark of cancer), Sir2 proteins have been implicated as important targets for chemotherapeutic agents. Indeed, a recent study on Sir2-activating compounds characterized a family of polyphenol compounds, several of which are currently being used as chemotherapeutic agents *(17)*. Interestingly, the most potent of these compounds is resveratrol, a natural plant product found in high abundance in red wine and correlated with increased life span and reduced cancer risk in humans *(17,18)*. The more recent studies implicating mammalian Sir2 homologs in insulin signaling and fat mobilization have also stimulated interest in modulating Sir2 function for the treatment of obesity and type II diabetes *(13)*.

To understand the underlying mechanism of Sir2 activity, several laboratories have determined the structures of different Sir2 proteins in various liganded forms. Together with associated biochemical work, these studies have addressed the following questions: (1) what is the overall fold of the Sir2 catalytic core domain and how is it used to recognize NAD^+ and acetyl-lysine-bearing protein substrates? (2) what is the conserved mode of catalysis by Sir2 enzymes? (3) how do nonconserved regions of the Sir2 enzymes mediate functions that distinguish the different homologs? and (4) how might different Sir2 proteins target their respective cognate substrates? The implications of these studies for the structure-based design of Sir2-specific small-molecule compounds that might modulate Sir2 function for therapeutic application are discussed.

OVERALL STRUCTURE OF THE SIR2 PROTEINS

A sequence alignment of the Sir2 proteins reveals that they contain a highly conserved catalytic core domain of about 270 residues and more variable N- and C-terminal extensions that are believed to play more protein-specific functions *(7)*. To date, several structures of the catalytic core domain of Sir2 proteins have been reported either alone *(19,20)* or in complex with various NAD^+ analog and/or acetyl-lysine-bearing peptide substrates *(21–23)*. A comparison of these structures reveals a structurally conserved elongated shape containing, at one end of the molecule, a large Rossmann fold domain characteristic of NAD^+/NADH binding proteins and, at the opposite end of the molecule, a smaller domain containing a structural zinc ion *(19,22,24–26)* (Fig. 1). The larger Rossmann fold domain shows greater structural supposition with a root-mean-square deviation between Cα atoms of 1.0 to 1.3 Å; the smaller domain shows significantly more variability, with a root-mean-square deviation between Cα

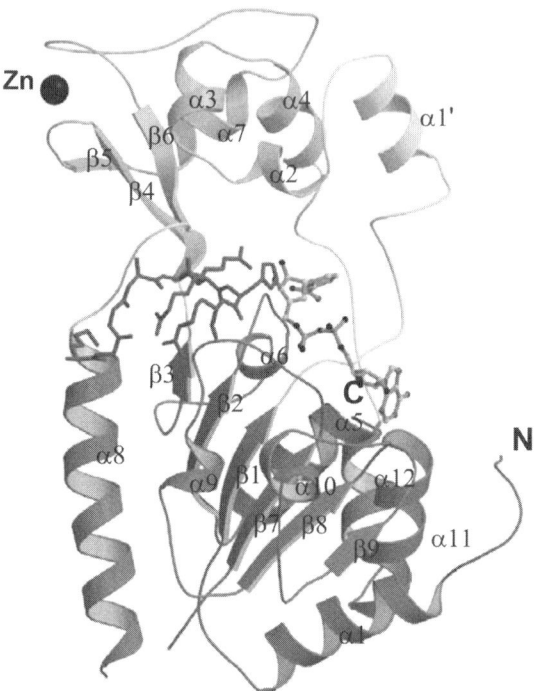

Fig. 1. Overall structure of the yeast Sir2 protein, Hst2, in ternary complex with acetyl-lysine-16 histone H4 and carba-NAD$^+$. Ribbon diagram of the complex highlighting the large domain (dark gray), small domain (light gray) and connecting loops (light gray) of the protein forming the cleft for substrate binding. The carba-NAD$^+$ (ball-and-stick model) and acetyl-lysine-16 histone H4 peptide (stick model) substrates as well as a Zn ion (black) are also highlighted.

atoms of 4.0 to 10.0 Å. A series of loops (called loops 1–4 here for their sequence order) traverse the space between the large and small domains, forming a pronounced extended cleft that is between the two protein domains and roughly perpendicular to the long axis of the molecule.

The liganded Sir2 structures reveal that the two substrates enter the protein through opposite sides of a cleft between the small and large domains of the catalytic core and that the functional groups of both the protein and substrates are buried within a protein tunnel that harbors the region of highest conservation within the Sir2 proteins *(27,28)* (Fig. 1). A comparison between the liganded and unliganded structures also reveals that whereas the large domain does not undergo significant conformational change upon the binding of ligands, the small domain and the connecting loops undergo more significant conformational changes upon the binding of substrates. In particular, connecting loops 1 and 4 (β1–α2 and β6–α8 in

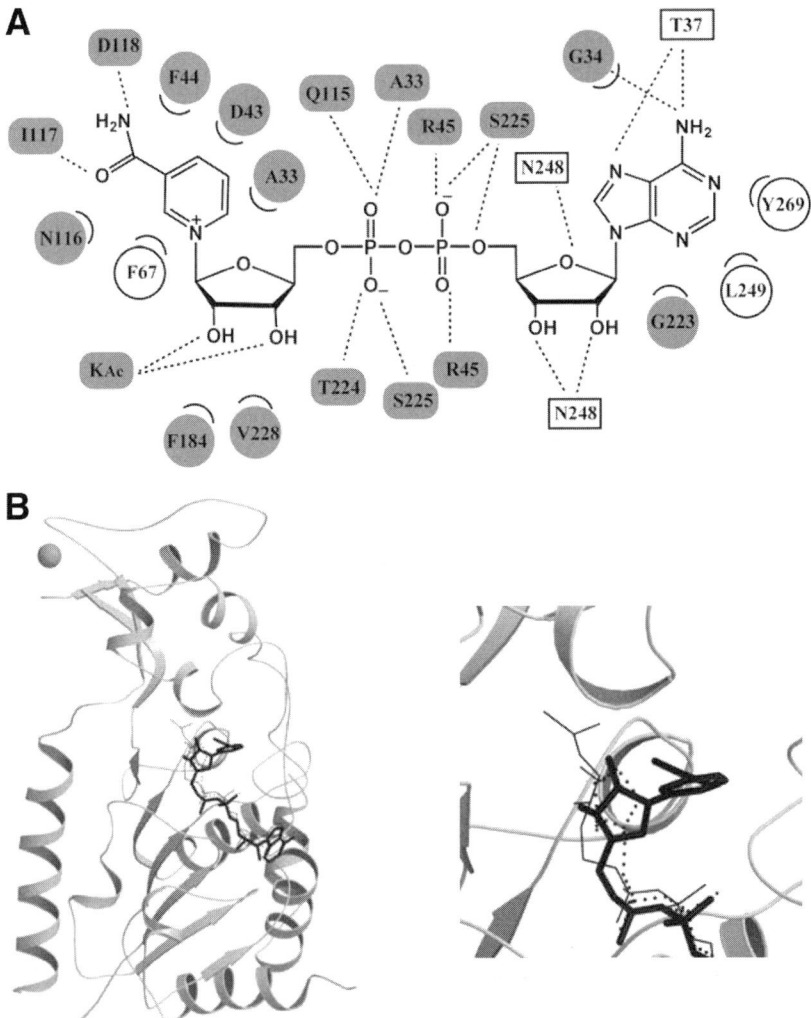

Fig. 2. The NAD$^+$ binding site of Sir2 proteins. **(A)** Schematic of the interactions between yHst2 and carba-NAD$^+$ in which conserved interactions with other Sir2/NAD$^+$ structures are indicated with gray boxes for hydrogen bonds and gray circles for hydrophobic bonds, respectively. **(B)** An overlay of different NAD$^+$ analogs bound to yHst2, highlighting the structural superposition of the ADP group and the structural variability of the nicotinamide-ribose group. The carba-NAD$^+$, 2'-O-acetyl-ADP-ribose, and ADP-ribose ligands are shown by solid thick, solid medium, and dotted lines, respectively.

the yHst2 structure) undergo significant structural movement upon the binding of ligands and play particularly important roles in binding NAD$^+$ (Fig. 2) and acetyl-lysine (Fig. 3) bearing substrates, respectively.

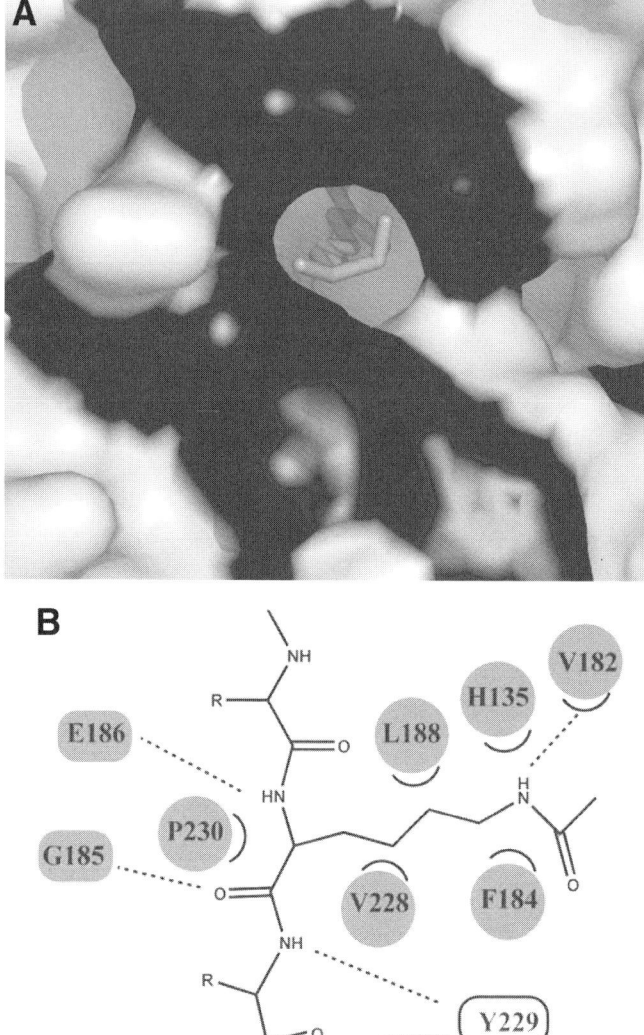

Fig. 3. The acetyl-lysine binding site of Sir2 proteins. (**A**) Surface representation of the yHst2/acetyl-lysine-16 histone H4/carba-NAD$^+$ structure showing the inter-action between yHst2 and acetyl-lysine and highlighting the residues that make

NAD⁺ BINDING BY SIR2 PROTEINS

Several Sir2 structures are available with bound NAD⁺ *(21,24)* or NAD⁺ analogs *(27,28)*, and a comparison of these structures reveals that the ADP group of NAD⁺ adopts a structurally conserved extended conformation that mediates conserved protein interactions with the large Rossmann fold domain of the Sir2 proteins in a way that is typical of NAD⁺/NADH bound to other Rossmann fold-containing proteins such as the dehydrogenases (Figs. 1 and 2A). In contrast, the nicotinamide-ribonucleotide group shows significant variability among the Sir2 structures, as highlighted by the structure of an archaeal Sir2 homolog cocrystallized with NAD⁺, which shows the nicotinamide-ribonucleotide moiety bound in two different conformations in the same crystal lattice *(21)* (Fig. 2A).

Interestingly, the ternary structure of the Sir2 homolog, yHst2 bound to acetyl-lysine-16 histone H4 and carba-NAD⁺ (in which a cyclopentane ring replaces the furanose of the nicotinamide-ribonucleotide moiety) suggests that the acetyl-lysine moiety helps lock the nicotinamide-ribonucleotide group into a distinct conformation that presumably promotes appropriate catalysis *(28)* (Fig. 2A). Specifically, the acetyl group of acetyl-lysine hydrogen binds to the 2′ and 3′ hydroxyl groups of the ribose ring and orients the nicotinamide-ribonucleotide group to interact with residues from the connection loops (mostly 1 and 4) and the zinc-bound small domain of the catalytic core. The nicotinamide group in particular is located in a pocket formed by residues from the Rossmann fold domain and loop 1. Strikingly, the residues that contact the nicotinamide-ribonucleotide moiety are highly conserved among the Sir2 enzymes, suggesting that the mode of NAD⁺ binding observed in the yHst2 structure extends to the other Sir2 enzymes (Fig. 2B).

ACETYL-LYSINE BINDING AND PROTEIN SPECIFICITY OF SIR2 PROTEINS

To date, three Sir2 structures have been reported with acetyl-lysine-containing peptides. These include the structures of an archaeal Sir2 protein (Sir2-Af2) bound to a p53 peptide *(22)*, as well as bacterial (CobB) *(23)* and yeast (yHst2) *(27,28)* Sir2 proteins bound to a histone H4 peptide. A comparison of these structures reveals conserved contacts between the

---

Fig. 3. (*Continued*) conserved acetyl-lysine peptide interactions in other Sir2/acetyl-lysine structures (black). **(B)** Schematic of the interactions between yHst2 and acetyl-lysine-16 histone H4 in which conserved interactions with other Sir2/acetyl-lysine peptide structures are indicated by gray boxes for hydrogen bonds and gray circles for hydrophobic bonds, respectively.

acetyl-lysine side chain and the one backbone residue just C-terminal to the acetyl-lysine (Fig. 3). Specifically, the aliphatic region of the acetyl-lysine is contacted by Sir2-conserved hydrophobic residues from the large domain of the Sir2 catalytic core and loop 4 (β6-α8 loop of yHst2) connecting the large and small domains. Residues from these protein regions also medicate conserved β-sheet-type interactions with the backbone residues of acetyl-lysine and one adjacent C-terminal residue. The conserved nature of these interactions suggests a common mode of acetyl-lysine recognition among all Sir2 proteins (Fig. 3B).

A comparison of the peptide-bound Sir2 structures also shows that interactions outside the acetyl-lysine and the one C-terminal residue are not conserved and that the peptides traverse in different directions (20,22,23). Although it should be noted that none of the reported peptide complexes with Sir2 proteins are bound to their "cognate" peptide sequences, these findings suggest that specificity for cognate substrates by Sir2 proteins may derive from target regions outside the local acetyl-lysine binding site. This conclusion is consistent with recent biochemical studies from our laboratory on the Sir2 homolog from bacteria, CobB (23). In these studies, the binding properties of cognate and noncognate 11-residue acetyl-lysine-bearing peptide substrates to CobB were quantitated using isothermal titration calorimetry (ITC) (23). Escalante-Semerena and coworkers had previously shown that CobB deacetylates Lys-609 of acetyl-CoA synthetase (Acs) in vivo to stimulate its enzymatic activity (29). The cognate peptide contained acetyl-lysine 609 of Acs, and the noncognate peptide contained acetyl-lysine-16 of histone H4 and acetyl-lysine Lys-382 of p53. The data reveal that the binding of each of these peptides is exothermic, which is indicative of hydrogen bond formation upon complexation. However, and quite surprisingly, CobB shows very little discrimination between these substrates, binding each with a dissociation constant between 0.44 and 3.7 μM, with the weakest binding constant for the cognate Acs peptide. Analogous binding studies employing intact Acs proteins specifically acetylated at lysine-609 yielded a dissociation constant of 14 μM but, surprisingly, showed an endothermic binding reaction indicative of an entropy-dominant contribution to binding involving a burial of hydrophobic surface and/or structural rearrangement involving CobB, Acs, or both proteins. Taken together, these results support the conclusion that substrate specificity determinants of bacterial CobB, and probably other Sir2 proteins, derive from regions outside the sequence local to the acetyl-lysine substrate.

CATALYSIS BY SIR2 PROTEINS

The laboratories of Schramm and Denu have investigated the catalytic mechanism of the Sir2 proteins and have proposed that the reaction proceeds through an oxocarbenium ion intermediate resulting in the formation of a novel metabolite in which the acetyl group from acetyl-lysine is transferred to the 2′ hydroxyl of the nicotinamide-ribose, 2′-O-acetyl-ADP-ribose *(4,5)*. A comparison of the ternary structures of yHst2, acetyl-lysine-16 histone H4 peptide bound to one of three NAD^+ analogs along the reaction pathway *(27,28)* has allowed our laboratory to propose a structural framework for this mechanism. The three structures analyzed contain carba-NAD^+, a nonhydrolyzable NAD^+ analog in which a cyclopentane ring replaces the furanose of the nicotinamide-ribonucleotide moiety; an intermediate analog complex containing ADP-ribose, a close mimic of a reaction intermediate, formed following cleavage of the glycosidic bond between nicotinamide and ADP-ribose (it differs only by the addition of a 1′ OH group); and a product analog complex containing 2′-O-acetyl-ADP-ribose, the NAD^+-derivatized product of the Sir2 reaction. A comparison of these structures reveals that whereas nearly 90% of the protein remains structurally invariant, the ribose ring of the cofactor and the highly conserved β1-α2 loop (loop 1) of the protein undergo significant structural rearrangements to facilitate the ordered NAD^+ reactions of nicotinamide cleavage and ADP-ribose transfer to acetate (Fig. 4).

The structure of the substrate mimic complex (with carba-NAD^+) shows that the carbonyl oxygen of the acetyl-lysine forms hydrogen bonds to the 2′ and 3′ hydroxyl groups of the nicotinamide ribose ring. This appears to position what would be the ribose ring oxygen of NAD^+ within hydrogen bonding distance of a water-mediated contact to the side chain carbonyl of a Sir2 conserved asparagine residue (Asn-116 in yHst2). This places the asparagine side chain carbonyl in position to help stabilize the oxocarbenium that has been proposed to form upon hydrolysis of the nicotinamide group *(4,5,30)* and is consistent with solution studies showing that this asparagine is essential for the nicotinamide exchange by Sir2 proteins *(24)*. It should be noted that the basicity of the asparagine side chain oxygen is probably insufficient to stabilize the oxocarbenium ion on its own and it is likely that other factors such as the proximity of the phosphate oxygens of the ADP ribose and the hydrophobic environment of the ribose binding pocket may also serve to stabilize the proposed intermediate.

The structure of the intermediate analog complex (with ADP-ribose) shows that the ribose ring of the intermediate complex is rotated by about 45° along the ring plane relative to the ribose ring of the substrate analog complex, to a position that now permits nucleophilic attack of the 1′ carbon of the ribose ring by the carbonyl oxygen of acetyl-lysine. The product analog complex (with 2′-O-acetyl-ADP ribose) reveals that the nicotinamide ribose ring is finally rotated by about 90° along the ring plane relative to the ribose ring of the substrate analog complex, to a position that now allows a Sir2 conserved histidine residue (His-135 in yHst2), a

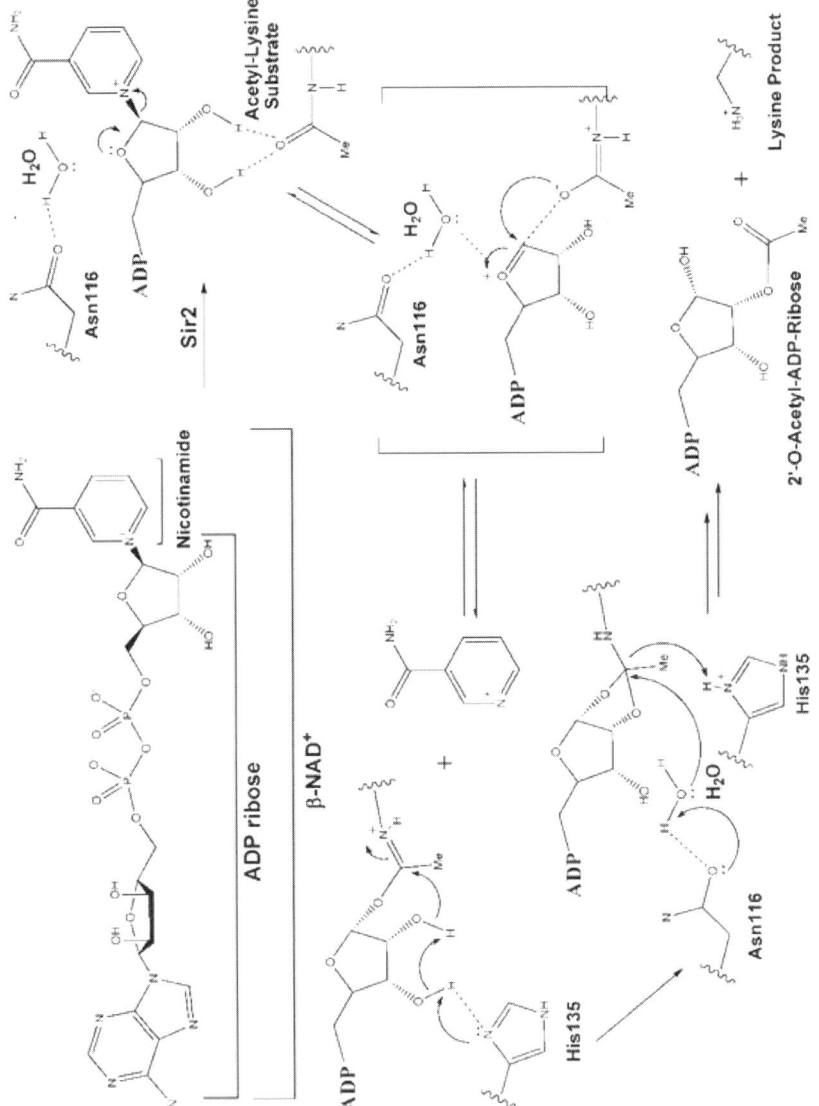

Fig. 4. Proposed catalytic mechanism for Sir2 proteins.

residue essential for the deacetylation reaction, to deprotonate the 3′ hydroxyl group of the nicotinamide ribose, nucleating formation of a cyclic acyldioxalane involving the 1′ and 2′ oxygens of the ribose ring. We then propose that a crystallographically well-ordered water molecule, which is held in place by the conserved asparagine residue, carries out nucleophilic attack of the cyclic acyldioxalane, resulting in the collapse of the cyclic intermediate to the 2′-O-ADP ribose and lysine reaction products (Fig. 4).

A comparison of the three ternary yHst2/acetyl-lysine-16 histone H4/NAD$^+$ analog complexes reveals that the β1-α2 loop (loop 1) also plays important roles in catalysis (27,28). Specifically, loop 1 mediates important NAD$^+$ interactions involving several Sir2 conserved loop residues (Ala-33, Gly-34, Thr-37, and Phe-44 in yHst2). The relatively open conformation of this loop in the product and intermediate analog complexes also suggests that the loop conformation facilitates NAD$^+$ substrate access as well. The more closed conformation of loop 1 in the product analog complex suggests that it may also play a role in nicotinamide release, as a Sir2 conserved phenylalanine (Phe-44 in yHst2) of the loop of the product analog complex partially occupies the binding site for nicotinamide, and it is also possible that the burial of the active site facilitates the acetyl-transfer reaction even more. Taking these date together, it appears that the nicotinamide ribose ring of the NAD$^+$ and loop 1 of the Sir2 proteins play dynamic roles in NAD$^+$ association and protein catalysis.

ROLES OF REGIONS N- AND C-TERMINAL TO THE SIR2 CATALYTIC DOMAIN

The variability in length and sequence of the regions N- and C-terminal to the eukaryotic Sir2 proteins suggests that these regions may play particularly important roles in the different biological processes with which the different Sir2 proteins are associated. To address the role these regions might play in Sir2 proteins, our laboratory has reported the structure of the full-length yHst2 protein (20). Interestingly, our results, along with related biochemical studies reveals that the regions N- and C-terminal to the catalytic core domain play autoregulatory roles (20). Specifically, a C-terminal helix overlaps with the NAD$^+$ binding site and thus autoregulates NAD$^+$ binding, and an N-terminal strand sits in the acetyl-lysine binding site of a symmetry-related subunit in the crystal lattice mediating formation of a homotrimer and thus autoregulating acetyl-lysine binding (Fig. 5). Solution studies in our laboratory correlate with these findings (20). Specifically, yHst2 constructs in which regions C-terminal to the catalytic core domain have been deleted bind NAD$^+$ about 3.5-fold more strongly. Moreover, whereas the full-length

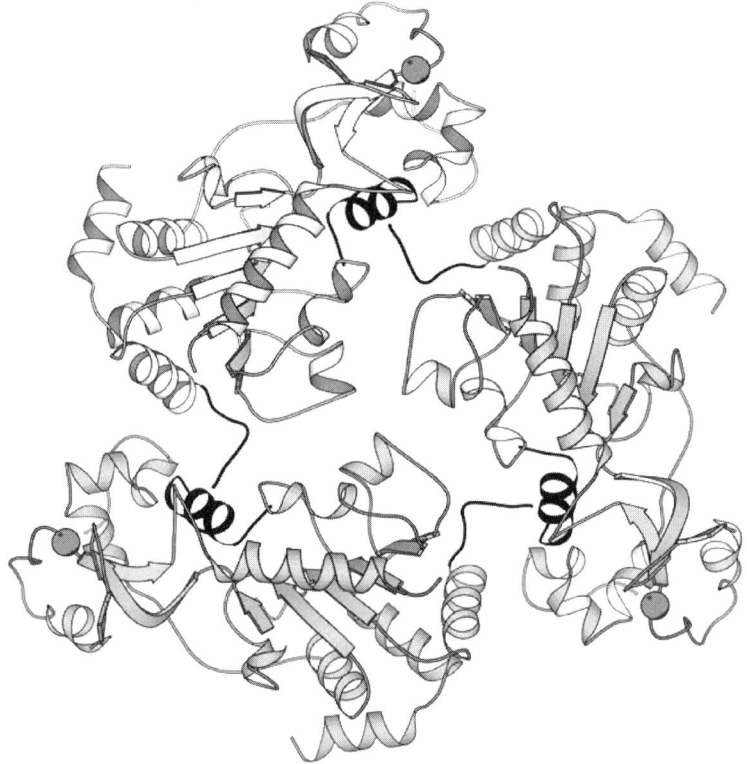

Fig. 5. Structure of the intact Hst2 homotrimer. The N- and C-terminal extensions that occupy the acetyl-lysine and NAD$^+$ binding sites, respectively, of the conserved Sir2 catalytic core domain are highlighted in black.

yHst2 protein forms a homotrimer in solution, with a dissociation constant in the low-micromolar range, an N-terminal deletion construct does not form detectable trimers and binds acetyl-lysine substrates two- to three-fold more avidly.

Whether or not this type of enzyme atoregulation occurs with other Sir2 proteins is unknown; however, the sequence divergence of regions N- and C-terminal to the catalytic core domain of the Sir2 proteins suggests that these interactions may differ in other Sir2 proteins, possibly also correlating with the substrate-specific roles of different Sir2 proteins.

PERSPECTIVE

Because of the possible association of Sir2 enzymes with human disease and life extension, there is an interest in the design of small-molecule compounds that might regulate the activity of Sir2 enzymes (1,7). Several inhibitors to Sir2 enzymes have been reported including sirtinol (31), split-omicin (32), and nicotinamide (6), a product of the Sir2 reaction. A short-coming of these inhibitors, however, is that they have relatively weak binding constants, with IC_{50} or K_m values in the midmicromolar range. The structural studies with yHst2 bound to NAD^+ analog suggest that a more fruitful avenue for inhibitor design should focus on a mimic of the reaction intermediate, such as ADP-ribose (28). Indeed, binding studies reveal that ADP-ribose binds to yHst2 with a dissociation constant of 0.4 μM, about 100-fold more avidly than previously characterized Sir2 inhibitors (28).

The possibility of generating Sir2-activating compounds has also gen-erated considerable interest (6). The structural studies with yHst2 (28) suggest a rational approach for developing Sir2-activating compounds that takes advantage of the observation that nicotinamide, a product of the Sir2 reaction, functions as a noncompetitive inhibitor of Sir2 by reacting with an ADP-ribosyl-enzyme-acetyl peptide intermediate with regeneration of NAD^+ (transglycosidation) (30,33). This mode of nicotinamide inhibition implies that nicotinamide binds to Sir2 at a site distinct from the nicoti-namide group of NAD^+ but still in a geometry that promotes the regenera-tion of NAD^+. Interestingly, if we assume that the conformation of ADP-ribose in the intermediate analog complex mimics the conformation of the NAD^+ intermediate that forms immediately after nicotinamide cleavage, it is particularly stricking that an entering nicotinamide group can be modeled onto the 1' carbon of the ADP-ribose ring with suitable geometry, without stereochemical clash with the protein, and in a binding site that is distinct from the binding site of the nicotinamide group of NAD^+. This suggests that compounds that block the binding site for free nicotinamide, as suggested from the structural modeling, might serve as potent activators of Sir2 with potential therapeutic applications.

Taken together, the structural studies on the catalytic core domain of the Sir2 proteins have provide important insights into the mode of NAD^+ and acetyl-lysine binding as well as the mode of catalysis; as described just above, these studies may contribute to the rational design of Sir2 regulatory molecules with therapeutic applications. However, it is also clear that Sir2 proteins mediate different biological processes, and it is likely that at least some of these differences are imparted by the more variable N- and C-terminal regions of the different Sir2 proteins. As described for yHst2, these regions may be involved in autoregulating catalytic activity (20), but they may also be associated with substrate selectivity and differential regulation by other proteins. Understanding the mechanistic basis for substrate discrimination by Sir2 proteins and the different biological processes that they are associated with will require structural analysis of other intact Sir2 proteins as well as their complexes with intact cognate protein substrates and associated regulatory factors. Ultimately, understanding what makes Sir2 proteins different might be at the heart of designing Sir2-specific regulatory compounds with therapeutic value.

ACKNOWLEDGMENTS

We thank William C. Ho for critically reading the manuscript.

REFERENCES

1. Guarente L. Sir2 links chromatin silencing, metabolism, and aging. Genes Dev 2000;14:1021–1026.
2. Imai S, Armstrong CM, Kaeberlein M, Guarente L. Transcriptional silencing and longevity protein Sir2 is an NAD-dependent histone deacetylase. Nature, 2000;403:795–800.
3. de Ruijter AJ, van Gennip AH, Caron HN, Kemp S, van Kuilenburg AB. Histone deacetylases (HDACs): characterization of the classical HDAC family. Biochem J 2003;370:737–749.
4. Sauve AA, Celic I, Avalos J, Deng H, Boek JD, Schramm VL. Chemistry of gene silencing: the mechanism of NAD+-dependent deacetylation reactions. Biochemistry 2001;40:15,456–15,463.
5. Jackson MD, Denu JM. Structural identification of 2′- and 3′-O-acetyl-ADP-ribose as novel metabolites derived from the Sir2 family of beta-NAD+-dependent histone/protein deacetylases. J Biol Chem 2002;277:18,535–18,544.
6. Bitterman KJ, Anderson RM, Cohen HY, Latorre-Esteves M, Sinclair D. Inhibition of silencing and accelerated aging by nicotinamide, a putative negative regulator of yeast Sir2 and human SIRT1. J Biol Chem 2002;277:45,099–45,107.
7. Buck SW, Gallo CM, Smith JS. Diversity in the Sir2 family of protein deacetylases. J Leukoc Biol 2004;75:939–950.
8. Luo J, Nikolaer AY, Imai S. Negative control of p53 by Sir2alpha promotes cell survival under stress. Cell 2001;107:137–148.
9. Vaziri H, Dessain SK, Ng Eaton E, et al. hSIR2(SIRT1) functions as an NAD-dependent p53 deacetylase. Cell 2001;107:149–159.
10. Brunet A, Sweeneg LB, Sturgill JF, et al. Stress-dependent regulation of FOXO transcription factors by the SIRT1 deacetylase. Science 2004;303:2011–2015.
11. Motta MC, Divecha N, Lemieu XM, et al. Mammalian SIRT1 represses forkhead transcription factors. Cell 2004;116:551–563.
12. Daitoku H, Natta M, Matsuzaki H, et al. Silent information regulator 2 potentiates Foxo1-mediated transcription through its deacetylase activity. Proc Natl Acad Sci U S A 2004;101:10,042–10,047.
13. Picard F, Kurtev M, Chung N, et al. Sirt1 promotes fat mobilization in white adipocytes by repressing PPAR-gamma. Nature 2004;429:771–776.
14. North BJ, Marshall BL, Borra MT, Denu JM, Verdin E. The human Sir2 ortholog, SIRT2, is a NAD+-dependent tubulin deacetylase. Mol Cell 2003;11:437–444.
15. Lin SJ, Defossez PA, Guarente L. Requirement of NAD and SIR2 for life-span extension by calorie restriction in *Saccharomyces cerevisiae*. Science 2000; 289:2126–2128.

16. Tissenbaum HA, Guarente L. Increased dosage of a sir-2 gene extends lifespan in *Caenorhabditis elegans*. Nature 2001;410:227–230.

17. Howitz KT, Bitterman KJ, Cohen HY, et al. Small molecule activators of sirtuins extend *Saccharomyces cerevisiae* lifespan. Nature 2003;425:191–196.

18. Wood JG, Rogina B, Lavu S, et al. Sirtuin activators mimic caloric restriction and delay ageing in metazoans. Nature 2004;430:686–689.

19. Finnin MS, Donigian JR, Pavletich NP. Structure of the histone deacetylase SIRT2. Nat Struct Biol 2001;8:621–625.

20. Zhao K, Chai X, Clements A, Marmorstein R. Structure and autoregulation of the yeast Hst2 homolog of Sir2. Nat Struct Biol 2003;10:864–871.

21. Avalos JL, Boeke JD, Wolberger C. Structural basis for the mechanism and regulation of Sir2 enzymes. Mol Cell 2004;13:639–648.

22. Avalos JL, Celic I, Muhammad S, Cosgrove MS, Boeke JD, Wolberger C. Structure of a Sir2 enzyme bound to an acetylated p53 peptide. Mol Cell 2002;10:523–535.

23. Zhao K, Chai X, Marmorstein R. Structure and substrate binding properties of cobB, a Sir2 homolog protein deacetylase from *Escherichia coli*. J Mol Biol 2004;337:731–741.

24. Min J, Landry J, Sternglanz R. Crystal structure of a SIR2 homolog-NAD complex. Cell 2001;105:269–279.

25. Jacobs SA, Harp JM, Devarakonda S, Kim Y, Rastinejad F, Khorasanizadeh S. The active site of the SET domain is constructed on a knot. Nat Struct Biol 2002;9:833–838.

26. Chang JH, Kim HC, Hwang KY, et al. Structural basis for the NAD-dependent deacetylase mechanism of Sir2. J Biol Chem 2002;277:34,489–34,498.

27. Zhao K, Chai X, Marmorstein R. Structure of the yeast Hst2 protein deacetylase in ternary complex with 2′-O-acetyl ADP ribose and histone peptide. Structure 2003;11:1403–1411.

28. Zhao K, Narshaw R, Chai X, Marmorstein R. Structural basis for nicotinamide cleavage and ADP-ribose transfer by NAD+-dependent Sir2 histone/protein deacetylases. Proc Natl Acad Sci U S A 2004;101:8563–8568.

29. Starai VJ, Celic I, Cole RN, Boeke JD, Escalante-Semerena JC. Sir2-dependent activation of acetyl-CoA synthetase by deacetylation of active lysine. Science 2002;298:2390–2392.

30. Sauve AA, Schramm VL. Sir2 regulation by nicotinamide results from switching between base exchange and deacetylation chemistry. Biochemistry 2003; 42:9249–9256.

31. Grozinger CM, Chao ED, Blackwell HE, Mozed D, Schreiber SL. Identification of a class of small molecule inhibitors of the sirtuin family of NAD-dependent deacetylases by phenotypic screening. J Biol Chem 2001;276:38,837–38,843.

32. Bedalov A, Gatbonton T, Irvine WP, Gottschling DE, Simon JA. Identification of a small molecule inhibitor of Sir2p. Proc Natl Acad Sci U S A 2001;98:15, 113–15,118.

33. Jackson MD, Schmidt MT, Oppenheimer NJ, Denu JM. Mechanism of nicotinamide inhibition and transglycosidation by Sir2 histone/protein deacetylases. J Biol Chem 2003;278:50,985–50,998.

10 The Enzymology of SIR2 Proteins

Margie T. Borra, PhD
and John M. Denu, PhD

CONTENTS

SUMMARY

Sir2 enzymes are NAD$^+$-dependent histone/protein deacetylases that tightly couple the cleavage of NAD$^+$ and protein deacetylation to produce nicotinamide, the deacetylated product, and O-acetyl-ADP-ribose. An increasing number of cellular processes including apoptosis, cell cycling, gene silencing, and longevity, have been shown to be dependent and regulated by these deacetylases. Several small molecules have been identified as regulators of Sir2 activity and related cellular processes. Understanding and modulating the cellular activities of these enzymes therefore necessitates an understanding of their enzymology. We review the enzymatic

From: *Cancer Drug Discovery and Development*
Histone Deacetylases: Transcriptional Regulation and Other Cellular Functions
Edited by: E. Verdin © Humana Press Inc., Totowa, NJ

activities, the crystal structures, the basic kinetic mechanism, and the regulation of Sir2 enzymes.

Key Words: Sir2, sirtuin, NAD$^+$, nicotinamide, deacetylation, aging, silencing.

INTRODUCTION

The dynamic balance between the activities of protein acetyltransferases and deacetylases has been shown to be a major regulatory mechanism in the control of cellular processes including transcription, metabolism, and DNA repair *(1)*. Acetyltransferases transfer the acetyl group of acetyl-CoA to the lysine residues of histones and nonhistone proteins. Generally, hyperacetylated histones are correlated with transcriptional activity. Deacetylases remove the acetyl group from these proteins and are linked to transcriptional silencing *(1)*. There are three classes of histone/protein deacetylases, which are classified on the basis of their similarity to the corresponding yeast enzymes *(2)*. The Rpd3-like (class I) and HDA1-like (class II) ones are commonly referred to as histone deacetylases (HDACs). Class III deacetylases are members of the silent information regulator 2 (Sir2) family *(2,3)* and are often referred to as sirtuins *(4)*.

The Sir2 proteins are conserved in all phyla of life *(4,5)*. There are five homologs in yeast (ySir2 and HST1–4) and seven in humans (SIRT1–7) *(5)*. Sir2 proteins have been implicated in DNA repair through nonhomologous end-joining *(6)*, cell cycle progression and chromosomal stability *(7)*, gene silencing *(8–11)*, and longevity *(12,13)*. The founding member of this family is ySir2, which is required for gene silencing at the three silent loci, the telomeres, ribosomal DNA (rDNA), and the mating-type loci *(8–11,14–19)*. At the telomeres and the mating-type loci, Sir2 is found in complex with Sir3 and Sir4, which are recruited by other DNA binding proteins *(9,14,20,21)*. At the rDNA, Sir2 forms a complex with Net1 and Cdc14 *(17,22)*, although the process of recruiting this complex to DNA is unknown. The presence of ySir2 at the rDNA has been linked to its role in longevity *(23–25)*. Sir2 prevents rDNA recombination, a cause of extra-chromosomal rDNA circle (ERC) formation *(12)*. ERCs have been shown to segregate to yeast mother cells and titrate transcription factors, resulting in cell mortality *(12)*.

Although the roles and cellular targets of many Sir2 proteins are unknown, reports concerning potential substrates are increasing. The human ortholog, SIRT2, has been shown to deacetylate α-tubulin, which is acetylated on lysine-40, suggesting a role in the cell cycle, cell division, and cellular structure *(26)*. The *Salmonella typhimurium* homolog, CobB, was shown to deacetylate, and thereby activate, acetyl-CoA synthetase, an important enzyme in the metabolism of small fatty acids *(27)*. The human homolog SIRT1 and its mouse counterpart, mSir2, deacetylate, in vitro and in vivo, the tumor suppressor protein, p53, which is acetylated by p300 in response to DNA damage *(28–30)*. Deacetylation of p53 has been proposed to block p53-dependent cell cycle arrest and apoptosis. Besides p53, SIRT1 has been shown to deacetylate and regulate p300 and forkhead transcription factors, including Foxo3a, Foxo1, and Foxo4 *(31,32)*. Foxo transcription factors regulate apoptosis, cell cycle arrest, differentiation, DNA repair, and oxidative stress resistance *(33–39)*, suggesting a wide range of cellular consequences for SIRT1 activity. SIRT1 has also been shown to promote fat mobilization in white adipocytes by binding to the nuclear receptor corepressor (NCoR) and the silencing mediator of retinoid and thyroid hormone receptors (SMRT), cofactors of peroxisome proliferator-activated receptor-γ. However, no evidence showing whether SIRT1 deacetylates either NCoR or SMRT has been presented *(40)*.

Over the last several years, it has become clear that Sir2 enzymes play a major role in many cellular functions including gene silencing, metabolism, and longevity. Recently, several small molecules have shown great promise in regulating Sir2-dependent processes *(28,30–32,40–47)*. Some of these regulators take advantage of the catalytic mechanism to mediate their effects *(45–47)*. Understanding the mode of regulation by these compounds would provide a specific mechanism for fine tuning Sir2 activity in the hope of developing therapeutics for such diseases as diabetes and cancer. To understand Sir2 regulation and function, however, one needs to understand the details of the reaction mechanism. In this chapter, we review the reactions catalyzed by Sir2 enzymes, the crystal structures, the kinetic mechanism, and investigations on activators and inhibitors, all of which have led to an important understanding of the molecular details of these unique enzymes.

SIR2 REACTIONS

Sir2 enzymes possess a robust NAD^+-dependent deacetylase activity, which tightly couples the cleavage of NAD^+ and the deacetylation of a substrate *(48–52)*. Attempts to identify the authentic reaction products led to the finding that acetate is not a product of the reaction; instead, a novel metabolite, *O*-acetyl-ADP-ribose (*O*AADPr) is produced *(53,54)*. The other two products are nicotinamide and the deacetylated product. The formation of *O*AADPr is conserved among homologs, and stoichiometric analysis revealed that for every molecule of NAD^+ cleaved and substrate deacetylated, one molecule of nicotinamide, deacetylated product, and *O*AADPr are formed *(52–55)*. Using a variety of approaches including rapid quench analysis, nuclear magnetic resonance (NMR), ^{18}O exchange, and mass spectrometry (MS), the acetyl group was found on the 2′ oxygen

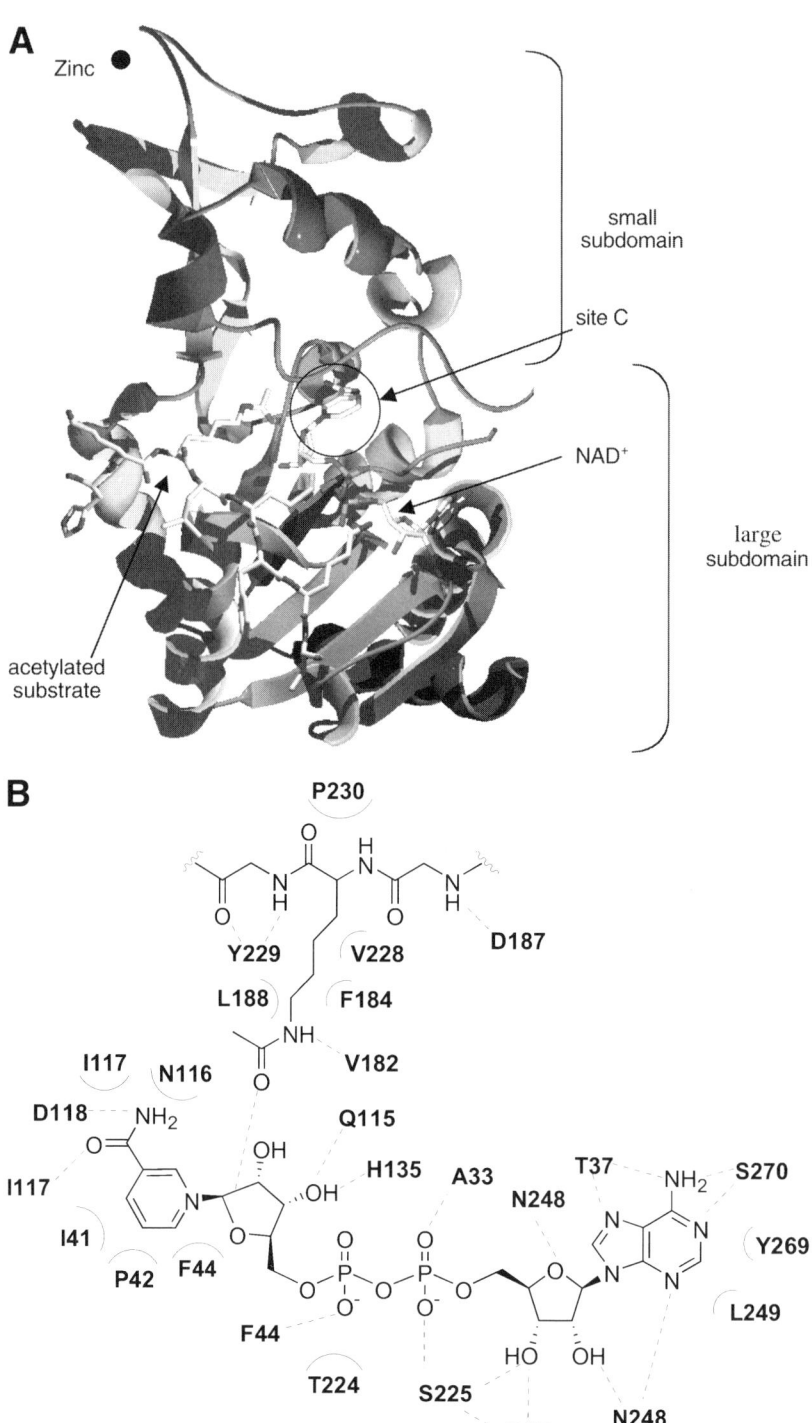

of the nicotinamide ribose *(56,57)*. The subsequent delineation of the crystal structures of Sir2 homologs showing enzymes in complex with 2′-*O*AADPr further supports the finding that 2′-*O*AADPr is the product formed at the enzyme surface *(58,59)*. Once released by the enzyme, an equilibrium between the 2′- and 3′-*O*AADPr is observed through a solution transesterification reaction *(56,57)*.

Besides the NAD$^+$-dependent deacetylase activity, a weak protein ADP-ribosyltransferase activity has been reported with some Sir2 homologs *(4,60,61)*. In fact, several of these findings were the first suggestion that Sir2 proteins harbored enzymatic activity. At this point, however, it is difficult to assess the importance of the observed ADP-ribosyltransferase activity, especially given the contradictory evidence seen in several different labs. It has been proposed that the observed ADP-ribosyltransferase activity may be caused by a small amount of uncoupling of the deacetylase reaction *(53)*. The deacetylase activity was estimated to be approx 1000-fold more efficient than the ADP-ribosyltransferase activity. Sir2 enzymes have been proposed to go through an enzyme-ADP-ribose-like intermediate, which, when exposed to nucleophiles other than the acetyl-substrate, could transfer the ADP-ribose to an alternate acceptor molecule *(53)*. To date, no detailed mechanistic analysis has compared the deacetylase and ADP-ribosyltransferase activities, leaving the biological importance of ADP-ribosylation an open question.

SIR2 CRYSTAL STRUCTURES

Crystal structures of bacterial, human, archaeal, and yeast Sir2 enzymes have been solved *(58,59,62–68)*. These crystal structures are in agreement with the general structure of the catalytic domain of the Sir2 enzymes (Fig. 1A). The catalytic domain consists of two subdomains. The large

---

Fig. 1. Structure of Sir2 and residues contacting the substrates. Residues are numbered based on the HST2 sequence. **(A)** A model of the Sir2-Af2 structure with bound p53 peptide and NAD$^+$. The structure of NAD$^+$ from Min et al. *(62)* was superimposed on the structure of Sir2-Af2 with bound p53 peptide from Avalos et al. *(64)*. Sir2 enzymes consist of two subdomains. The large subdomain contains the Rossmann fold, which is present in many NAD$^+$-binding proteins. The smaller subdomain contains the zinc-binding module, which holds the zinc ion through two pairs of cysteine residues. The acetylated substrate and NAD$^+$ bind in a cleft between the two domains. **(B)** Residues contacting the NAD$^+$ and the acetyl-lysine. The NAD$^+$ molecule is bound in an extended conformation, with the nicotinamide moiety bound in a hydrophobic portion of the enzyme, referred to as site C. The acetyl-lysine group of the acetylated substrate inserts into a hydrophobic pocket and positions the carbonyl group in proximity to the nicotinamide ribose. Only a few residues of the residues flanking the acetyl-lysine are depicted in the figure because interactions between these residues and the enzyme are predominantly nonspecific, backbone interactions.

subdomain is composed of six β-strands surrounded by α-helices on each side, forming an inverted Rossman fold. The smaller subdomain consists of three antiparallel β-strands and two α-helices, with the zinc-binding module held by two pairs of cysteine residues. The NAD^+ and the acetylated substrate bind in a cleft between the two domains.

As with many NAD^+ binding proteins, NAD^+ binds to the Rossman fold in an inverted and extended orientation *(58,59,62,67,68)* (Fig. 1B). In Sir2, NAD^+ binds extensively to a pocket formed by several conserved residues at the interface between the large and the small subdomains. The large subdomain forms the floor, where most of the conserved residues reside, and the small subdomain forms the ceiling of the NAD^+ binding pocket. All the crystal structures have consistently observed the ADP-ribose portion of NAD^+. However, the nicotinamide moiety was not clearly visible in the early crystal structures *(51,52,55)*. One report originally postulated that the nicotinamide portion binds in a hydrophobic pocket, referred to as site C *(62)* (Fig. 1A). This C pocket appeared to be quite inaccessible and somewhat distant from the position of the observed ADP-ribose portion of NAD^+, although several polar, conserved residues are found here. Mutation of these residues affects enzymatic activity *(62)*, but these alterations were suggested to result from structural perturbations that decreased or abolished NAD^+ binding *(58)*.

The nicotinamide binding site in the context of an intact NAD^+ molecule was recently identified in the crystal structures of Sir2-Af2 *(67)* and the C-terminal deletion construct of yHST2 *(68)*. These structures clearly demonstrated that the nicotinamide moiety binds to the C site *(67,68)* (Fig. 1A) and that a 150° rotation about the glycosidic bond, resulting in loss of coplanarity of the ribose and the nicotinamide group, is required for nicotinamide to bind to the previously reported inaccessible site. Rotation of the nicotinamide group indicates destabilization of the NAD^+ molecule, which may permit the formation of the oxocarbenium ion, a proposed reactive intermediate. With the contorted NAD^+ molecule, the acetyl-lysine would be in the proximity of the C_1 position of the nicotinamide ribose and would be capable of performing a nucleophilic attack on the α-face of the molecule *(67,68)*. Also, binding of the acetylated substrate was predicted to promote binding of the NAD^+ coenzyme.

A binding site for the acetylated substrate has been observed in the bacterial *(66)*, yeast *(59)*, and archaeal *(64)* Sir2 enzymes (Fig. 1B). These crystal structures show a similar location of the acetyl-lysine group and the interactions between the enzyme and the substrate. The acetylated substrate binds to the enzyme by forming a β-sheet-like interaction with two flanking strands from the enzyme. The extended acetyl-lysine group from the acetylated substrate inserts into a hydrophobic tunnel, positioning the carbonyl group in close proximity to the nicotinamide ribose ring. Peptide backbone interactions predominate between the enzyme and the residues flanking the acetyl-lysine, leading the authors to postulate that the catalytic domain offers little substrate specificity and that specificity may be conferred by domains outside the catalytic core *(64)*. It is important to point out, however, that no evidence exists showing that the acetylated substrates used in the crystal structures are the in vivo substrates for the enzymes investigated.

SUBSTRATE SPECIFICITY

With a possible abundance of acetylated proteins in the cell, how do Sir2 enzymes identify their cellular targets? Can Sir2 enzymes alone discriminate between acetylated proteins or do they require accessory proteins for targeting to their physiological substrates? Because Sir2 enzymes are critical players in many diverse cellular processes, it is imperative that these enzymes find and discriminate their physiological targets during the appropriate cellular signals.

Evidence indicates that some Sir2 homologs have the capability of deacetylating several substrates in vitro. For example, the yeast homolog HST2 deacetylates histone peptides *(51–53,65,69)* as well as tubulin peptides *(26,69)*. Sir2-Af1, Sir2-Af2, ySir2, and SIRT2 were shown to deacetylate histones as well as p53 peptides *(64)*. The bacterial homolog cobB was shown to have a similar affinity for the histone H4 peptide, the p53 peptide, and acetyl-CoA synthetase peptides *(66)*. Several Sir2 crystal structures with bound acetylated peptide suggested that the catalytic core harbors little specificity *(64)*.

Although few quantitative studies have examined the substrate specificity of Sir2 enzymes, there is growing evidence that these enzymes do exhibit preferences among substrates. The archaea homolog, Sir2-Af1 can deacetylate bovine serum albumin, but not chicken core histones *(62)*. SIRT5, which was shown previously to deacetylate a histone H4 peptide *(26)*, was incapable of deacetylating a p53 peptide *(28)*. Overexpression of SIRT1 resulted in deacetylation of p53, but not histone H3, acetylated at Lys-9, suggesting substrate preference in vivo *(29)*. A quantitative study on the ability of the achaeal homologs to deacetylate p53 peptides showed that Sir2-Af2 exhibits higher catalytic efficiency and is, therefore, a better enzyme for the p53 peptide compared with Sir2-Af1 *(64)*, although p53 is not a physiological substrate for either enzyme.

A more recent quantitative analysis of the substrate specificity of ySir2, SIRT2, and HST2 showed that the three enzymes exhibit varying catalytic efficiency among monoacetylated histone H3 and H4 peptide substrates *(69)*. HST2 displayed the highest catalytic efficiency for all the histone peptides examined. Each enzyme also showed a preference for the location of the acetyl group within a given histone substrate. For example, ySir2 demonstrated the highest preference for the histone H4 peptide acetylated at Lys-16 (69), which is consistent with previous cellular studies (70).

Besides ySir2, SIRT1, SIRT2, and cobB, very little is known about the physiological substrates and specificity of other Sir2 homologs. Although some homologs have been shown to deacetylate various acetylated substrates in vitro, it is possible that in vivo, some Sir2 enzymes are targeted to their physiological substrates. For example, ySir2 is found in complex with DNA binding proteins (9,14,20,21), which most likely recruit ySir2 to the histones of heterochromatic chromatin, thereby increasing the effective substrate concentration and increasing the catalytic efficiency of deacetylation. Substrate specificity has been postulated to be conferred by domains outside the catalytic core (59,64,66). Sir2 proteins have varying C- and N-terminal extensions, which may be involved in substrate recognition and binding (65). Further studies are needed to determine the factors involved in substrate selectivity among the Sir2 proteins.

KINETIC MECHANISM

Among the deacetylase families, Sir2 enzymes catalyze a unique reaction that requires NAD^+ and produces a newly discovered product. Several mechanisms have been proposed for the Sir2 reaction (45,46,53,54, 56–59,67,68), but the basic kinetic mechanism and the order of substrate binding and product release were not elucidated until recently. Bisubstrate kinetic analysis indicated that Sir2 enzymes follow a sequential mechanism, in which both NAD^+ and the acetylated substrate must bind and form a ternary complex for catalysis to proceed (69) (Fig. 2). This means that no chemical reactions occur and no covalent enzyme intermediate is formed in the absence of one of the substrates. The [^{14}C]nicotinamide-NAD^+ exchange reaction, which was first described by R. Sternglanz and co-workers (51,52), is consistent with a ternary complex mechanism. In the exchange reaction, NAD^+ and acetylated substrate react with the enzyme, and the subsequent enzyme-ADP-ribose-like intermediate condenses with the exogenous [^{14}C]nicotinamide to form [^{14}C]NAD^+. The exchange reaction does not occur in the absence of the acetylated substrate (51,52), indicating that no cleavage of the nicotinamide ribosyl bond occurs without the acetylated substrate.

The complete order of substrate binding and product release has been determined (69) (Fig. 2). The exchange reaction is consistent with nicotinamide being the first product released, as this reaction occurs in the absence of the deacetylated product and OAADPr. Product inhibition analysis of nicotinamide versus NAD^+ and an acetylated substrate showed noncompetitive inhibition, which is consistent with the conclusion that

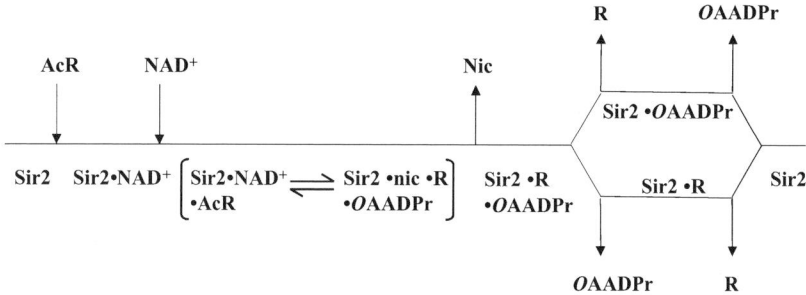

Fig. 2. Kinetic mechanism of the Sir2 family of enzymes. Sir2 enzymes follow a sequential mechanism, in which both the acetylated substrate and NAD⁺ must bind prior to catalysis. The acetylated substrate is the preferred first substrate to bind, followed by NAD⁺, forming a ternary complex. After catalysis, nicotinamide is the first product released, followed by a random release of the deacetylated product and O-acetyl-ADP-ribose (OAADPr).

nicotinamide is the first product released *(69)*. Additional product and dead-end inhibition studies suggested a random release of the deacetylated product and OAADPr *(69)*.

Several lines of evidence indicate that the acetylated substrate is the first to bind. First, a product inhibition analysis of a deacetylated product vs the acetylated substrate displayed competitive inhibition *(69)*. Second, a recent crystal structure of Sir2-Af2 in ternary complex with NAD⁺ and an acetylated substrate mimic indicated that NAD⁺ binding may be facilitated by the acetylated substrate binding *(67)*. Equilibrium binding studies also showed that the acetylated substrate can bind independently to the free enzyme *(68,69)*. Although NAD⁺ binding has been observed with Sir2-Af1 *(58)*, no significant binding was observed with HST2 and SIRT2 *(69)*. Even though NAD⁺ binding to the free enzyme was shown, whether this complex is productive is unknown. Alternatively, some Sir2 enzymes might bind the two substrates in a random fashion.

REGULATION OF SIR2

Because Sir2 enzymes are important for various cellular processes including gene silencing/activation, metabolism, apoptosis, and longevity *(3,24,25,48,71–75)*, understanding the regulation of Sir2 enzymes would pave the way for identifying therapeutic interventions that can modulate these pathways. Numerous small molecules have been shown to inhibit and activate Sir2 enzymes.

To date, nicotinamide has been shown to be the most potent inhibitor of Sir2 activity *(41,45–47,69)*. It was first postulated that nicotinamide binds to an allosteric site and consequently inhibits Sir2 activity *(41)*. However, a detailed kinetic analysis indicated that the effectiveness of nicotinamide inhibition arises from the fact that it can condense with an enzyme/ADP-ribose-like/acetylated-substrate intermediate and drive the reverse reaction, forming NAD^+ and inhibiting product formation *(45,46)*. Nicotinamide decreases the forward reaction at a rate similar to that at which it increases this partial reverse reaction. Sensitivity to nicotinamide inhibition has been postulated to be enzyme dependent, as the overall rate of deacetylation in comparison with the rate of the exchange reaction has been shown to vary between enzymes. The potency of nicotinamide inhibition has been reported to depend on the relative rates of the deacetylation and exchange reactions *(45,46)*.

Given the requirement for NAD^+ and the potency of nicotinamide inhibition, several NAD^+ and nicotinamide analogs were tested as possible substrates or inhibitors of Sir2 reaction *(45,47)*. NAD^+ analogs, with substitution at either the nicotinamide ring or the adenine base, were poor substrates for the Sir2 reaction, suggesting deficient binding and/or catalysis *(47)*. Some pyridine derivatives were shown to support the Sir2-catalyzed exchange reaction, suggesting that these compounds can bind to the nicotinamide binding site and promote the transglycosidation reaction *(45)*. However, inhibition analyses using these pyridine derivatives, as well as NAD^+ analogs with an altered nicotinamide ring, indicated that these compounds are at least an order of magnitude less efficient compared with nicotinamide. Collectively, these data demonstrate an exquisitely specific nicotinamide binding site *(45,47)*.

The cellular NAD^+/NADH ratio has also been implicated in the regulation of Sir2 activity. Contradicting reports have been presented regarding the role of the NAD^+/NADH ratio in Sir2 regulation. Anderson et al. *(76)* reported a lack of NAD^+ fluctuation as well as a lack of change in NADH levels, for calorie-restricted yeast cells. Lin et al. *(77)* reported that Sir2-mediated life span extension during calorie restriction results from decreased NADH levels. Kinetic analyses, however, indicated that NADH levels may not be a factor in regulating Sir2 activity, as NADH is a poor inhibitor of Sir2 enzymes, with IC_{50} values in high millimolar range *(47)*. In comparison, the K_m values for NAD^+ fall typically between 10 and 100 μM *(69)*. Therefore, changes in NAD^+ levels, but not NADH levels, would likely be a factor in Sir2 regulation.

A number of small molecules are reported to inhibit or activate Sir2 enzymes. High-throughput chemical screens have identified splitomicin *(78)* and sirtinol *(44)* as inhibitors of Sir2 enzymes. Splitomicin analogs also have inhibitory effects on Sir2 enzymes *(42)*. It is, however, important to point out that of all the inhibitors tested to date, none have shown comparable potency to that seen with nicotinamide. Additionally, the mode of inhibition by these molecules has not been established. It is possible that these compounds bind to allosteric sites on the enzyme, although no such sites are obvious from the available crystal structures. Competition for binding to the NAD^+ binding site is another possibility, as these compounds have ring structures that may be accommodated. Further studies are needed to evaluate the mechanism of inhibition and to improve the efficacy of these compounds.

A few plant polyphenols, including quercetin, piceatoannol, and resveratrol activate some Sir2 enzymes *(43)*. Demonstrating the best activation of the compounds tested, resveratrol lowers the K_m for NAD^+ and for acetylated substrate but does not affect the turnover rate of the enzyme. Life span extension and increased cell survival upon DNA damage were observed in the presence of resveratrol *(43)*, making this polyphenol found in red wine an excellent tool for future studies on Sir2 regulation. Recent studies have shown that the previously observed resveratrol activation, in vitro, was dependent on the use of fluorophore-containing peptides as substrates *(43a,b)*. Peptide substrates lacking the fluorophore exhibited no activation. Activation was also largely specific to SIRT1. Therefore, unclear at this point is the mechanism of resveratrol-mediated Sir2 activation in vivo. Resveratrol has known antioxidant properties, and it is not clear whether the observed Sir2 activation is due to antioxidant effects indirectly or whether activation occurs by direct binding to Sir2, perhaps at a remote allosteric site in the enzyme.

CATALYTIC MECHANISM

From the available evidence, acetylated substrate binds first and NAD^+ second, with no chemical step occurring until the formation of the ternary complex *(67–69)*. Data from rapid quench analysis indicate that cleavage of the nicotinamide ribosyl bond precedes the transfer of the acetyl group from the acetylated substrate to the ADP-ribose portion of NAD^+ *(69)*. Formation of an initial oxocarbenium ion-like species after elimination of nicotinamide has been suggested previously as the initial step in the reaction *(45)* (Fig. 3). Following oxocarbenium ion formation, the carbonyl oxygen of the acetyl-lysine performs a nucleophilic attack on the C_1 of the nicotinamide ribose, forming an iminium ion intermediate. The 2′-OH of the nicotinamide ribose attacks the carbonyl carbon of the acetyl-lysine, probably activated by deprotonation through the involvement of a conserved histidine residue, forming a cyclic intermediate. The conserved histidine appears to be involved in this step of the reaction but is not critical in the initial elimination of nicotinamide *(45)*. A water molecule can then perform a nucleophilic attack on the cyclized intermediate, to form the 2′-OAADPr. Water attack at the C_1 is also possible and would generate the identical product.

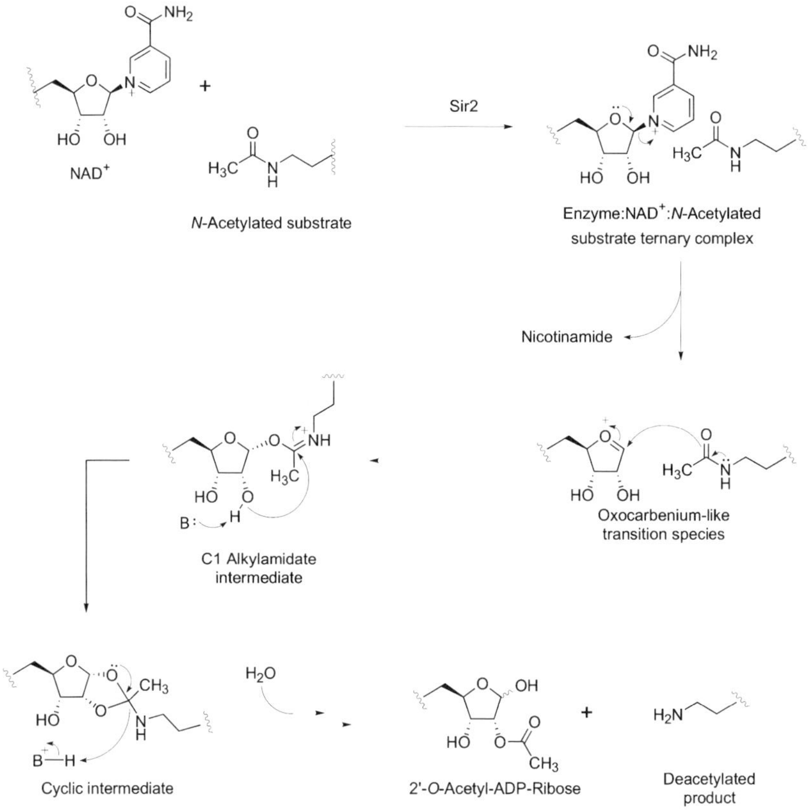

Fig. 3. Sir2 catalytic mechanism. After formation of the ternary complex, nicotinamide cleavage precedes the acetyl transfer step. The carbonyl oxygen of the acetyl group then performs a nucleophilic attack on the C_1 position of the nicotinamide ribose. Activation of the 2'-OH of the nicotinamide ribose, possibly by the conserved histidine residue, allows the nucleophilic attack on the carbonyl carbon, leading to the formation of a cyclic intermediate. Attack of a water molecule collapses the cyclic intermediate and allows formation of the 2'-OAADPr.

Formation of a covalent enzyme-ADP-ribose intermediate was proposed by Min et al. *(62)*; however, there are no data to support this hypothesis. Although the mechanism outlined above and in Fig. 3 is consistent with the latest findings *(45,46,67,68)*, several important questions remain: Can the formation of a 1'-OAADPr intermediate be ruled out? Can the imine adduct be isolated and proved to exist? Where and when does water attack the proposed intermediate? What are the roles of the conserved active site residues? Can these enzymes function as viable ADP-ribosyltransferases? What is the mechanistic basis for the difference between protein deacetylation and ADP ribosylation? Further studies are needed to address these and other important mechanistic questions.

ACKNOWLEDGMENTS

We thank Brian C. Smith for his expertise in generating Figure 1. This work was supported by American Cancer Society grant RSG-01-029-01 and NIH grant RO1 GM65386 to J.M.D. and NIH predoctoral fellowship F31 GM66366 to M.T.B.

REFERENCES

1. Roth SY, Denu JM, Allis CD. Histone acetyltransferases. Annu Rev Biochem 2001;70:81–120.
2. Gray SG, Ekstrom TJ. The human histone deacetylase family. Exp Cell Res 2001;262:75–83.
3. Blander G, Guarente L. The sir2 family of protein deacetylases. Annu Rev Biochem 2004;73:417–435.
4. Frye RA. Characterization of five human cDNAs with homology to the yeast SIR2 gene: Sir2-like proteins (sirtuins) metabolize NAD and have protein ADP-ribosyltransferase activity. Biochem Biophys Res Commun 1999;260: 273–279.
5. Frye RA. Phylogenetic classification of prokaryotic and eukaryotic Sir2-like proteins. Biochem Biophys Res Commun 2000;273:793–798.
6. Tsukamoto Y, Kato J, Ikeda H. Silencing factors participate in DNA repair and recombination in Saccharomyces cerevisiae. Nature 1997;388:900–903.
7. Brachmann CB, Sherman JM, Devine SE, Cameron EE, Pillus L, Boeke JD. The SIR2 gene family, conserved from bacteria to humans, functions in silencing, cell cycle progression, and chromosome stability. Genes Dev 1995;9:2888–2902.
8. Rine J, Herskowitz I. Four genes responsible for a position effect on expression from HML and HMR in Saccharomyces cerevisiae. Genetics 1987;116:9–22.
9. Aparicio OM, Billington BL, Gottschling DE. Modifiers of position effect are shared between telomeric and silent mating-type loci in S. cerevisiae. Cell 1991;66:1279–1287.
10. Bryk M, Banerjee M, Murphy M, Knudsen KE, Garfinkel DJ, Curcio MJ. Transcriptional silencing of Ty1 elements in the RDN1 locus of yeast. Genes Dev 1997;11:255–269.
11. Smith JS, Boeke JD. An unusual form of transcriptional silencing in yeast ribosomal DNA. Genes Dev 1997;11:241–254.
12. Sinclair DA, Guarente L. Extrachromosomal rDNA circles—a cause of aging in yeast. Cell 1997;91:1033–1042.
13. Kaeberlein M, McVey M, Guarente L. The SIR2/3/4 complex and SIR2 alone promote longevity in Saccharomyces cerevisiae by two different mechanisms. Genes Dev 1999;13:2570–2580.

14. Strahl-Bolsinger S, Hecht A, Luo K, Grunstein M. SIR2 and SIR4 interactions differ in core and extended telomeric heterochromatin in yeast. Genes Dev 1997;11:83–93.

15. Gottschling DE, Aparicio OM, Billington BL, Zakian VA. Position effect at *S. cerevisiae* telomeres: reversible repression of Pol II transcription. Cell 1990;63:751–762.

16. Shou W, Sakamoto KM, Keener J, et al. Net1 stimulates RNA polymerase I transcription and regulates nucleolar structure independently of controlling mitotic exit. Mol Cell 2001;8:45–55.

17. Shou W, Seol JH, Shevchenko A, et al. Exit from mitosis is triggered by Tem1-dependent release of the protein phosphatase Cdc14 from nucleolar RENT complex. Cell 1999;97:233–244.

18. Fritze CE, Verschueren K, Strich R, Easton Esposito R. Direct evidence for SIR2 modulation of chromatin structure in yeast rDNA. EMBO J 1997;16:6495–6509.

19. Loo S, Rine J. Silencing and heritable domains of gene expression. Annu Rev Cell Dev Biol 1995;11:519–548.

20. Hecht A, Laroche T, Strahl-Bolsinger S, Gasser SM, Grunstein M. Histone H3 and H4 N-termini interact with SIR3 and SIR4 proteins: a molecular model for the formation of heterochromatin in yeast. Cell 1995;80:583–592.

21. Moazed D, Kistler A, Axelrod A, Rine J, Johnson AD. Silent information regulator protein complexes in *Saccharomyces cerevisiae*: a SIR2/SIR4 complex and evidence for a regulatory domain in SIR4 that inhibits its interaction with SIR3. Proc Natl Acad Sci U S A 1997;94:2186–2191.

22. Straight AF, Shou W, Dowd GJ, et al. Net1, a Sir2-associated nucleolar protein required for rDNA silencing and nucleolar integrity. Cell 1999;97:245–256.

23. Sinclair DA, Mills K, Guarente L. Accelerated aging and nucleolar fragmentation in yeast sgs1 mutants. Science 1997;277:1313–1316.

24. Guarente L. Sir2 links chromatin silencing, metabolism, and aging. Genes Dev 2000;14:1021–1026.

25. Guarente L. SIR2 and aging—the exception that proves the rule. Trends Genet 2001;17:391, 392.

26. North BJ, Marshall BL, Borra MT, Denu JM, Verdin E. The human Sir2 ortholog, SIRT2, is an NAD+-dependent tubulin deacetylase. Mol Cell 2003;11:437–444.

27. Starai VJ, Celic I, Cole RN, Boeke JD, Escalante-Semerena JC. Sir2-dependent activation of acetyl-CoA synthetase by deacetylation of active lysine. Science 2002;298:2390–2392.

28. Luo J, Nikolaev AY, Imai S, et al. Negative control of p53 by Sir2alpha promotes cell survival under stress. Cell 2001;107:137–148.

29. Vaziri H, Dessain SK, Eaton EN, et al. hSIR2(SIRT1) functions as an NAD-dependent p53 deacetylase. Cell 2001;107:149–159.

30. Langley E, Pearson M, Faretta M, et al. Human SIR2 deacetylates p53 and antagonizes PML/p53-induced cellular senescence. EMBO J 2002;21:2383–2396.

31. Motta MC, Divecha N, Lemieux M, et al. Mammalian SIRT1 represses forkhead transcription factors. Cell 2004;116:551–563.

32. Brunet A, Sweeney LB, Sturgill JF, et al. Stress-dependent regulation of FOXO transcription factors by the SIRT1 deacetylase. Science 2004;303:2011–2015.

33. Brunet A, Bonni A, Zigmond MJ, et al. Akt promotes cell survival by phosphorylating and inhibiting a Forkhead transcription factor. Cell 1999;96:857–868.
34. Nakamura N, Ramaswamy S, Vazquez F, Signoretti S, Loda M, Sellers WR. Forkhead transcription factors are critical effectors of cell death and cell cycle arrest downstream of PTEN. Mol Cell Biol 2000;20:8969–8982.
35. Dijkers PF, Medema RH, Pals C, et al. Forkhead transcription factor FKHR-L1 modulates cytokine-dependent transcriptional regulation of p27(KIP1). Mol Cell Biol 2000;20:9138–9148.
36. Kops GJ, Medema RH, Glassford J, et al. Control of cell cycle exit and entry by protein kinase B-regulated forkhead transcription factors. Mol Cell Biol 2002;22:2025–2036.
37. Hribal ML, Nakae J, Kitamura T, Shutter JR, Accili D. Regulation of insulin-like growth factor-dependent myoblast differentiation by Foxo forkhead transcription factors. J Cell Biol 2003;162:535–541.
38. Tran H, Brunet A, Grenier JM, et al. DNA repair pathway stimulated by the forkhead transcription factor FOXO3a through the Gadd45 protein. Science 2002;296:530–541.
39. Murphy CT, McCarroll SA, Bargmann CI, et al. Genes that act downstream of DAF-16 to influence the lifespan of *Caenorhabditis elegans*. Nature 2003;424:277–283.
40. Picard F, Kurtev M, Chung N, et al. Sirt1 promotes fat mobilization in white adipocytes by repressing PPAR-gamma. Nature 2004;429:771–776.
41. Bitterman KJ, Anderson RM, Cohen HY, Latorre-Esteves M, Sinclair DA. Inhibition of silencing and accelerated aging by nicotinamide, a putative negative regulator of yeast sir2 and human SIRT1. J Biol Chem 2002;277:45,099–45,107.
42. Posakony J, Hirao M, Stevens S, Simon JA, Bedalov A. Inhibitors of Sir2: evaluation of splitomicin analogues. J Med Chem 2004;47:2635–2644.
43. Howitz KT, Bitterman KJ, Cohen HY, et al. Small molecule activators of sirtuins extend *Saccharomyces cerevisiae* lifespan. Nature 2003;425:191–196.
43a. Kaeberlein M, McDonagh T, Heltweg B, et al. Substrate-specific activation of sirtuins by resveratrol. J Biol Chem 2005;280:17,038–17,045.
43b. Borra MT, Smith BC, Denu JM. Mechanism of human SIRT1 activation by resveratrol. J Biol Chem 2005;280:17,187–17,195.
44. Grozinger CM, Chao ED, Blackwell HE, Moazed D, Schreiber SL. Identification of a class of small molecule inhibitors of the sirtuin family of NAD-dependent deacetylases by phenotypic screening. J Biol Chem 2001;276:38,837–38,843.
45. Jackson MD, Schmidt MT, Oppenheimer NJ, Denu JM. Mechanism of nicotinamide inhibition and transglycosidation by Sir2 histone/protein deacetylases. J Biol Chem 2003;278:8807–8814.
46. Sauve AA, Schramm VL. Sir2 regulation by nicotinamide results from switching between base exchange and deacetylation chemistry. Biochemistry 2003;42:9249–9256.
47. Schmidt MT, Smith BC, Jackson MD, Denu JM. Co-enzyme specificity of SIR2 protein deacetylases: implications for physiological regulation. J Biol Chem 2004;279:40,122–40,129.
48. Sauve AA, Schramm VL. SIR2: the biochemical mechanism of NAD(+)-dependent protein deacetylation and ADP-ribosyl enzyme intermediates. Curr Med Chem 2004;11:807–826.

49. Smith JS, Brachmann CB, Celic I, et al. A phylogenetically conserved NAD+-dependent protein deacetylase activity in the Sir2 protein family. Proc Natl Acad Sci U S A 2000;97:6658–6663.

50. Imai S, Armstrong CM, Kaeberlein M, Guarente L. Transcriptional silencing and longevity protein Sir2 is an NAD- dependent histone deacetylase. Nature 2000;403:795–800.

51. Landry J, Sutton A, Tafrov ST, et al. The silencing protein SIR2 and its homologs are NAD-dependent protein deacetylases. Proc Natl Acad Sci U S A 2000;97: 5807–5811.

52. Landry J, Slama JT, Sternglanz R. Role of NAD(+) in the deacetylase activity of the SIR2-like proteins. Biochem Biophys Res Commun 2000;278:685–690.

53. Tanner KG, Landry J, Sternglanz R, Denu JM. Silent information regulator 2 family of NAD- dependent histone/protein deacetylases generates a unique product, 1-O-acetyl-ADP-ribose. Proc Natl Acad Sci U S A 2000;97:14,178–14,182.

54. Tanny JC, Moazed D. Coupling of histone deacetylation to NAD breakdown by the yeast silencing protein Sir2: evidence for acetyl transfer from substrate to an NAD breakdown product. Proc Natl Acad Sci U S A 2001;98:415–420.

55. Borra MT, O'Neill FJ, Jackson MD, et al. Conserved enzymatic production and biological effect of O-acetyl-ADP-ribose by silent information regulator 2-like NAD+-dependent deacetylases. J Biol Chem 2002;277:12,632–12,641.

56. Jackson MD, Denu JM. Structural identification of 2′- and 3′-O-acetyl-ADP-ribose as novel metabolites derived from the Sir2 family of beta-NAD+-dependent histone/protein deacetylases. J Biol Chem 2002;277:18,535–18,544.

57. Sauve AA, Celic I, Avalos J, Deng H, Boeke JD, Schramm VL. Chemistry of gene silencing: the mechanism of NAD+-dependent deacetylation reactions. Biochemistry 2001;40:15,456–15,463.

58. Chang JH, Kim HC, Hwang KY, et al. Structural basis for the NAD-dependent deacetylase mechanism of Sir2. J Biol Chem 2002;277:34,489–34,498.

59. Zhao K, Chai X, Marmorstein R. Structure of the yeast Hst2 protein deacetylase in ternary complex with 2′-O-acetyl ADP ribose and histone peptide. Structure (Camb) 2003;11:1403–1411.

60. Tanny JC, Dowd GJ, Huang J, Hilz H, Moazed D. An enzymatic activity in the yeast Sir2 protein that is essential for gene silencing. Cell 1999;99:735–745.

61. Garcia-Salcedo JA, Gijon P, Nolan DP, Tebabi P, Pays E. A chromosomal SIR2 homologue with both histone NAD-dependent ADP-ribosyltransferase and deacetylase activities is involved in DNA repair in *Trypanosoma brucei*. EMBO J 2003;22:5851–5962.

62. Min J, Landry J, Sternglanz R, Xu RM. Crystal structure of a SIR2 homolog-NAD complex. Cell 2001;105:269–279.

63. Finnin MS, Donigian JR, Pavletich NP. Structure of the histone deacetylase SIRT2. Nat Struct Biol 2001;8:621–625.

64. Avalos JL, Celic I, Muhammad S, Cosgrove MS, Boeke JD, Wolberger C. Structure of a Sir2 enzyme bound to an acetylated p53 peptide. Mol Cell 2002;10:523–535.

65. Zhao K, Chai X, Clements A, Marmorstein R. Structure and autoregulation of the yeast Hst2 homolog of Sir2. Nat Struct Biol 2003;10:864–871.

66. Zhao K, Chai X, Marmorstein R. Structure and substrate binding properties of cobB, a Sir2 homolog protein deacetylase from *Escherichia coli*. J Mol Biol 2004;337:731–741.

67. Avalos JL, Boeke JD, Wolberger C. Structural basis for the mechanism and regulation of Sir2 enzymes. Mol Cell 2004;13:639–648.

68. Zhao K, Harshaw R, Chai X, Marmorstein R. Structural basis for nicotinamide cleavage and ADP-ribose transfer by NAD+-dependent Sir2 histone/protein deacetylases. Proc Natl Acad Sci U S A 2004;101:8563–8568.

69. Borra MT, Langer MR, Slama JT, Denu JM. Substrate specificity and kinetic mechanism of the Sir2 family of NAD+-dependent histone/protein deacetylases. Biochemistry 2004;43:9877–9887.

70. Braunstein M, Sobel RE, Allis CD, Turner BM, Broach JR. Efficient transcriptional silencing in *Saccharomyces cerevisiae* requires a heterochromatin histone acetylation pattern. Mol Cell Biol 1996;16:4349–4356.

71. Denu JM. Linking chromatin function with metabolic networks: Sir2 family of NAD(+)-dependent deacetylases. Trends Biochem Sci 2003;28:41–48.

72. Moazed D. Enzymatic activities of Sir2 and chromatin silencing. Curr Opin Cell Biol 2001;13:232–238.

73. Moazed D. Common themes in mechanisms of gene silencing. Mol Cell 2001;8:489–498.

74. Starai VJ, Takahashi H, Boeke JD, Escalante-Semerena JC. A link between transcription and intermediary metabolism: a role for Sir2 in the control of acetyl-coenzyme A synthetase. Curr Opin Microbiol 2004;7:115–119.

75. Gottschling DE. Gene silencing: two faces of SIR2. Curr Biol 2000;10: R708–R711.

76. Anderson RM, Bitterman KJ, Wood JG, et al. Manipulation of a nuclear NAD+ salvage pathway delays aging without altering steady-state NAD+ levels. J Biol Chem 2002;277:18,881–18,890.

77. Lin SJ, Ford E, Haigis M, Liszt G, Guarente L. Calorie restriction extends yeast life span by lowering the level of NADH. Genes Dev 2004;18:12–16.

78. Bedalov A, Gatbonton T, Irvine WP, Gottschling DE, Simon JA. Identification of a small molecule inhibitor of Sir2p. Proc Natl Acad Sci U S A 2001;98: 15,113–15,118.

11 The Class III Protein Deacetylases

Homologs of Yeast Sir2p

Bjoern Schwer, MD,
Brian J. North, PhD,
Nidhi Ahuja, PhD, Brett Marshall,
and Eric Verdin, MD

SUMMARY

Sirtuins are NAD-dependent protein deacetylases found in organisms ranging from bacteria to humans that share sequence homology with the yeast transcriptional regulator Sir2. In eukaryotes, sirtuins regulate

The first two authors contributed equally to this review.

From: *Cancer Drug Discovery and Development*
Histone Deacetylases: Transcriptional Regulation and Other Cellular Functions
Edited by: E. Verdin © Humana Press Inc., Totowa, NJ

237

Acronyms and Abbreviations

Abf1	ARS-binding factor 1 protein
Age-1	AGEing alteration family member 1
Bax	BCL2-associated X protein
Daf-2	Abnormal dauer formation family member 2
GCN5	General control of amino-acid synthesis 5
Hap4	Subunit of the heme-activated, glucose-repressed Hap2p/3p/4p/5p CCAAT-binding complex
HES1	Hairy and enhancer of split 1
HEY2	Hairy/enhancer-of-split related with YRPW motif 2
HRAS1	Harvey rat sarcoma virus oncogene 1
MyoD	Myogenic differentiation 1
Net1p	Nucleolar protein involved in exit from mitosis; protein 1
Orc	Origin recognition complex
PGC-1-α	Peroxisome proliferative activated receptor, gamma, coactivator 1, α
PML	Promyelocytic leukemia
PNC1	Pyrazinamidase/nicotinamidase 1
Rap1	Repressor activator protein 1
RelA	v-rel reticuloendotheliosis viral oncogene homolog A
SRC-1	Steroid receptor coactivator-1
TAF	TBP-associated transcription factor family member
Tat	Transactivating regulatory protein

transcriptional repression, recombination, cell cycle division, microtubule organization, and cellular responses to DNA-damaging agents. Sir2 proteins have also been implicated in regulating the molecular mechanisms of aging. Eukaryotic sirtuins contain a core catalytic domain and variable amino- and carboxyl-terminal extensions that regulate their subcellular localizations and catalytic activity. This review focuses on the diverse subcellular distribution, substrate specificity, and cellular functions of sirtuins with particular emphasis on the biology of mammalian sirtuins.

Key Words: Sirtuins, aging, metabolism, mitochondria.

INTRODUCTION

The silent information regulator (Sir) gene family was first identified in the yeast *Saccharomyces cerevisiae*, in which a mutation in Sir1, *sir1-1*, suppressed the mating and sporulation defects of all mutations present in the mating-type loci *(1)*. In further studies, four separate genes named

Sir1, Sir2, Sir3, and Sir4 were isolated that complemented Sir mutations in vivo *(2–4)*. Two decades following their initial characterization, the enzymatic activity of Sir2p was identified as a histone deacetylase, an activity required for the silencing observed for Sir2p-controlled loci *(5–7)*. A uniquely intriguing aspect of Sir2p-mediated histone deacetylase activity is the requirement of the cofactor nicotinamide adenine dinucleotide (NAD) for Sir2p action. Here we review what has been learned in past years about the biology of Sir2 proteins in several experimental model systems.

S. CEREVISIAE SIR2 AND HOMOLOGS OF SIR2

The yeast genome contains Sir2 and four other closely related open reading frames, called homolog of sir2 (HST). These proteins play critical roles in transcriptional silencing at several unique loci in the yeast genome.

Sir2p at the HML/HMR *Locus*

Haploid *S. cerevisiae* can be one of two different mating types. The genetic determinants that define the mating type for a given yeast cell are found in the mating-type locus (*MAT* locus). Cells with the *MAT*α allele have the α mating type, and cells with the *MAT*a allele have the a mating type. Cells of different mating types can mate or fuse, to generate a diploid cell. When diploid cells are starved, they sporulate, forming four haploid spores, each of which can germinate when supplied with sufficient nutrients, regenerating haploid cells. Two additional loci are found on chromosome III of the *S. cerevisiae* genome, termed *HML* and *HMR*, which contain the necessary and sufficient genetic information required to direct each of the two different mating types. The *HML* and *HMR* loci are nontranscribed and are thus termed silent mating-type loci. These loci can be transferred to the *MAT* locus via a unique type of recombination termed gene conversion, allowing cells to change mating types during each generation *(8)*. The *sir1-1* suppressor mutant was identified because of its ability to suppress the mating and sporulation defects of all mutations found in the *MAT* loci, suggesting that it was involved in repression of the cryptic silent mating type loci *(1)*.

The Sir proteins were further characterized for their ability to mediate transcriptional repression at *HMR* and *HML (4)*. Strains harboring mutations in *SIR2*, *SIR3*, and *SIR4* are defective in silencing at both *HML* and *HMR*, whereas mutations in *SIR1* only partially reduce silencing at these loci. A heteromeric protein complex containing Sir1p, Sir2p, Sir3p, and Sir4p is localized at the silent mating-type loci and is recruited via an interaction with a complex of DNA binding proteins comprising Rap1, Orc, and Abf1 *(9–11)*. A model has been proposed in which the Sir2/3/4 complex is recruited for nucleation by DNA binding factors and Sir1p, upon which Sir2p will deacetylate histones within the neighboring nucleosome, allowing for recruitment of a new Sir2/3/4 complex to this nucleosome via the Sir3p/Sir4p interaction with the newly hypoacetylated histones *(12–16)*. This cycle of deacetylation followed by recruitment continues across the loci *(17,18)*. The silenced region is associated with nucleosome hypoacetylation and displays features of a heterochromatin-like structure *(15,19,20)*.

Telomeres

Telomeres are protein-DNA complexes formed at the ends of chromosomes that are important for chromosomal end stability; they also promote organization of chromosomes within the nucleus *(21)*. In *S. cerevisiae*, telomeric DNA consists of $C_{1–3}A/TG_{1–3}$ repeats that are approx 300 bp in length. These repeats are organized into a nonnucleosomal chromatin structure termed the telosome *(22)*. A transient form of silencing termed telomere position effect, characterized as a stochastic alternation between transcriptional silencing and activation in a telomere distal distance-dependent manner, is found at yeast telomeres *(23)*. Similar to the silent mating-type loci, telomeric silencing requires Sir2p, Sir3p, and Sir4p but not Sir1p *(23)*. Sir proteins are components of the telosome and may be recruited by Sir4p interaction with $C_{1–3}A/TG_{1–3}$ repeats *(24)*.

Another mechanism mediating Sir complex recruitment to the telomeres involves interaction with the telomere-repeat binding protein Rap1p *(11,25,26)*. The stepwise model of spreading heterochromatin across the telomere is thought to be similar to what is observed at the silent mating-type loci. Telomeric silencing also requires Ku70/80, a DNA binding protein involved in nonhomologous end joining (NHEJ) during DNA double-strand break repair *(27)*. In yeast, Ku is localized primarily at telomeres, and Ku-deficient strains lose telomere silencing by relocalization of the Sir complex *(27–30)*. The Ku proteins are a component of the DNA-dependent protein kinase, which is involved in NHEJ. Upon DNA damage, the Sir proteins relocalize to the sites of DNA damage in a Ku70/80-dependent manner *(28,29)*. The role of Sir protein-mediated histone deacetylation during NHEJ is not clear. The heterochromatic environment surrounding a DNA break and created under the influence of Sir proteins may enhance the accuracy of the repair process. Further studies in both yeast and higher organisms are necessary to define the Ku70/80/Sir complex interaction more completely.

rDNA

The nucleolus, the site of rRNA transcription and ribosomal assembly, is the third known site of action of Sir2p function in yeast *(31,32)*. The nucleolus contains the ribosomal DNA (rDNA) array, encoding the 35S and the

5S ribosomal RNA, and consists of a 9-kb unit tandemly repeated 100 to 200 times on chromosome 12. Sir2p-mediated alterations in chromatin structure at the rDNA array suppress homologous recombination among the tandemly repeated rDNA copies. In addition, Sir2p silences transcription of RNA polymerase II-dependent marker genes inserted within the rDNA array (31–34). Sir2p is recruited to the nucleolus independently of Sir3p and Sir4p via its interaction with the regulator of nucleolar silencing and telophase exit (RENT) complex, containing Net1p, and a telophase-regulating phosphatase, Cdc14p, which is released in late metaphase (35,36).

Homologs of Sir2 (HST)

In addition to *SIR2*, *S. cerevisiae* has four homologs of Sir2 (HST) genes. Of these, Hst1p is the most closely related to Sir2p and also localizes predominantly in the nucleus. HST1 overexpression restores transcriptional silencing in a sir2 mutant, suggesting that the homology is significant enough for Hst1p to be incorporated into the same complexes as Sir2p (37). However, Hst1p represses the expression of genes involved in NAD biosynthesis via its NAD-dependent histone deacetylase activity, a gene subset that is not targeted by Sir2p. A decrease in cellular NAD levels leads to reduced enzymatic activity of Hst1p, therefore allowing the derepression of genes involved in NAD biosynthesis and a subsequent increase in cellular NAD levels (38).

Hst2p is distinct from Sir2p and Hst1p in yeast, and phylogenetic analysis suggests that it is the closest homolog to the human SIRT2 and SIRT3 proteins. Hst2p, which also possesses NAD-dependent deacetylase activity, shows a predominantly cytoplasmic localization, similar to the human SIRT2 protein (39–41). However, although Hst2p is found in the cytoplasm, it functions as a transcriptional silencer (39). In contrast to Hst1p, Hst2p does not restore silencing in a Sir2 deletion mutant. However, overexpression of Hst2p leads to a derepression of telomeric silencing while increasing silencing at the rDNA locus (39). Hst2p and Sir2p could compete for a substrate or ligand required for Sir2p to perform silencing functions at the telomere but not the rDNA array (39).

Hst3p and Hst4p are more distantly related to Sir2p and do not have any close orthologs in mammals. In yeast, Hst3/Hst4 double mutants are defective in telomeric silencing (37). In addition, HST3 and HST4 together contribute to proper cell cycle progression, radiation resistance, and genomic stability, thereby establishing new connections between silencing and these fundamental cellular processes (37).

Role in Yeast Aging

Aging in *S. cerevisiae* occurs, at least in part, as a result of recombination between rDNA repeats, which can lead to the excision of extrachromosomal rDNA circles (ERCs). An autonomous replicating sequence (ARC) within the rDNA array allows ERCs to replicate. In addition, ERCs are preferentially segregated to mother cells during cell division. ERCs can accumulate in old cells, causing a DNA content greater than that of the entire yeast genome, and are thought to cause cell death by titrating out essential transcription and/or replication factors (42). As described earlier, Sir2p functions in S. cerevisiae in transcriptional repression at the telomeres, silent mating-type loci, and both transcriptional and recombinational repression at the rDNA array. This latter activity, i.e., suppression of recombination at the rDNA array, might be how Sir2p modulates yeast aging (33,34).

A screen search for long-lived yeast cells identified a mutant form of Sir4, termed Sir4-42. This mutant caused a relocalization of the Sir2/3/4 complex from the telomeres and silent mating-type loci to the rDNA array, in effect locally increasing the dosage of Sir2p at the rDNA array (43). Relocalization of the Sir2/3/4 complex to the nucleolus occurs naturally in aging wild-type cells; however, the Sir4-42 allele caused a premature relocalization of the Sir complex in young yeast cells (43). Deletion of Sir2 eliminates rDNA silencing, increases the frequency with which a marker gene is recombined out of the rDNA, and results in a shortened life span (44). Furthermore, recent work suggests that the Sir2/3/4 complex also suppresses ERCs via the transcriptional repression of α mating-type genes. Deletion of Sir3 or Sir4 results in transcriptional derepression at the silencing mating-type loci and coexpression of genes responsible for the a and α mating-types. This results in an increase in RAD52-mediated recombination at the rDNA array (44). These data suggest that both nucleolar Sir2p (the RENT complex) and the Sir2/3/4 complex at the mating-type loci function to increase life span by regulation of rDNA recombination and ERC formation.

Calorie Restriction

For more than 60 years, reduction of caloric intake has been known to extend life span in a wide variety of organisms. Calorie restriction is a dietary regimen in which organisms are fed 30 to 50% less calories than normal. The mechanism underlying the increased life span in response to calorie restriction remains elusive, although a reduction in reactive oxygen species and decreased blood glucose and insulin levels have been proposed as potential mechanisms (45). Growth of yeast cells in 0.5% glucose, instead of the routine 2% glucose, results in a significant life span extension (46). In addition, a yeast strain carrying a deletion of hexokinase, HXK2, which carries one of the first steps of glycolysis, also shows life span extension, even when grown in normal glucose concentrations (46). The observed life span extension mediated by low glucose levels (i.e., caloric restriction) is not found in a strain lacking Sir2p (47).

Furthermore, life span extension mediated by caloric restriction also requires NAD, as strains lacking NPT1 and other components of the NAD synthesis pathway do not display life span extension *(47)*. Caloric restriction also leads to an increase in respiration, which drives NAD production through the electron transport chain *(46)*. More NAD, or a higher NAD/NADH ratio, will result in an increase in Sir2 activity. In support of this model, strains of yeast having high levels of HAP4, a transcription factor that activates a number of respiratory genes, show both an increase in respiration and an increase in life span *(46)*. Similar to caloric restriction, this life span extension is also dependent on Sir2p *(46)*. Further complicating this issue, a recent study has demonstrated the existence of a Sir2-independent pathway responsible for most of the longevity benefit associated with calorie restriction *(48,49)*.

NAD/NADH Ratio

Caloric restriction presumably alters Sir2p activity via changes in the cellular NAD/NADH ratio. As discussed above, the extension of life span induced by caloric restriction appears to be dependent on increased respiration. Calorie restriction is associated with a shunting of carbon metabolism from fermentation to the mitochondrial TCA cycle with a concomitant increase in respiration leading to the oxidation of NADH to NAD. Measurement of NAD and NADH levels in cells grown on either 2.0% or 0.5% glucose showed decreased NADH levels and unchanged NAD levels, increasing the NAD/NADH ratio *(50)*. Furthermore, NADH is a competitive inhibitor of Sir2, implying that a reduction in NADH levels would also result in increased Sir2p activity *(50)*. Overexpression of two NADH dehydrogenases, Nde1 and Nde2, specifically lowered NADH levels without influencing NAD levels but still resulted in an extended life span *(50)*. These observations indicate that the NAD/NADH ratio, rather than the absolute NAD level, controls Sir2 activity.

Nicotinamide

A second model for how caloric restriction results in altered levels of Sir2p activity is by regulating cellular nicotinamide levels. Nicotinamide is produced from NAD by cleavage of the glycosidic bond by Sir2 proteins *(51)*. Nicotinamide acts as a strong noncompetitive inhibitor by binding to a site near NAD in the Sir2 enzyme, thereby blocking NAD hydrolysis. Thus, changes in nicotinamide levels could alter the level of Sir2p activity *(51,52)*. Cells grown in the presence of nicotinamide show a loss of Sir2p-mediated silencing and a life span decrease that mimicks that found in a *Sir2* mutant *(52)*. Nicotinamide is converted back into NAD in a multistep process during an NAD-salvage pathway (Fig. 1) The enzyme PNC1 functions in this NAD salvage pathway to convert nicotinamide

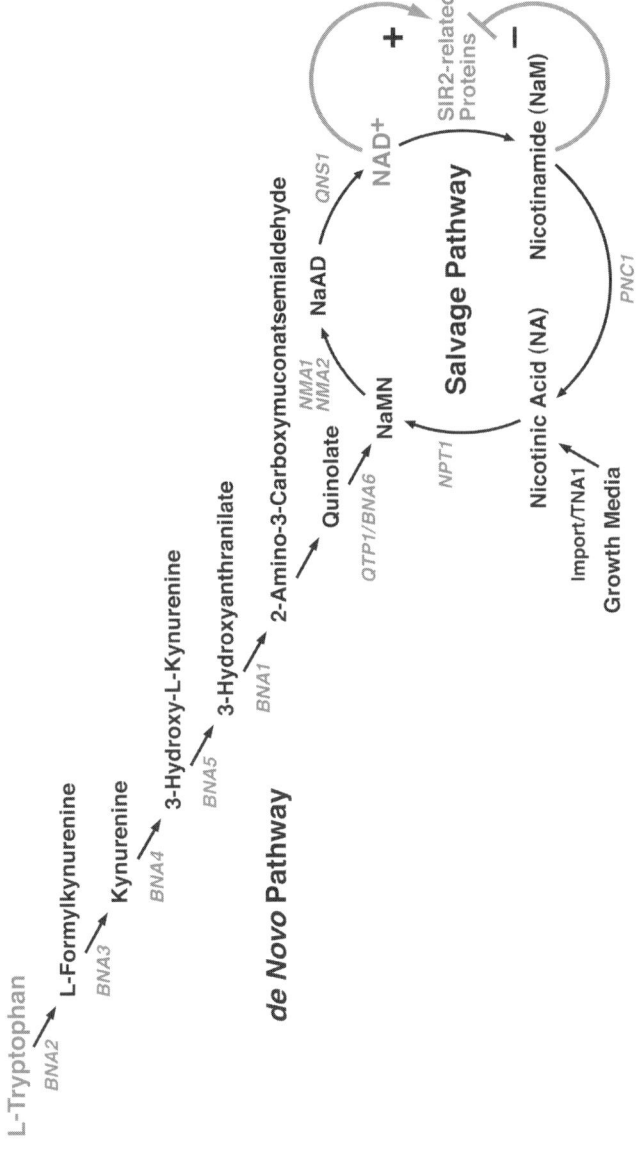

into nicotinic acid. Overexpression of *PNC1* is associated with an increase in life span that is dependent on Sir2 *(53)*. Furthermore, a strain lacking PNC1, which should have increased levels of nicotinamide and low Sir2 activity, showed no extended life span in response to caloric restriction *(53)*. Interestingly, calorie restriction leads to increased PNC1 levels, decreased cellular levels of nicotinamide, and increased Sir2p activity *(53)*. These experiments strengthened the hypothesis that both NAD and nicotinamide levels control life span, at least in part via Sir2 activity *(53,54)*.

SIRTUINS IN BACTERIA AND ARCHAE

As discussed in Chapter 8, sirtuin orthologs are found in bacteria and archae. Although this review focuses primarily on other organisms, these proteins are briefly discussed below.

Acetate and propionate are short-chain fatty acids, which are used as carbon and energy sources by prokaryotes. CobB, a bacterial sirtuin, controls the activity of both acetyl- and propionyl-coenzyme A synthetase in *Salmonella*. CobB-deficient strains of *Salmonella enterica* undergo growth arrest when grown in the presence of acetate *(55)*. In the absence of CobB, residue K609 of the *S. enterica* acetyl-CoA synthetase (ACS) is acetylated. Since acetylation of Lys-609 inhibits the adenylating activity of this enzyme, the CobB-deficient strains cannot produce acetyl-CoA from acetate. CobB deacetylates ACS on Lys-609 and thereby activates ACS in an NAD-dependent fashion. Both human SIRT1 and yeast Sir2 protein restore the ability of Sir2-deficient *S. enterica* to grow on acetate and propionate *(56)*. Like acetate, propionate has to be activated before

---

Fig. 1. Biosynthetic pathways for NAD. NAD can be synthesized *de novo* starting from tryptophan or recycled in a salvage pathway. When NAD is utilized as a cofactor by a sirtuin, nicotinamide is produced and recycled using the salvage pathway. Several enzymes that control distinct steps of the salvage pathway play a role in the genetic control of life span. Enzymes involved in the *de novo* pathway convert L-tryptophan to nicotinic acid mononucleotide (NaMN). These reactions are catalyzed by several enzymes in the BNA (biosynthesis of nicotinic acid) group. Specific names for individual BNA enzymes are: BNA2, tryptophan 2,3-dioxygenase; BNA3, arylformamidase; BNA4, kynurenine 3-monooxygenase; BNA5, kynureninase; BNA1, 3-hydroxyanthranilic acid dioxygenase; and QTP1/BNA6, quinolinate phosphoryibosyl transferase. Enzymes involved in the salvage pathway are called NMA1 and NMA2 (nicotinic acid mononucleotide adenylyltransferase 1 and 2); QNS1, glutamine-dependent NAD+ synthase; TNA1, transporter of nicotinic acid; NPT1, nicotinate phosphoribosyl transferase; and PNC1, nicotinamidase. Intermediates in the NAD biosynthesis pathway are NaMN and NaAD (nicotinic acid adenine dinucleotide).

it can be converted into metabolites suitable for central metabolism. This reaction is performed by propionyl-CoA synthetase, and acetylation of Lys592 of this enzyme abrogates the adenylation activity of the enzyme *(55,57)*.

The crenarchaeon *Sulfolobus solfataricus* P2 genome also encodes a sirtuin homolog, called ssSir2, which doubles as an NAD-dependent deacetylase and a mono-ADP-ribosyltransferase *(58,59)*. The acetylated archaeal chromatin protein Alba interacts with ssSir2. The deacetylation of Alba by ssSir2 results in increased DNA binding activity and transcriptional repression in a reconstituted in vitro transcription system *(58)*.

C. ELEGANS SIRTUINS

There are four orthologs to Sir2p in the nematode *C. elegans*. Genetic studies have implicated Sir-2.1, the closest ortholog to yeast Sir2p, in the insulin/insulin-like growth factor 1 (IGF-1)-like endocrine system.

IGF-1 Pathway/Sir2.1

Upon induction of insulin signaling, activation of the insulin/IGF-1 receptor daf-2 activates the phosphatidylinositol-3-OH kinase/phosphoinositide-dependent kinase-1/Akt signal transduction pathway (Fig. 2). Activation of this pathway leads to phosphorylation of Daf-16, a Forkhead transcription factor, resulting in its sequestration in the cytoplasm *(25)*. Sir-2.1 appears to play a role in the Daf-2 pathway, and its effect requires a functional Daf-16; however, the molecular interplay between Sir-2.1 and the Daf pathway is not clear *(60)*. The mammalian Sir2 protein SIRT1 also regulates the activity of forkhead transcription factors in mammalian cells (*see* Mammalian Sirtuins below), suggesting that these interactions are conserved across species.

Role in C. elegans *Aging*

A link between aging and the IGF-1 pathway has been demonstrated at many levels (Fig. 2). Knock-down experiments utilizing RNA interference (RNAi) for the suspected ligand for Daf-2 (Ceinsulin-1) cause an extension of life span *(61)*. Mutations in Daf-2 leading to a reduction in expression, and reduced signaling through the receptor, also result in extended life span *(62,63)*. Reduction-of-function mutations within the insulin/IGF-1 signaling cascade including age-1 (a phosphatidylinositol-3-OH kinase) and phosphoinositide-dependent kinase-1 result in a significant extension in life span *(64,65)*. As observed in yeast, an extra copy of Sir-2.1 in *C. elegans* significantly extends the span, which also requires a functional Daf-16 *(60)* (Fig. 2). By regulating the insulin-like signaling pathway, Sir-2.1 may also enhance dauer formation *(60)*. The dauer larvae are a specialized

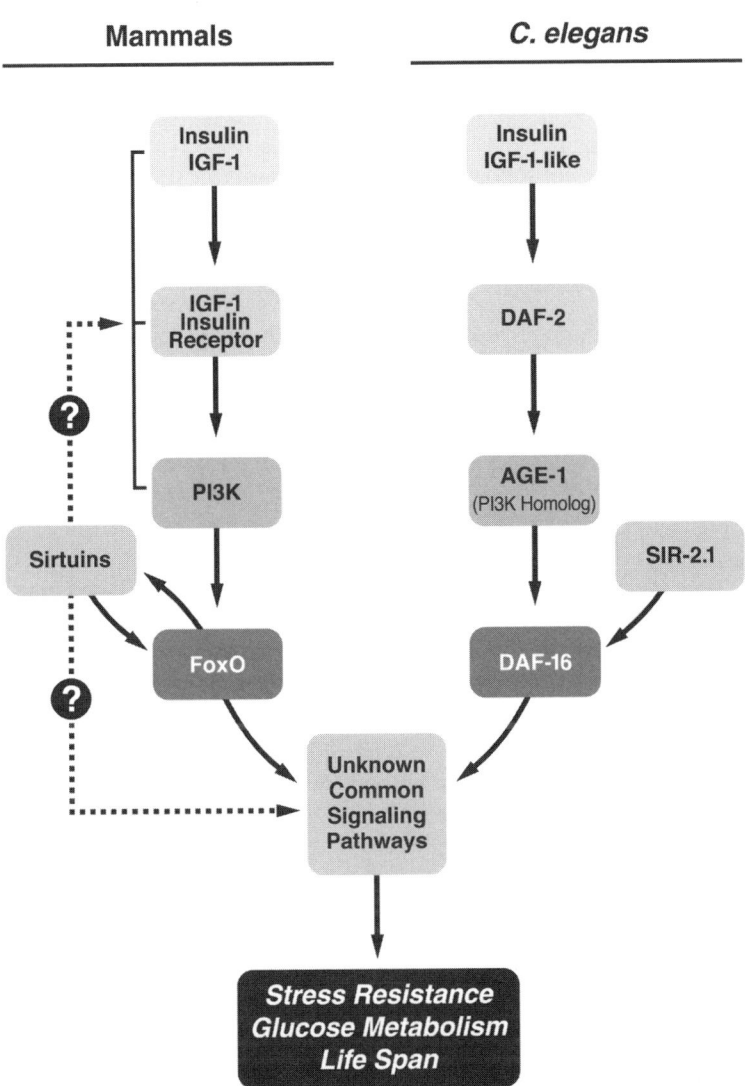

Fig. 2. Conserved genetic pathways could impact life span and age-related diseases in *C. elegans* and mammals. The insulin-like growth factor-1 (IGF-1) like pathway has been defined in *C. elegans* as a major pathway controlling aging in this organism. Sirtuins might control aging by modifying factors in this pathway, including DAF-16 and the FOXO proteins. PI3K, phosphatidylinositol 3'-kinase; FOXO, forkhead box-containing protein, O subfamily; DAF-2, abnormal dauer formation family member 2; SIR-2.1, silent information regulator 2.1; AGE-1, AGEing alteration family member 1.

survival form of the worm; however, the molecular mechanisms by which Sir-2.1 controls dauer formation remains to be elucidated.

DROSOPHILA SIRTUINS

There are five homologs to Sir2p in *Drosophila*. dSir2 is the closest homolog to yeast Sir2p and functions as a histone deacetylase toward all four acetylatable K residues of histone H4 *(66)*. Unlike Sir2p in yeast, dSir2 is not required for silencing at telomeres but is required for heterochromatic silencing *(67)*. dSir2 interacts genetically and physically with members of the Hairy/Deadpan/E(Spl) family of basic helix-loop-helix (bHLH) euchromatin repressors, which are key regulators of *Drosophila* development *(67)*. dSir2 also interacts with the histone acetyltransferase cyclic AMP-responsive element binding protein (CBP) *(68)*. However, contradictory reports have been published on the role of dSir2 in various physiological processes. dSir2 may be an essential gene whose loss of function results in both segmentation defects and skewed sex ratios, associated with reduced activities of the Hairy and Deadpan bHLH repressors *(67)*. In a contrasting report, knockout of dSir2 has no developmental or sex ratio defects; however, these mutants do have reduced life span *(69)*. In a third report, dSir2 had a minor role in position effect variegation, similar to its yeast counterpart; however, this study indicates that dSir2 does not appear to have a function in regulation of life span *(68)*. Further studies of the role for dSir2 are needed to understand the role of Sir2 in *Drosophila* transcriptional silencing and development.

MAMMALIAN SIRTUINS

Seven distinct Sir2 homologs have been identified in humans and are called SIRT1 to 7. Protein deacetylase activity has been reported for SIRT1, -2, -3, and -5, whereas SIRT4, -6, and -7 have no detectable enzymatic activity on a histone peptide substrate *(41)*.

SIRT1

SUBCELLULAR LOCALIZATION

SIRT1 is the most homologous mammalian sirtuin to yeast Sir2p and is also an NAD-dependent deacetylase primarily found in the nucleus *(7,70–74)*. A uniform nuclear localization is observed, but the endogenous and overexpressed SIRT1 is partially recruited to PML bodies upon overexpression of PML IV protein or expression of oncogenic Ras, an upstream regulator of PML *(75)*. Although the direct role of PML bodies in nuclear activity is presently unclear, they are implicated in the regulation of transcription, tumor suppression, and apoptosis. In some cell types, however, the endogenous SIRT1 displays a cytoplasmic localization, indicating that the functions of SIRT1 may not be entirely restricted to the nucleus (S. Imai, personal communication).

INTERACTING FACTORS
TAF$_I$68

TAF$_I$68, a subunit of the promoter selectivity factor TIF-IB/SL1, was the first target to be reported for murine SIRT1 *(76)*. The TIF-IB/SL1 complex mediates the recruitment of RNA polymerase I to the rDNA promoter and transcription initiation. TAF$_I$68 is acetylated in vitro by p300/CBP-associated factor (PCAF), a modification that enhances its binding to the rDNA promoter and stimulates rDNA transcription. SIRT1 deacetylates TAF$_I$68 in an NAD-dependent manner in vitro and in the context of the purified TIF-IB complex. SIRT1 interaction with TAF$_I$68 leads to the repression of RNA polymerase I transcription, a situation similar to that in yeast, in which Sir2p is involved in gene silencing at mating-type loci, telomeres, and the rDNA locus *(77)*.

p53

The tumor suppressor protein p53 is acetylated by the coactivator CBP/p300 on multiple Ks (positions 370, 372, 373, 381, and 382) *(78,79)*. Acetylation stimulates the transcriptional activation activity of p53 by enhancing protein stability, cofactor recruitment, and DNA binding *(80)*. Human and mouse SIRT1 can specifically deacetylate K382 of p53 *(71,72,75)*. SIRT1 physically interacts with p53 in the nucleus *(72)*, and this interaction is enhanced after induction of DNA damage *(71)*. Acetylation of p53 results in the activation of p53 target genes such as p21, resulting in cell cycle arrest, apoptosis, or senescence. Conversely, deacetylation of p53 by SIRT1 decreases p53-mediated transcriptional activation *(71,72,75)*. The consequence of SIRT1 action is the suppression of apoptosis induced by DNA damage or oxidative stress. Accordingly, mice homozygous for a deleted SIRT1 allele show hyperacetylated p53 after DNA damage and increased ionizing radiation-induced thymocyte apoptosis *(81)*. A separately derived SIRT1 knockout mouse strain showed defects in spermatogenesis with increased apoptosis in the testes *(82)*, possibly through modulation of p53 function.

PML IV

PML, a tumor suppressor implicated in leukemia and cancer pathogenesis and a structural component of nuclear bodies (or PODs, PML bodies), is critical to the recruitment of a number of proteins to nuclear bodies, including SIRT1 and p53 *(75)*. SIRT1 overexpression overcomes the growth arrest induced by PML IV overexpression, whereas overexpression of a catalytically inactive SIRT1 mutant (H363Y) partially relieves the PML IV-induced growth arrest *(75)*.

RelA/p65

The nuclear factor-κB (NFκB) complex is composed of p50 and RelA/p65 subunits and is sequestered in the cytoplasm through its interaction with the inhibitory family of IκB proteins *(83)*. Stimulus-induced phosphorylation of the IκBs results in translocation of the NF-κB heterodimer to the nucleus *(83)*. NF-κB controls the expression of genes involved in the cell cycle, apoptosis, and other important cellular processes *(84)*. NF-κB interacts with several acetyltransferases such as CBP, its homolog p300, and PCAF *(85–87)*. The acetyltransferases SRC-1 and p300 acetylate the p50 and RelA/p65 subunits of NF-κB *(71,85,88)* and modify its DNA binding activity and transcriptional activity *(89,90)*. SIRT1 directly interacts with RelA/p65 and inhibits its transcriptional activity by deacetylating K310 *(91)*. Since NF-κB exerts an antiapoptotic effect during tumor necrosis factor-α (TNF-α) activation, inhibition of NF-κB-mediated gene activation by SIRT1 sensitizes cells to apoptosis during TNF-α treatment. RelA/p65 can also be deacetylated by HDAC1, HDAC2, and HDAC3. Deacetylation of RelA/p65 by these class I histone deacetylases increases its interaction with the inhibitory IκBα and reduces the transcactivation potential of RelA/p65 *(71,88,92)*.

CTIP2

Endogenous SIRT1 and chicken ovalbumin upstream promotor transcription-factor-interacting protein 2 (CTIP2) copurify from human nuclear extracts, and both proteins interact directly in vivo and in vitro *(93)*. CTIP2 represses transcription through its sequence-specific DNA binding activity. The transcriptional repression and deacetylation of promoter-bound histones H3/H4 observed upon CTIP2 transfection is reversed by nicotinamide treatment. Exogenous SIRT1 increases both transcriptional repression and histone H3/H4 deacetylation in CTIP2-transfected cells. These observations indicate that specific transcription factors such as CTIP2 can recruit SIRT1 to promoters where it mediates gene silencing via histone deacetylation *(93)*.

HES1 and HEY2

Members of the bHLH transcription factor family are important developmental activators or repressors *(94,95)*. Two members of the bHLH family, HES1 and HEY2, interact with SIRT1 *(96)*. HES1 is the mammalian ortholog of the *Drosophila* Hairy protein, which interacts with the *Drosophila* Sir2 protein *(67)*. SIRT1 enhances the transcriptional repression activities of HES1 and HEY2, but the mechanism accounting for this effect is not understood.

Histone H1

Immunopurification of overexpressed SIRT1 from nuclear extracts led to the copurification of histone H1b *(73)*. This interaction is mediated by the N terminus of SIRT1. Histone H1 is acetylated in vivo on K26 and can be specifically deacetylated by SIRT1 in vitro *(73)*. The interaction between histone H1 and SIRT1 may participate in the establishment of heterochromatin.

PCAF, p300, and GCN5

SIRT1 directly interacts with the acetyltransferases p300 and PCAF *(97,98)* and reduces the acetylation of PCAF *(97)*. The conserved domain of SIRT1 is necessary and sufficient for its interaction with PCAF *(97)*. SIRT1 can be coimmunoprecipitated with both forms of hGCN5 (hGCN5-L and hGCN5-S) *(97)*. It remains to be established whether SIRT1 interacts with CBP, a transcriptional cofactor related to p300; however, the *Drosophila* Sir2 protein associates with the *Drosophila* CBP ortholog *(68)*.

Ku70

Ku70 is a subunit of the Ku protein complex involved in nonhomologous repair of DNA double-strand breaks *(99)*. Ku70 also serves as a cytosolic retention factor for the proapoptotic Bax protein *(100)*. Ku70 is acetylated in vivo by CBP and PCAF at *K*s 539 and 542 in response to cell damage or stress. This acetylation causes Bax to dissociate from Ku70 and to translocate to mitochondria, where it participates in the induction of the apoptotic cascade *(101)*. SIRT1 and Ku70 physically interact in vivo, and overexpression of SIRT1 decreases the acetylation level of Ku70, thereby promoting the antiapoptotic Bax-Ku70 interaction *(102)*.

FOXO1, 3, and 4

Members of the FOXO family of transcription factors (Forkhead box-containing protein, O subfamily) are involved in cellular processes that range from longevity, metabolism, and reproduction in *C. elegans* to regulation of gene transcription downstream from insulin, cell cycle arrest, apoptosis, and stress responses in mammalian cells. Mammalian cells have four FOXO protein: FOXO1, FOXO3, FOXO4, and FOXO6. The acetyltransferases p300 and CBP interact with FOXO proteins (FOXO1, 3, and 4), mediate their acetylation, and function as their transcriptional coactivators *(98,103–107)*. SIRT1 interacts with FOXO proteins and deacetylates FOXO1, FOXO3, and FOXO4 *(98,104–106)*.

NCoR/SMRT

The recent observation that SIRT1 interacts with and represses peroxisome proliferator-activated receptor-γ (PPAR-γ) establishes a functional link between SIRT1 and lipid metabolism *(108)*. PPAR-γ is a member of the nuclear receptor superfamily and integrates the control of energy, lipid metabolism, and glucose homeostasis. Both nuclear receptor corepressor (NCoR) and silencing mediator of retinoid and thyroid hormone receptors (SMRT) are PPAR-γ corepressors and interact with SIRT1. These interactions suggest that SIRT1 represses PPAR-γ activity by interacting with its corepressors. Whether SIRT1 deacetylates PPAR-γ directly is presently unclear *(108)*.

HIV Tat Transactivator

The human immunodeficiency virus (HIV) Tat protein is a transcriptional activator of the HIV promoter. Tat is acetylated on a single residue, lysine-50, by the transcriptional coactivator p300, and Tat and p300 synergize to activate the HIV promoter *(109–116)*. The opposite reaction, Tat deacetylation, is mediated by human SIRT1 in vitro and in vivo *(117)*. Tat and SIRT1 coimmunoprecipitate, and, paradoxically, SIRT synergistically activates the HIV promoter with Tat. Conversely, knockdown of SIRT1 via small interfering RNAs (siRNAs) inhibits Tat-mediated transactivation of the HIV long terminal repeat. Treatment with a splitomicin analog (HR73) that specifically inhibits SIRT1 also inhibits Tat-mediated transactivation *(117)*. Tat transactivation is defective in SIRT1-null mouse embryonic fibroblasts and can be rescued by expression of SIRT1. A model is proposed that involves a role for SIRT1 in the recycling of Tat to its unacetylated state, a form of Tat that is necessary to initiate its transcriptional activity on the HIV promoter *(117)*.

BIOLOGY OF SIRT1

Transcriptional Regulation by SIRT1

SIRT1 directly deacetylates K16 of histone H4 and K9 of histone H3, and inhibition of SIRT1 expression leads to hyperacetylation of both residues *(73)*. Acetylated K16 is a mark for euchromatin, whereas heterochromatin is hypoacetylated in K16 *(118,119)*. SIRT1 also interacts with histone H1, deacetylates its K26, and leads to heterochromatin formation *(73)*.

Several transcription factors appear to target SIRT1 to chromatin. Chromatin immunoprecipitation experiments indicate that SIRT1 is bound to the promoters of genes involved in skeletal muscle differentiation *(97)*. There, SIRT1 probably mediates the deacetylation of K9 and K14 of histone H3, the same residues that are targeted by SIRT1 in vitro *(7)*. MyoD, a transcriptional regulator of muscle gene expression and differentiation, is regulated by acetyltransferases and deacetylases *(120,121)*. A MyoD mutant that cannot be modified by acetylation is transcriptionally inactive and fails to promote muscle conversion of murine fibroblasts *(122)*.

MyoD interacts indirectly with SIRT1 via the acetyltransferase PCAF, and all three proteins form a ternary complex in vivo. In the presence of PCAF, SIRT1 deacetylates both PCAF and MyoD *(97)*. SIRT1 inhibits muscle differentiation, an activity that is dependent on its enzymatic activity. Furthermore, inhibition of SIRT1 activity by sirtinol, a small-molecule inhibitor of SIRT1, activates the expression of muscle specific-reporters *(97)*.

SIRT1 has also been implicated in the repression of genes that drive white adipocyte differentiation and fat storage *(108)*. SIRT1 is recruited to PPAR-γ binding sites in the aP2 and PPAR-γ promoters in the white adipocyte tissue of fasted mice, where it represses target genes regulating fat storage *(108)*. Since increased fat mass, especially visceral fat, is associated with the metabolic syndrome of aging, these results point to a possible role of SIRT1 in mammalian aging. The metabolic syndrome of aging is associated with hyperinsulinemia, dyslipidemia, type 2 diabetes mellitus, atherosclerosis, hypercoagulability, and hypertension *(123)*. In addition, fat tissue secretes several metabolically active factors that are potentially responsible for the development of insulin resistance *(124)*. Remarkably, a reduced fat mass can extend murine life span *(125)*. 3T3-L1 cells that overexpress SIRT1 accumulate less fat after induction of adipogenesis, suggesting a protective effect of SIRT1. Furthermore, SIRT1 also activates the mobilization of fat in differentiated fat cells *(108)*.

FOXO transcription factors induce the transcription of genes related to the oxidative stress response (MnSOD), cell cycle arrest (p27kip1), DNA repair (GADD45), and apoptosis (Bim, Fas ligand). Currently, the functional consequences of FOXO-SIRT1 interactions are not entirely clear. Recent studies found a SIRT1-mediated repression or no effect on the expression of genes involved in cell death induction (Bim, Fas ligand) *(98,105)*. GADD45 expression and MnSOD expression are induced through SIRT1 *(104–106)*. Depending on the experimental system, expression of p27kip1 is either decreased by SIRT1 *(98)* or increased *(104–106)*. As a net effect, it appears that SIRT1 shifts FOXO-mediated processes from apoptosis induction to cell cycle arrest and cellular survival.

Regulation of Apoptosis and Cellular Senescence

p53 hyperactivity has been proposed to mediate premature aging *(126)*. Depending on cell type and stress/damage stimulus, p53 can cause cell cycle arrest or apoptotic cell death. This cell cycle arrest can be either transient, giving the cell the opportunity to repair itself, or permanent. The permanent cell cycle arrest is also called cellular senescence and appears to function as a cellular cancer prevention mechanism *(127)*. The level of acetylated p53 in primary fibroblasts is increased by the Ras oncogene and by PML, two proteins that induce premature senescence in a p53-dependent manner *(128,129)*. SIRT1 deacetylates p53 and thereby antagonizes the induction of cellular senescence by p53.

SIRT1 may also regulate apoptosis in a pathway-specific manner. Indeed, SIRT1 inhibits p53-mediated apoptosis, whereas it promotes TNF-α-mediated apoptosis through inhibition of NF-κB transcription *(71,72,75,81,91)*. SIRT1 may also regulate apoptosis via its interaction with Ku70 *(102)*. In healthy cells, the Ku70 protein prevents the proapoptotic factor Bax from translocating to the mitochondrial outer membrane. In response to apoptotic stimuli, such as ultraviolet (UV) irradiation, Ku70 becomes acetylated and dissociates from Bax. Ku hyperacetylation is induced by inhibition of either class I/II HDACs or class III HDACs (sirtuins). Deacetylation of Ku70 by SIRT1 promotes the Ku70/Bax interaction and increases cellular survival after DNA damage.

Overexpression of SIRT1 inhibits FOXO3-induced cell death in response to stress *(105)* and protects cardiac myocytes from apoptosis induction by serum starvation *(74)*. These observations point to a general protective activity of SIRT1 against apoptosis, with the exception of TNF-induced apoptosis.

SIRT1 and Metabolism

Loss-of-function mutations in genes coding for components of the insulin and/or IGF signaling pathway extend life span in *C. elegans*, *Drosophila*, and mice *(130–132)* (Fig. 2). Life span extension by Sir2 in *C. elegans* requires Daf-16, the only *C. elegans* FOXO homolog *(60)*. Daf-16 is also required for the extension of life span mediated by reduced IGF signaling in *C. elegans (62)*. Metabolic studies suggest that FOXO1 could be the insulin-regulated transcription factor that translates insulin action into gene expression. FOXO1 promotes transcription of genes that increase glucose production in concert with the PPAR-γ coactivator PGC-1α *(133)*. Mice overexpressing a constitutively active FOXO1 mutant in the liver develop diabetes, most likely as a result of increased glucose production *(134)*. An early report indicated that SIRT1 represses FOXO1 *(98)*, suggesting that SIRT1 could suppress the development of type II diabetes. However, SIRT1 can also potentiate FOXO1-mediated transcription by deacetylation of three lysine residues in another experimental system, indicating that the effect of SIRT1 on FOXO1 is likely to be context dependent *(104)*.

Epidemiological studies suggest that cancer prevalence increases with body mass in humans *(135)*. FOXO factors are involved in the regulation of both metabolism and cellular differentiation, and one of the FOXO target genes, p21cip, is critical for both transforming growth factor-β (TGF-β)-dependent transformation and insulin-dependent adipogenesis. Alteration of FOXO function by SIRT1 could therefore influence the balance between differentiation and cancer development. However, the situation is further complicated by the observation that class I/II deacetylases also participate in the control of FOXO acetylation levels *(98,105)*.

SIRT2

SUBCELLULAR LOCALIZATION

The human SIRT2 protein is a closer homolog to the yeast Hst2p than to yeast Sir2p. Both proteins are localized to the cytoplasmic compartment *(39,40)*, and human SIRT2 localizes along the microtubule network *(41)*. Microtubules are a component of the cytoskeleton, along with actin and intermediate filaments. Microtubules are formed by the polymerization of α- and β-tubulin heterodimers. During interphase, microtubules form an array within the cytoplasm termed the microtubule network. This network plays an important role in the regulation of cell shape, intracellular transport, and cell motility. During cell division, the interphase microtubule network depolymerizes, followed by a repolymerization into microtubules, forming the spindle fibers. Spindle fibers are involved in the essential role of chromosomal separation during mitosis. Following mitosis, the interphase microtubule network re-forms polymerizing microtubules in each new daughter cell. Although the primary localization of SIRT2 is within the cytoplasm, a role for SIRT2 in the nucleus is likely, given that SIRT2 appears to shuttle continuously between the nucleus and the cytoplasm (B.J. North and E. Verdin, unpublished observations).

BIOLOGICAL FUNCTIONS

Tubulin Deacetylation

SIRT2 colocalizes with the microtubule network and deacetylates K40 of α-tubulin *(41)*. α-Tubulin can also be deacetylated by HDAC6, a class II HDAC, and this activity can regulate cellular motility *(136)*. Both SIRT2 and HDAC6 are found along microtubules and deacetylate α-tubulin independently of one another; however, they are found within the same macromolecular complex as demonstrated by their coimmunoprecipitation *(41)*. Interestingly, the closely related Hst2p in yeast, although localized in the cytoplasm, has a preference for a histone peptide as substrate over an α-tubulin peptide, whereas SIRT2 shows a preference for an α-tubulin peptide over a histone peptide, suggesting that SIRT2 has evolved to carry out the deacetylation of tubulin *(41)*.

Mitotic Exit

SIRT2 levels are upregulated prior to mitosis, and SIRT2 is phosphorylated during mitosis, suggesting a role for SIRT2 in cell cycle regulation *(137)*. Coexpression of SIRT2 with the phosphatase CDC14B, but not CDC14A, leads to lower abundance of SIRT2, which is reversed with proteosome inhibitors *(137)*. Cells overexpressing mutant forms of SIRT2 have a delay in mitotic exit *(137)*. Whether SIRT2-dependent regulation of α-tubulin acetylation is related to the cell cycle delay phenotype, and how SIRT2 may be regulated in a cell cycle manner, remain to be determined. However, these observations could explain why SIRT2 may function as a tumor suppressor (*see* that section below).

Transcriptional Regulation and HOXA10

The nuclear-cytoplasmic shuttling of SIRT2 suggests that it may also have nuclear activities. SIRT2 interacts with the homeobox (HOX) transcription factor HOXA10 in vitro and in vivo and may modulate its transcriptional activity *(138)*. HOXA10 plays a role in myeloid and B-lymphoid progenitor cell differentiation and in the adult uterus during periimplantation events *(139,140)*. HOX proteins are evolutionarily conserved transcription factors that play pivotal roles in developmental regulation through pattern formation. This regulation is mediated via the homeodomain, a conserved protein motif that is responsible for sequence-specific DNA binding *(141)*. Differential cofactor binding to HOX proteins can modify their activities from activation to repression *(142,143)*.

Tumor Suppressor

The gene for SIRT2 is located at chromosome 19q13.2, a region frequently deleted in human gliomas *(144)*. Expression of SIRT2 mRNA is reduced in human glioma cell lines *(144)*. Furthermore, forced expression of SIRT2 in these glioblastoma cell lines suppressed colony formation and modified their microtubule network *(144)*. These results indicate that SIRT2 may act as a tumor suppressor.

SIRT3

SIRT3 is phylogenetically closely related to SIRT2 and is highly expressed in the brain, heart, kidney, liver, and muscle *(145,146)*. The telomeric terminal chromosomal region, 11p15.5, where the SIRT3 gene is located, harbors four genes potentially associated with longevity. These are HRAS1, IGF-2, proinsulin, and tyrosine hydroxylase. To investigate the relationship between longevity and polymorphism of the SIRT3 gene, a silent G/T transversion at position 477 in the evolutionarily conserved exon 3 of the SIRT3 gene was used as a marker. Analysis of the genotype-specific survival function relevant to this marker revealed that, in males, the TT genotype increases and GT genotype decreases survival in the elderly. These studies indicate that SIRT3 variability may modulate human aging *(147)*.

The SIRT3 cDNA encodes a protein of 43.6 kDa. However, in cultured cells, most of the protein exists as a 28-kDa protein *(148)*. SIRT3 is present in mitochondria, and its first 100 amino acids are removed after the protein reaches the mitochondrial matrix *(146,148)*. Proteolytic processing of SIRT3 can be recapitulated in vitro by treating full-length SIRT3 with mitochondrial processing peptidase. The unprocessed, full-length SIRT3 is enzymatically inactive and becomes active after proteolytic processing *(148)*. Biological targets of SIRT3 in the mitochondria are unknown, but, given the central role of mitochondria in the control of metabolism, it is likely that SIRT3 will participate in metabolic control. Mouse SIRT3 is also mitochondrial and is expressed at high levels in the brain, heart, testis, kidney, brown adipose tissue, and liver *(149,150)*.

SIRT4

The gene encoding SIRT4 is located in the chromosomal region 12q24.31. The SIRT4 expression profile indicates the strongest expression in muscle, kidney, testis, and liver *(150)*. SIRT4, like SIRT3, is found predominantly in the mitochondrial matrix (N. Ahuja and E. Verdin, unpublished observations). The SIRT4 cDNA encodes for a 35-kDa protein, and SIRT4 is processed in the mitochondrial matrix to a 30-Kda protein. SIRT4 shows no detectable histone deacetylase activity, and its biological target in cells is yet to be determined.

SIRT5

SIRT5 is phylogenetically closest to prokaryotic sirtuins. The gene encoding SIRT5 is located in the chromosomal region 6p23. Reverse transcriptase-polymerase chain reaction analysis of SIRT5 expression profiles indicated that SIRT5 is broadly expressed in adult and fetal tissues, with the highest expression in the kidney, brown adipose tissue, and heart *(70,145)*. SIRT5 shows low deacetylase activity in vitro *(41)*. It is predominantly found in the cytoplasm and its function and biological targets are not known.

SIRT6 and SIRT7

The SIRT6 gene is located on chromosome 19p13.3, and the SIRT7 gene has been mapped to chromosome 17q. The SIRT6 and SIRT7 cDNAs encode proteins with predicted molecular weights of 39.1 and 44.9 kDa, respectively. The SIRT6 and SIRT7 sequences are much more similar to each other than they are to Sir2 *(145)*. Both proteins have no detectable histone deacetylase activity in vitro *(41)*. SIRT6 is expressed in all tissues at comparable levels *(150)*, whereas SIRT7 shows the highest expression in the brain, kidney, white adipose tissue, liver, and lung *(150)*.

SIRTUIN INHIBITORS

Small-molecule inhibitors of sirtuins were identified using a high-throughput cell-based screen of 1600 unbiased compounds *(151)*. The primary screen was for inhibitors of Sir2p-mediated silencing of a URA3

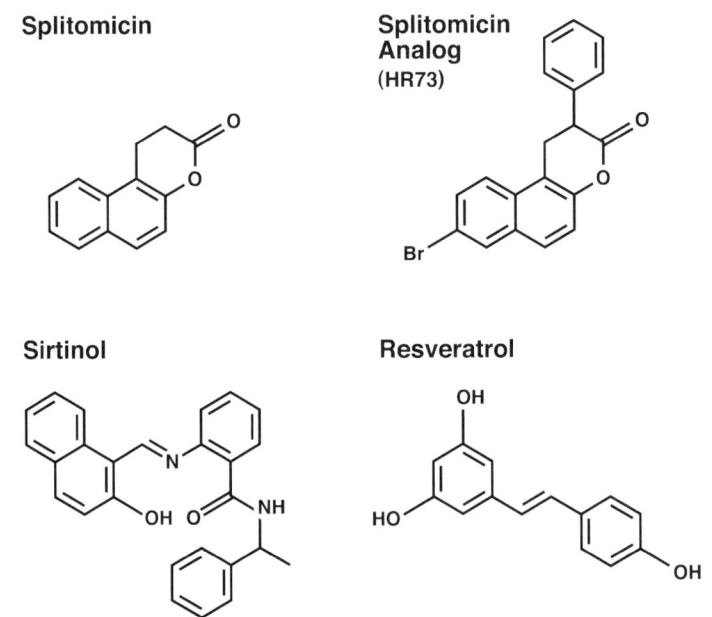

Fig. 3. Chemical structure of sirtuin activators and inhibitors. *See* text for details.

reporter gene integrated into a telomeric locus. This yeast strain grows in the presence of 5-fluoroorotic acid (5-FOA), but addition of sir2p inhibitors resulted in the expression of the URA3 gene and death in the presence of 5-FOA. Three compounds out of 1600 scored positively in this screen: A3, sirtinol, and M15 (Fig. 3). All three compounds are planar and aromatic and similar in structure to the adenine and nicotinamide moieties of NAD. Both sirtinol and M15 contain substructures derived from 2-hydroxy-1-napthaldehyde. These inhibitors inhibit both yeast and human sirtuins in vitro and inhibit transcriptional silencing in yeast in vivo. Preliminary studies show that sirtinol inhibition of sirtuins interferes with body axis formation in *Arabidopsis (151)*. Sirtinol also can activate the expression of muscle-specific reporters *(97)*, in agreement with the proposed role of SIRT1 in the modulation of MyoD and PCAF activities (discussed above in the section Transcriptional Regulation by SIRT1) *(97)*.

Another phenotypic screen was conducted using a yeast strain carrying the URA3 gene in close proximity to telomeric chromatin *(152)*. This URA3 gene is repressed, and the yeast strain carrying it requires uracil in the media for growth. Inhibition of silencing activates URA3 expression and enables the cells to grow in the absence of uracil. Six thousand compounds from the National Cancer Institute Repository were screened, and 11 structurally unrelated compounds were selected. These compounds were tested in a secondary screen based on silencing at HML and HMR loci. A single compound, 1,2-hydro-^{3}H-naptho [2,1-b]pyran-3-one, called splitomicin, was selected that also disrupted silencing at both the HMR and HML loci (Fig. 3). Splitomicin inhibits the deacetylase activity of Sir2p in vitro. Additional studies on the structure-function relationship of splitomicin and its analogs reveals that the lactone ring or some naphthalene substituents (positions 7–9) decrease activity, whereas other napthalene substitutions (positions 5 and 6) are well tolerated *(153)*.

The hydrolytically unstable aromatic lactone is important for activity. Lactone hydrolysis rates, used as a measure of reactivity of the compounds, correlate with inhibitory activity. The most potent sir2 inhibitors are structurally similar to and have hydrolysis rates similar to that of splitomicin *(153)*. A novel inhibitor of mammalian sirtuins was recently developed based on the splitomicin structure *(117)*. This compound, called HR73, inhibits SIRT1 enzymatic activity and leads to p53 hyper-acetylation (E. Verdin and W. Gu, unpublished observations; Fig. 3). HR73 blocks Tat deacetylation and inhibits its transcriptional activity on the HIV promoter *(117)*.

Another potent inhibitor of sirtuin activity both in vivo and in vitro is nicotinamide, a product of the sirtuin deacetylation reaction. It has been proposed that this inhibition occurs by chemical reversal of a covalent reaction intermediate. Nicotinamide inhibits SIRT1 and promotes p53/dependent apoptosis in mammalian cells *(51,71,72)*. Moreover, in yeast cells, nicotinamide derepresses all three Sir2 target loci, increases recombination at the rDNA loci, and shortens life span, comparable to that of the Sir2 mutant *(52)*. Further studies have revealed that PNCI, which encodes enzymes that deaminate nicotinamide, depletes nicotinamide and promotes life span extension *(53)*.

Small-molecule inhibitors of sirtuins are powerful tools for dissecting the functional roles of sirtuin proteins in vivo. Further studies are under way to identify specific and potent inhibitors of sirtuins that could be used to study the roles of these proteins in transcriptional regulation, DNA damage repair, cell cycle control, and developmental biology. These drugs could also pave the way for the therapeutic use of small-molecule inhibitors and activators of sirtuins in a variety of metabolic and neoplastic disorders.

SIRTUIN ACTIVATORS

The observation that calorie restriction increases life span by increasing the activity of sirtuins prompted investigators to screen small-molecule libraries to identify molecules capable of modulating sirtuin activity *(154)*.

Two structurally related compounds, quercetin and piceatannol, stimulate SIRT1 activity by five- and eight-fold, respectively. Both quercetin and piceatannol are polyphenols, plant secondary metabolites. The most potent activator is resveratrol (3,5,4′-trihydrostilbene), a polyphenol found in the skin of red grapes *(154)* (Fig. 3). Resveratrol has no significant effect on the V_{max} and lowers the K_m of the acetylated peptide 35-fold and that for NAD more than 5-fold. Resveratrol reduces the frequency of rDNA recombination by about 60% in a Sir2-dependent manner and increases average yeast life span by 70%, also in a Sir2-dependent manner. Resveratrol and other sirtuin-activating compounds also activate sirtuins from *C. elegans* and *Drosophila* and extend the life span of these animals without reducing fecundity. Life span extension is dependent on a functional Sir2 and is not observed when nutrients are restricted *(155)*. These data indicate that sirtuin-activating compounds slow metazoan aging by mechanisms that may be related to caloric restriction.

REFERENCES

1. Rine J, Strathern JN, Hicks JB, Herskowitz I. A suppressor of mating-type locus mutations in *Saccharomyces cerevisiae*: evidence for and identification of cryptic mating-type loci. Genetics 1979;93:877–901.
2. Ivy JM, Hicks JB, Klar AJ. Map positions of yeast genes SIR1, SIR3 and SIR4. Genetics 1985;111:735–744.
3. Ivy JM, Klar AJ, Hicks JB. Cloning and characterization of four SIR genes of *Saccharomyces cerevisiae*. Mol Cell Biol 1986;6:688–702.
4. Rine J, Herskowitz I. Four genes responsible for a position effect on expression from HML and HMR in *Saccharomyces cerevisiae*. Genetics 1987; 116:9–22.
5. Landry J, Sutton A, Tafrov ST, et al. The silencing protein SIR2 and its homologs are NAD-dependent protein deacetylases. Proc Natl Acad Sci U S A 2000;97: 5807–5811.
6. Smith JS, Brachmann CB, Celic I, et al. A phylogenetically conserved NAD+-dependent protein deacetylase activity in the Sir2 protein family. Proc Natl Acad Sci U S A 2000;97:6658–6663.
7. Imai S, Armstrong CM, Kaeberlein M, Guarente L. Transcriptional silencing and longevity protein Sir2 is an NAD-dependent histone deacetylase. Nature 2000;403:795–800.
8. Kupiec M, Byers B, Esposito RE, Mitchell AP. Meiosis and sporulation in *Saccharomyces cerevisiae*. In: Pringle JR, Broach JR, Jones EW, eds. The Molecular and Cellular Biology of the Yeast *Saccharomyces*: Cell Cycle and Cell Biology. Cold Spring Harbor, NY: Cold Spring Harbor Laboratory Press, 1997:889–1036.
9. Triolo T, Sternglanz R. Role of interactions between the origin recognition complex and SIR1 in transcriptional silencing. Nature 1996;381:251–253.
10. Boscheron C, Maillet L, Marcand S, Tsai-Pflugfelder M, Gasser SM, Gilson E. Cooperation at a distance between silencers and proto-silencers at the yeast HML locus. EMBO J 1996;15:2184–2195.

11. Moretti P, Freeman K, Coodly L, Shore D. Evidence that a complex of SIR proteins interacts with the silencer and telomere-binding protein RAP1. Genes Dev 1994;8:2257–2269.

12. Rusche LN, Kirchmaier AL, Rine J. Ordered nucleation and spreading of silenced chromatin in *Saccharomyces cerevisiae*. Mol Biol Cell 2002;13: 2207–2222.

13. Hecht A, Laroche T, Strahl-Bolsinger S, Gasser SM, Grunstein M. Histone H3 and H4 N-termini interact with SIR3 and SIR4 proteins: a molecular model for the formation of heterochromatin in yeast. Cell 1995;80:583–592.

14. Braunstein M, Sobel RE, Allis CD, Turner BM, Broach JR. Efficient transcriptional silencing in *Saccharomyces cerevisiae* requires a heterochromatin histone acetylation pattern. Mol Cell Biol 1996;16:4349–4356.

15. Braunstein M, Rose AB, Holmes SG, Allis CD, Broach JR. Transcriptional silencing in yeast is associated with reduced nucleosome acetylation. Genes Dev 1993;7:592–604.

16. Hoppe GJ, Tanny JC, Rudner AD, et al. Steps in assembly of silent chromatin in yeast: Sir3-independent binding of a Sir2/Sir4 complex to silencers and role for Sir2-dependent deacetylation. Mol Cell Biol 2002;22:4167–4180.

17. Moazed D, Rudner AD, Huang J, Hoppe GJ, Tanny JC. A model for step-wise assembly of heterochromatin in yeast. Novartis Found Symp 2004;259:48–56; discussion 56–62, 163–169.

18. Rusche LN, Kirchmaier AL, Rine J. The establishment, inheritance, and function of silenced chromatin in *Saccharomyces cerevisiae*. Annu Rev Biochem 2003;72:481–516.

19. Bi X, Broach JR. DNA in transcriptionally silent chromatin assumes a distinct topology that is sensitive to cell cycle progression. Mol Cell Biol 1997;17: 7077–7087.

20. Loo S, Rine J. Silencers and domains of generalized repression. Science 1994;264:1768–1771.

21. Bryan TM, Cech TR. Telomerase and the maintenance of chromosome ends. Curr Opin Cell Biol 1999;11:318–324.

22. Wright JH, Gottschling DE, Zakian VA. *Saccharomyces* telomeres assume a non-nucleosomal chromatin structure. Genes Dev 1992;6:197–210.

23. Gottschling DE, Aparicio OM, Billington BL, Zakian VA. Position effect at *S. cerevisiae* telomeres: reversible repression of Pol II transcription. Cell 1990; 63:751–762.

24. Bourns BD, Alexander MK, Smith AM, Zakian VA. Sir proteins, Rif proteins, and Cdc13p bind *Saccharomyces* telomeres in vivo. Mol Cell Biol 1998; 18:5600–5608.

25. Liu C, Lustig AJ. Genetic analysis of Rap1p/Sir3p interactions in telomeric and HML silencing in *Saccharomyces cerevisiae*. Genetics 1996;143:81–93.

26. Cockell M, Palladino F, Laroche T, et al. The carboxy termini of Sir4 and Rap1 affect Sir3 localization: evidence for a multicomponent complex required for yeast telomeric silencing. J Cell Biol 1995;129:909–924.

27. Laroche T, Martin SG, Gotta M, et al. Mutation of yeast Ku genes disrupts the subnuclear organization of telomeres. Curr Biol 1998;8:653–656.

28. Martin SG, Laroche T, Suka N, Grunstein M, Gasser SM. Relocalization of telomeric Ku and SIR proteins in response to DNA strand breaks in yeast. Cell 1999;97:621–633.

29. Mills KD, Sinclair DA, Guarente L. MEC1-dependent redistribution of the Sir3 silencing protein from telomeres to DNA double-strand breaks. Cell 1999;97: 609–620.

30. Gravel S, Larrivee M, Labrecque P, Wellinger RJ. Yeast Ku as a regulator of chromosomal DNA end structure. Science 1998;280:741–744.

31. Bryk M, Banerjee M, Murphy M, Knudsen KE, Garfinkel DJ, Curcio MJ. Transcriptional silencing of Ty1 elements in the RDN1 locus of yeast. Genes Dev 1997;11:255–269.

32. Smith JS, Boeke JD. An unusual form of transcriptional silencing in yeast ribosomal DNA. Genes Dev 1997;11:241–254.

33. Fritze CE, Verschueren K, Strich R, Easton Esposito R. Direct evidence for SIR2 modulation of chromatin structure in yeast rDNA. EMBO J 1997;16:6495–6509.

34. Gottlieb S, Esposito RE. A new role for a yeast transcriptional silencer gene, SIR2, in regulation of recombination in ribosomal DNA. Cell 1989;56:771–776.

35. Straight AF, Shou W, Dowd GJ, et al. Net1, a Sir2-associated nucleolar protein required for rDNA silencing and nucleolar integrity. Cell 1999;97:245–256.

36. Shou W, Seol JH, Shevchenko A, et al. Exit from mitosis is triggered by Tem1-dependent release of the protein phosphatase Cdc14 from nucleolar RENT complex. Cell 1999;97:233–244.

37. Brachmann CB, Sherman JM, Devine SE, Cameron EE, Pillus L, Boeke JD. The SIR2 gene family, conserved from bacteria to humans, functions in silencing, cell cycle progression, and chromosome stability. Genes Dev 1995;9: 2888–2902.

38. Bedalov A, Hirao M, Posakony J, Nelson M, Simon JA. NAD+-dependent deacetylase Hst1p controls biosynthesis and cellular NAD+ levels in *Saccharomyces cerevisiae*. Mol Cell Biol 2003;23:7044–7054.

39. Perrod S, Cockell MM, Laroche T, et al. A cytosolic NAD-dependent deacetylase, Hst2p, can modulate nucleolar and telomeric silencing in yeast. EMBO J 2001;20:197–209.

40. Afshar G, Murnane JP. Characterization of a human gene with sequence homology to *Saccharomyces cerevisiae* SIR2. Gene 1999;234:161–168.

41. North BJ, Marshall BL, Borra MT, Denu JM, Verdin E. The human Sir2 ortholog, SIRT2, is an NAD+-dependent tubulin deacetylase. Mol Cell 2003;11: 437–444.

42. Sinclair DA, Guarente L. Extrachromosomal rDNA circles—a cause of aging in yeast. Cell 1997;91:1033–1042.

43. Kennedy BK, Gotta M, Sinclair DA, et al. Redistribution of silencing proteins from telomeres to the nucleolus is associated with extension of life span in *S. cerevisiae*. Cell 1997;89:381–391.

44. Kaeberlein M, McVey M, Guarente L. The SIR2/3/4 complex and SIR2 alone promote longevity in *Saccharomyces cerevisiae* by two different mechanisms. Genes Dev 1999;13:2570–2580.

45. Masoro EJ. Caloric restriction and aging: an update. Exp Gerontol 2000;35: 299–305.

46. Lin SJ, Kaeberlein M, Andalis AA, et al. Calorie restriction extends *Saccharomyces cerevisiae* life span by increasing respiration. Nature 2002;418: 344–348.

47. Lin SJ, Defossez PA, Guarente L. Requirement of NAD and SIR2 for life-span extension by calorie restriction in *Saccharomyces cerevisiae*. Science 2000;289: 2126–2128.

48. Kaeberlein M, Kirkland KT, Fields S, Kennedy BK. Sir2-independent life span extension by calorie restriction in yeast. PLoS Biol 2004;2:E296.

49. Kaeberlein M, Andalis AA, Liszt GB, Fink GR, Guarente L. *Saccharomyces cerevisiae* SSD1-V confers longevity by a Sir2p-independent mechanism. Genetics 2004;166:1661–1672.

50. Lin SJ, Ford E, Haigis M, Liszt G, Guarente L. Calorie restriction extends yeast life span by lowering the level of NADH. Genes Dev 2004;18:12–16.

51. Landry J, Slama JT, Sternglanz R. Role of NAD(+) in the deacetylase activity of the SIR2-like proteins. Biochem Biophys Res Commun 2000;278:685–690.

52. Bitterman KJ, Anderson RM, Cohen HY, Latorre-Esteves M, Sinclair DA. Inhibition of silencing and accelerated aging by nicotinamide, a putative negative regulator of yeast sir2 and human SIRT1. J Biol Chem 2002;277: 45,099–45,107.

53. Anderson RM, Bitterman KJ, Wood JG, Medvedik O, Sinclair DA. Nicotinamide and PNC1 govern life span extension by calorie restriction in *Saccharomyces cerevisiae*. Nature 2003;423:181–185.

54. Anderson RM, Bitterman KJ, Wood JG, et al. Manipulation of a nuclear NAD+ salvage pathway delays aging without altering steady-state NAD+ levels. J Biol Chem 2002;277:18,881–18,890.

55. Starai VJ, Celic I, Cole RN, Boeke JD, Escalante-Semerena JC. Sir2-dependent activation of acetyl-CoA synthetase by deacetylation of active lysine. Science 2002;298:2390–2392.

56. Starai VJ, Takahashi H, Boeke JD, Escalante-Semerena JC. Short-chain fatty acid activation by acyl-coenzyme A synthetases requires SIR2 protein function in *Salmonella enterica* and *Saccharomyces cerevisiae*. Genetics 2003;163: 545–555.

57. Horswill AR, Escalante-Semerena JC. Characterization of the propionyl-CoA synthetase (PrpE) enzyme of *Salmonella enterica*: residue Lys592 is required for propionyl-AMP synthesis. Biochemistry 2002;41:2379–2387.

58. Bell SD, Botting CH, Wardleworth BN, Jackson SP, White MF. The interaction of Alba, a conserved archaeal chromatin protein, with Sir2 and its regulation by acetylation. Science 2002;296:148–151.

59. She Q, Singh RK, Confalonieri F, et al. The complete genome of the crenarchaeon *Sulfolobus solfataricus* P2. Proc Natl Acad Sci U S A 2001;98:7835–7840.

60. Tissenbaum HA, Guarente L. Increased dosage of a sir-2 gene extends life span in *Caenorhabditis elegans*. Nature 2001;410:227–230.

61. Kawano T, Ito Y, Ishiguro M, Takuwa K, Nakajima T, Kimura Y. Molecular cloning and characterization of a new insulin/IGF-like peptide of the nematode *Caenorhabditis elegans*. Biochem Biophys Res Commun 2000;273:431–436.

62. Kenyon C, Chang J, Gensch E, Rudner A, Tabtiang R. A *C. elegans* mutant that lives twice as long as wild type. Nature 1993;366:461–464.

63. Kimura KD, Tissenbaum HA, Liu Y, Ruvkun G. daf-2, an insulin receptor-like gene that regulates longevity and diapause in *Caenorhabditis elegans*. Science 1997;277:942–946.

64. Paradis S, Ailion M, Toker A, Thomas JH, Ruvkun G. A PDK1 homolog is necessary and sufficient to transduce AGE-1 PI3 kinase signals that regulate diapause in *Caenorhabditis elegans*. Genes Dev 1999;13:1438–1452.

65. Friedman DB, Johnson TE. Three mutants that extend both mean and maximum life span of the nematode, *Caenorhabditis elegans*, define the age-1 gene. J Gerontol 1988;43:B102–B109.

66. Barlow AL, van Drunen CM, Johnson CA, Tweedie S, Bird A, Turner BM. dSIR2 and dHDAC6: two novel, inhibitor-resistant deacetylases in *Drosophila melanogaster*. Exp Cell Res 2001;265:90–103.

67. Rosenberg MI, Parkhurst SM. *Drosophila* Sir2 is required for heterochromatic silencing and by euchromatic Hairy/E(Spl) bHLH repressors in segmentation and sex determination. Cell 2002;109:447–458.

68. Newman BL, Lundblad JR, Chen Y, Smolik SM. A *Drosophila* homologue of Sir2 modifies position-effect variegation but does not affect life span. Genetics 2002;162:1675–1685.

69. Astrom SU, Cline TW, Rine J. The *Drosophila melanogaster* sir2+ gene is nonessential and has only minor effects on position-effect variegation. Genetics 2003;163:931–937.

70. Frye RA. Characterization of five human cDNAs with homology to the yeast SIR2 gene: Sir2-like proteins (sirtuins) metabolize NAD and may have protein ADP-ribosyltransferase activity. Biochem Biophys Res Commun 1999;260: 273–279.

71. Luo J, Nikolaev AY, Imai S, et al. Negative control of p53 by Sir2alpha promotes cell survival under stress. Cell 2001;107:137–148.

72. Vaziri H, Dessain SK, Ng Eaton E, et al. hSIR2(SIRT1) functions as an NAD-dependent p53 deacetylase. Cell 2001;107:149–159.

73. Vaquero A, Scher M, Lee D, Erdjument-Bromage H, Tempst P, Reinberg D. Human SirT1 interacts with histone H1 and promotes formation of facultative heterochromatin. Mol Cell 2004;16:93–105.

74. Alcendor RR, Kirshenbaum LA, Imai S, Vatner SF, Sadoshima J. Silent information regulator 2α, a longevity factor and class III histone deacetylase, is an essential endogenous apoptosis inhibitor in cardiac myocytes. Circ Res 2004;95: 971–980.

75. Langley E, Pearson M, Faretta M, et al. Human SIR2 deacetylates p53 and antagonizes PML/p53-induced cellular senescence. EMBO J 2002;21:2383–2396.

76. Muth V, Nadaud S, Grummt I, Voit R. Acetylation of TAF(I)68, a subunit of TIF-IB/SL1, activates RNA polymerase I transcription. EMBO J 2001;20: 1353–1362.

77. Guarente L. Diverse and dynamic functions of the Sir silencing complex. Nat Genet 1999;23:281–285.

78. Luo J, Li M, Tang Y, Laszkowska M, Roeder RG, Gu W. Acetylation of p53 augments its site-specific DNA binding both in vitro and in vivo. Proc Natl Acad Sci U S A 2004;101:2259–2264.

79. Luo J, Su F, Chen D, Shiloh A, Gu W. Deacetylation of p53 modulates its effect on cell growth and apoptosis. Nature 2000;408:377–381.

80. Ito A, Lai CH, Zhao X, et al. p300/CBP-mediated p53 acetylation is commonly induced by p53-activating agents and inhibited by MDM2. EMBO J 2001;20: 1331–1340.

81. Cheng HL, Mostoslavsky R, Saito S, et al. Developmental defects and p53 hyperacetylation in Sir2 homolog (SIRT1)-deficient mice. Proc Natl Acad Sci U S A 2003;100:10,794–10,799.

82. McBurney MW, Yang X, Jardine K, et al. The mammalian SIR2alpha protein has a role in embryogenesis and gametogenesis. Mol Cell Biol 2003;23:38–54.

83. Baldwin AS Jr. The NF-kappa B and I kappa B proteins: new discoveries and insights. Annu Rev Immunol 1996;14:649–683.

84. Mayo MW, Baldwin AS. The transcription factor NF-kappaB: control of onco-genesis and cancer therapy resistance. Biochim Biophys Acta 2000;1470: M55–M62.

85. Na SY, Lee SK, Han SJ, Choi HS, Im SY, Lee JW. Steroid receptor coactivator-1 interacts with the p50 subunit and coactivates nuclear factor kappaB-mediated transactivations. J Biol Chem 1998;273:10,831–10,834.

86. Sheppard KA, Phelps KM, Williams AJ, et al. Nuclear integration of glucocorti-coid receptor and nuclear factor-kappaB signaling by CREB-binding protein and steroid receptor coactivator-1. J Biol Chem 1998;273:29,291–29,294.

87. Sheppard KA, Rose DW, Haque ZK, et al. Transcriptional activation by NF-kappaB requires multiple coactivators. Mol Cell Biol 1999;19:6367–6378.

88. Zhong H, May MJ, Jimi E, Ghosh S. The phosphorylation status of nuclear NF-kappa B determines its association with CBP/p300 or HDAC-1. Mol Cell 2002;9:625–636.

89. Chen LF, Mu Y, Greene WC. Acetylation of RelA at discrete sites regulates distinct nuclear functions of NF-kappaB. EMBO J 2002;21:6539–6548.

90. Kiernan R, Bres V, Ng RW, et al. Post-activation turn-off of NF-kappa B-dependent transcription is regulated by acetylation of p65. J Biol Chem 2003;278:2758–2766.

91. Yeung F, Hoberg JE, Ramsey CS, et al. Modulation of NF-kappaB-dependent transcription and cell survival by the SIRT1 deacetylase. EMBO J 2004;23: 2369–2380.

92. Ashburner BP, Westerheide SD, Baldwin AS Jr. The p65 (RelA) subunit of NF-kappaB interacts with the histone deacetylase (HDAC) corepressors HDAC1 and HDAC2 to negatively regulate gene expression. Mol Cell Biol 2001;21:7065–7077.

93. Senawong T, Peterson VJ, Avram D, et al. Involvement of the histone deacetylase SIRT1 in chicken ovalbumin upstream promoter transcription factor (COUP-TF)-interacting protein 2-mediated transcriptional repression. J Biol Chem 2003;278: 43,041–43,050.

94. Massari ME, Murre C. Helix-loop-helix proteins: regulators of transcription in eucaryotic organisms. Mol Cell Biol 2000;20:429–440.

95. Kageyama R, Nakanishi S. Helix-loop-helix factors in growth and differentia-tion of the vertebrate nervous system. Curr Opin Genet Dev 1997;7:659–665.

96. Takata T, Ishikawa F. Human Sir2-related protein SIRT1 associates with the bHLH repressors HES1 and HEY2 and is involved in HES1- and HEY2-mediated tran-scriptional repression. Biochem Biophys Res Commun 2003;301:250–257.

97. Fulco M, Schiltz RL, Iezzi S, et al. Sir2 regulates skeletal muscle differentiation as a potential sensor of the redox state. Mol Cell 2003;12:51–62.

98. Motta MC, Divecha N, Lemieux M, et al. Mammalian SIRT1 represses fork-head transcription factors. Cell 2004;116:551–563.

99. Walker JR, Corpina RA, Goldberg J. Structure of the Ku heterodimer bound to DNA and its implications for double-strand break repair. Nature 2001;412: 607–614.

100. Sawada M, Sun W, Hayes P, Leskov K, Boothman DA, Matsuyama S. Ku70 suppresses the apoptotic translocation of Bax to mitochondria. Nat Cell Biol 2003;5:320–329.

101. Cohen HY, Lavu S, Bitterman KJ, et al. Acetylation of the C terminus of Ku70 by CBP and PCAF controls Bax-mediated apoptosis. Mol Cell 2004;13:627–638.

102. Cohen HY, Miller C, Bitterman KJ, et al. Calorie restriction promotes mammalian cell survival by inducing the SIRT1 deacetylase. Science 2004;305:390–392.

103. Nasrin N, Ogg S, Cahill CM, et al. DAF-16 recruits the CREB-binding protein coactivator complex to the insulin-like growth factor binding protein 1 promoter in HepG2 cells. Proc Natl Acad Sci U S A 2000;97:10,412–10,417.

104. Daitoku H, Hatta M, Matsuzaki H, et al. Silent information regulator 2 potentiates Foxo1-mediated transcription through its deacetylase activity. Proc Natl Acad Sci U S A 2004;101:10,042–10,047.

105. Brunet A, Sweeney LB, Sturgill JF, et al. Stress-dependent regulation of FOXO transcription factors by the SIRT1 deacetylase. Science 2004;303:2011–2015.

106. van der Horst A, Tertoolen LG, de Vries-Smits LM, Frye RA, Medema RH, Burgering BM. FOXO4 is acetylated upon peroxide stress and deacetylated by the longevity protein hSir2(SIRT1). J Biol Chem 2004;279:28,873–28,879.

107. Fukuoka M, Daitoku H, Hatta M, Matsuzaki H, Umemura S, Fukamizu A. Negative regulation of forkhead transcription factor AFX (Foxo4) by CBP-induced acetylation. Int J Mol Med 2003;12:503–508.

108. Picard F, Kurtev M, Chung N, et al. Sirt1 promotes fat mobilization in white adipocytes by repressing PPAR-gamma. Nature 2004;429:771–776.

109. Kaehlcke K, Dorr A, Hetzer-Egger C, et al. Acetylation of Tat defines a cyclinT1-independent step in HIV transactivation. Mol Cell 2003;12:167–176.

110. Dorr A, Kiermer V, Pedal A, et al. Transcriptional synergy between Tat and PCAF is dependent on the binding of acetylated Tat to the PCAF bromodomain. EMBO J 2002;21:2715–2723.

111. Mujtaba S, He Y, Zeng L, et al. Structural basis of lysine-acetylated HIV-1 Tat recognition by PCAF bromodomain. Mol Cell 2002;9:575–586.

112. Ott M, Schnolzer M, Garnica J, et al. Acetylation of the HIV-1 Tat protein by p300 is important for its transcriptional activity. Curr Biol 1999;9:1489–1492.

113. Bres V, Tagami H, Peloponese JM, et al. Differential acetylation of Tat coordinates its interaction with the co-activators cyclin T1 and PCAF. EMBO J 2002;21:6811–6819.

114. Benkirane M, Chun RF, Xiao H, et al. Activation of integrated provirus requires histone acetyltransferase. p300 and P/CAF are coactivators for HIV-1 Tat. J Biol Chem 1998;273:24,898–24,905.

115. Kiernan RE, Vanhulle C, Schiltz L, et al. HIV-1 tat transcriptional activity is regulated by acetylation. EMBO J 1999;18:6106–6118.

116. Marzio G, Tyagi M, Gutierrez MI, Giacca M. HIV-1 tat transactivator recruits p300 and CREB-binding protein histone acetyltransferases to the viral promoter. Proc Natl Acad Sci U S A 1998;95:13,519–13,524.

117. Pagans S, Pedal A, North BJ, et al. SIRT1 Regulates HIV transcription via Tat deacetylation. PLoS Biol 2005;3:e41.

118. Jeppesen P, Turner BM. The inactive X chromosome in female mammals is distinguished by a lack of histone H4 acetylation, a cytogenetic marker for gene expression. Cell 1993;74:281–289.

119. Johnson CA, O'Neill LP, Mitchell A, Turner BM. Distinctive patterns of histone H4 acetylation are associated with defined sequence elements within both heterochromatic and euchromatic regions of the human genome. Nucleic Acids Res 1998;26:994–1001.

120. Sartorelli V, Puri PL. The link between chromatin structure, protein acetylation and cellular differentiation. Front Biosci 2001;6:D1024–D1047.

121. McKinsey TA, Zhang CL, Olson EN. Signaling chromatin to make muscle. Curr Opin Cell Biol 2002;14:763–772.

122. Sartorelli V, Puri PL, Hamamori Y, et al. Acetylation of MyoD directed by PCAF is necessary for the execution of the muscle program. Mol Cell 1999;4:725–734.

123. Das M, Gabriely I, Barzilai N. Caloric restriction, body fat and ageing in experimental models. Obes Rev 2004;5:13–19.

124. Gabriely I, Ma XH, Yang XM, et al. Removal of visceral fat prevents insulin resistance and glucose intolerance of aging: an adipokine-mediated process? Diabetes 2002;51:2951–2958.

125. Bluher M, Kahn BB, Kahn CR. Extended longevity in mice lacking the insulin receptor in adipose tissue. Science 2003;299:572–574.

126. Tyner SD, Venkatachalam S, Choi J, et al. p53 mutant mice that display early ageing-associated phenotypes. Nature 2002;415:45–53.

127. Campisi J. Cellular senescence as a tumor-suppressor mechanism. Trends Cell Biol 2001;11:S27–S31.

128. Ferbeyre G, de Stanchina E, Querido E, Baptiste N, Prives C, Lowe SW. PML is induced by oncogenic ras and promotes premature senescence. Genes Dev 2000;14:2015–2027.

129. Pearson M, Carbone R, Sebastiani C, et al. PML regulates p53 acetylation and premature senescence induced by oncogenic Ras. Nature 2000;406:207–210.

130. Liang H, Masoro EJ, Nelson JF, Strong R, McMahan CA, Richardson A. Genetic mouse models of extended life span. Exp Gerontol 2003;38:1353–1364.

131. Dillin A, Crawford DK, Kenyon C. Timing requirements for insulin/IGF-1 signaling in *C. elegans*. Science 2002;298:830–834.

132. Clancy DJ, Gems D, Harshman LG, et al. Extension of life-span by loss of CHICO, a *Drosophila* insulin receptor substrate protein. Science 2001;292: 104–106.

133. Puigserver P, Rhee J, Donovan J, et al. Insulin-regulated hepatic gluconeogenesis through FOXO1-PGC-1alpha interaction. Nature 2003;423:550–555.

134. Nakae J, Biggs WH 3rd, Kitamura T, et al. Regulation of insulin action and pancreatic beta-cell function by mutated alleles of the gene encoding forkhead transcription factor Foxo1. Nat Genet 2002;32:245–253.

135. Calle EE, Rodriguez C, Walker-Thurmond K, Thun MJ. Overweight, obesity, and mortality from cancer in a prospectively studied cohort of U.S. adults. N Engl J Med 2003;348:1625–1638.

136. Hubbert C, Guardiola A, Shao R, et al. HDAC6 is a microtubule-associated deacetylase. Nature 2002;417:455–458.

137. Dryden SC, Nahhas FA, Nowak JE, Goustin AS, Tainsky MA. Role for human SIRT2 NAD-dependent deacetylase activity in control of mitotic exit in the cell cycle. Mol Cell Biol 2003;23:3173–3185.

138. Bae NS, Swanson MJ, Vassilev A, Howard BH. Human histone deacetylase SIRT2 interacts with the homeobox transcription factor HOXA10. J Biochem (Tokyo) 2004;135:695–700.

139. Benson GV, Lim H, Paria BC, Satokata I, Dey SK, Maas RL. Mechanisms of reduced fertility in Hoxa-10 mutant mice: uterine homeosis and loss of maternal Hoxa-10 expression. Development 1996;122:2687–2696.

140. Thorsteinsdottir U, Sauvageau G, Humphries RK. Hox homeobox genes as regulators of normal and leukemic hematopoiesis. Hematol Oncol Clin North Am 1997;11:1221–1237.

141. Capecchi MR. Hox genes and mammalian development. Cold Spring Harbor Symp Quant Biol 1997;62:273–281.

142. McGinnis W, Krumlauf R. Homeobox genes and axial patterning. Cell 1992;68: 283–302.

143. Saleh M, Rambaldi I, Yang XJ, Featherstone MS. Cell signaling switches HOX-PBX complexes from repressors to activators of transcription mediated by histone deacetylases and histone acetyltransferases. Mol Cell Biol 2000;20:8623–8633.

144. Hiratsuka M, Inoue T, Toda T, et al. Proteomics-based identification of differentially expressed genes in human gliomas: down-regulation of SIRT2 gene. Biochem Biophys Res Commun 2003;309:558–566.

145. Frye RA. Phylogenetic classification of prokaryotic and eukaryotic Sir2-like proteins. Biochem Biophys Res Commun 2000;273:793–798.

146. Onyango P, Celic I, McCaffery JM, Boeke JD, Feinberg AP. SIRT3, a human SIR2 homologue, is an NAD- dependent deacetylase localized to mitochondria. Proc Natl Acad Sci U S A 2002;99:13,653–13,658.

147. Rose G, Dato S, Altomare K, et al. Variability of the SIRT3 gene, human silent information regulator Sir2 homologue, and survivorship in the elderly. Exp Gerontol 2003;38:1065–1070.

148. Schwer B, North BJ, Frye RA, Ott M, Verdin E. The human silent information regulator (Sir)2 homologue hSIRT3 is a mitochondrial nicotinamide adenine dinucleotide-dependent deacetylase. J Cell Biol 2002;158:647–657.

149. Yang YH, Chen YH, Zhang CY, Nimmakayalu MA, Ward DC, Weissman S. Cloning and characterization of two mouse genes with homology to the yeast Sir2 gene. Genomics 2000;69:355–369.

150. Shi T, Wang F, Stieren E, Tong Q. SIRT3, a mitochondrial sirtuin deacetylase, regulates mitochondrial function and thermogenesis in brown adipocytes. J Biol Chem 2005;280:13,560–13,567.

151. Grozinger CM, Chao ED, Blackwell HE, Moazed D, Schreiber SL. Identification of a class of small molecule inhibitors of the sirtuin family of NAD-dependent deacetylases by phenotypic screening. J Biol Chem 2001;276:38,837–38,843.

152. Bedalov A, Gatbonton T, Irvine WP, Gottschling DE, Simon JA. Identification of a small molecule inhibitor of Sir2p. Proc Natl Acad Sci U S A 2001;98: 15,113–15,118.

153. Posakony J, Hirao M, Stevens S, Simon JA, Bedalov A. Inhibitors of Sir2: evaluation of splitomicin analogues. J Med Chem 2004;47:2635–2644.

154. Howitz KT, Bitterman KJ, Cohen HY, et al. Small molecule activators of sirtuins extend *Saccharomyces cerevisiae* life span. Nature 2003;425:191–196.

155. Wood JG, Rogina B, Lavu S, et al. Sirtuin activators mimic caloric restriction and delay ageing in metazoans. Nature 2004;430:686–689.

IV HISTONE DEACETYLASE INHIBITORS

12 HDAC Inhibitors

Discovery, Development, and Clinical Impacts

Akihiro Ito, PhD,
Norikazu Nishino, PhD,
and Minoru Yoshida, PhD

CONTENTS

SUMMARY

Natural and synthetic inhibitors of histone deacetylases (HDACs) have not only contributed to the discovery of HDAC enzyme molecules and the elucidation of their functions but have also developed as attractive therapeutic agents for diseases including cancer. After the disclosure of the crystal structure of the HDAC-like protein bound to the inhibitor, the

From: *Cancer Drug Discovery and Development*
Histone Deacetylases: Transcriptional Regulation and Other Cellular Functions
Edited by: E. Verdin © Humana Press Inc., Totowa, NJ

momentum of research on HDAC inhibitors increased, and several inhibitors are currently under clinical trials. This chapter focuses on the current knowledge of all classes of HDACs inhibitors and the most recent progress in their clinical development.

Key Words: Cancer therapy, chemical biology, catalytic mechanism, drug design.

INTRODUCTION

Reversible acetylation is generally accepted as a posttranslational modification that regulates diverse protein activity such as phosphorylation. The best established protein target for reversible acetylation is core histones, which have been known for almost 30 years. A correlation between acetylation and transcriptional activity has been well established, and the recent discovery that certain enzymes control the acetylation status of core histones showed that acetylation of histones plays a critical role in the regulation of chromatin structure and transcriptional activity. Both acetylation and deacetylation of histones are catalyzed by histone acetyltransferases (HATs) and histone deacetylases (HDACs), respectively.

Histone acetylation appears to constitute a signal that may function in combination with other covalent modifications to generate an epigenetic code. This specific signal is reversed by a mechanism involving HDACs, which were found as transcriptional regulators related to reduced potassium dependency 3 yeast (Rpd3), histone deacetylase-A1 (Hda1) *(1)*, and silent information regulator 2 (Sir2) *(2)*. One of the most important developments in this field of research was the isolation of specific HDAC inhibitors from natural sources. In the early 1990s, trichostatin A (TSA) and other fungal antibiotics such as trapoxin (TPX) were shown to inhibit HDACs at nanomolar concentrations and to allow the induction of histone hyperacetylation in living cells *(3,4)*. These HDAC inhibitors played important roles not only in biochemical analyses of the role of histone acetylation but also in cloning the HDAC cDNA *(5)*. In addition, it is becoming increasingly clear that reversible acetylation of proteins other than histones is one of the key posttranslational modifications controlling the activity of proteins. The HDAC inhibitors have been widely used as powerful tools for identification and functional analysis of the acetylated nonhistone proteins. More recently, the clinical importance of the HDAC inhibitors has been emphasized, in particular for cancer treatment.

STRUCTURE AND FUNCTION OF HDACs

Three classes of HDACs have been identified to date *(6)*. Class I HDACs exhibit a domain organization similar to that in the yeast protein

RPD3 and include HDAC1, -2, -3, -8, and -11. This family of enzymes appears to cleave the acetamide bond by activating a water molecule with a zinc atom coupled to a histidine-aspartate charge-relay system *(7)*. Members of this class possess 400 to 500 amino acids and are primarily located in the nucleus. Class II HDACs include HDAC4, -5, -6, -7, -9, and -10 and have a catalytic domain similar to that in the yeast HDA1 protein. Members of this class have approx 1000 amino acids and the ability to shuttle in a regulated fashion between the nucleus and the cytoplasm *(6)*. Class II HDACs are further divided into two subclasses, class IIa including HDAC4, -5, -7, and -9 and class IIb including HDAC6 and -10 *(8)*. HDCA6 is an atypical enzyme that contains two catalytic domains *(9,10)* and is essentially localized in the cytoplasm *(11)*, whereas HDAC10 possesses an N-terminal catalytic domain and a C-terminal incomplete catalytic domain *(12)*. Although the specific roles and target proteins of these enzymes remain largely elusive, it has been shown that they have diverse cellular biological functions in addition to transcriptional regulation. Moreover, class I/II HDAC enzymes are emerging as therapeutic agents for the treatment of cancer (*see* the mechanism of antitumor activity section below) *(13–15)*.

Class III HDACs are homologus to the yeast Sir2 and have no significant sequence similarity to class I/II HDACs. The Sir2 family of enzymes is collectively called sirtuins. The *Saccharomyces cerevisiae* genome encodes five sirtuins (SIR2 and HST1–4) and the human genome encodes seven sirtuins (SIRT1–7), which are divided into four classes *(16)*. The sirtuin members are nicotinamide adenine dinucleotide (NAD)-dependent-proteins, and some of them are required for gene silencing at the telomerase *(17–19)*, the silent mating-type loci *(17,20)*, and ribosomal DNA loci *(21–23)*. Sir2 is also implicated in chromosomal stability and cell cycle progression in yeast *(24)*. In addition, it has been shown that Sir2 plays an essential role in the regulation of aging in both *S. cerevisiae* and *Caenorhabditis elegans (25,26)*. Although the first enzymatic function was ADP-ribosyltransferase activity *(27,28)*, NAD-dependent deacetylase activity was subsequently demonstrated as a primary activity of Sir2 *(2,29,30)*. The mechanism of enzymatic reaction of sirtuins is completely different from that of class I/II HDACs. Upon formation of ternary complex containing the sirtuin, NAD, and acetylated substrate, nicotinamide is expelled from NAD to generate an oxocarbenium-like transition in which the carbonyl oxygen of the acetyl group attacks the C1 carbon of ADP ribose to form 1′-*O*-alkyl amidate intermediate *(31)*. The final products formed are nicotinamide, the deacetylated protein, and 2′-*O*-acetyl-ADP-ribose. The 2′-*O*-acetyl-ADP-ribose is released into solution where it equilibrates with 3′-*O*-acetyl-ADP-ribose. Accordingly, the mechanism of inhibition and the nature of the inhibitors of this class are different from those of the other classes of HDACs.

In addition to chromatin-related functions, protein acetylation seems to be a signal that directly controls the activity of key cellular regulators *(32)*. Indeed, HATs and HDACs have been shown to control the state of acetylation of many nonhistone proteins *(33)*. In 1997, p53, a tumor suppressor protein, was reported to be acetylated by p300, thereby enhancing the DNA binding activity *(34)*, suggesting that acetylation is a key event in the signaling of DNA damage to p53. In vivo and in vitro deacetylation of p53 was shown to be mediated by the HDAC1-containing complex *(35)* and SIRT1, a member of the sirtuin family *(36,37)*, which downregulate the p53 transcriptional activity and apoptosis-inducing activity. Ito et al. *(38)* showed that acetylation in p53 shares common sites with ubiquitination, indicating that acetylation competes with ubiquitination and inhibits p53 degradation by the ubiquitin-proteasome pathway. Following the discovery of p53 acetylation, a number of nonhistone nuclear proteins were identified as in vitro substrates for p300/cyclic AMP-responsive element binding protein (CREB)-binding protein (CBP) or p300/CBP-associated factor (PCAF), most of which are involved in transcriptional regulation.

Recently, regulation by protein acetylation has also been shown to work in the cytoplasm. By using the differential sensitivity of HDAC6 to TSA and TPX (*see* the next section), the proteins that are acetylated in cells treated with TSA but not TPX were screened, and α-tubulin was identified as one of the in vivo substrates for HDAC6 *(39,40)*. HDAC6 deacetylated α-tubulin both in vivo and in vitro. HDAC6 controls the stability of a dynamic pool of microtubules. Indeed, overexpression of HDAC6 enhanced cell motility, whereas highly acetylated microtubules were observed after TSA treatment exhibited delayed drug-induced depolymerization. The biological role of HDAC6 was further confirmed by a recent report showing that tubacin, a specific inhibitor of HDAC6, caused tubulin acetylation and decreased cell motility *(41)*. Recently, SIRT2, one of the human sirtuin members, was also shown to be an NAD-dependent tubulin deacetylase *(42)*. Thus, protein acetylation, like phosphorylation, serves as a variety of signals that modulate the protein functions in both the nucleus and the cytoplasm, and both class I/II and class III enzymes are involved in the deacetylation of the nonhistone acetylated proteins.

INHIBITORS OF CLASS I/II HDACs

The first compound described as an inhibitor of HDAC activity was sodium butyrate (Fig. 1) *(43)*. The effect of butyrate as a noncompetitive inhibitor was shown with a partially purified enzyme *(44)*. However, its effective concentration exceeds milimolar levels, which raised the possibility that it affects other enzymes, the cytoskeleton, and membranes. Therefore, butyrate should be used with caution. A natural product, TSA,

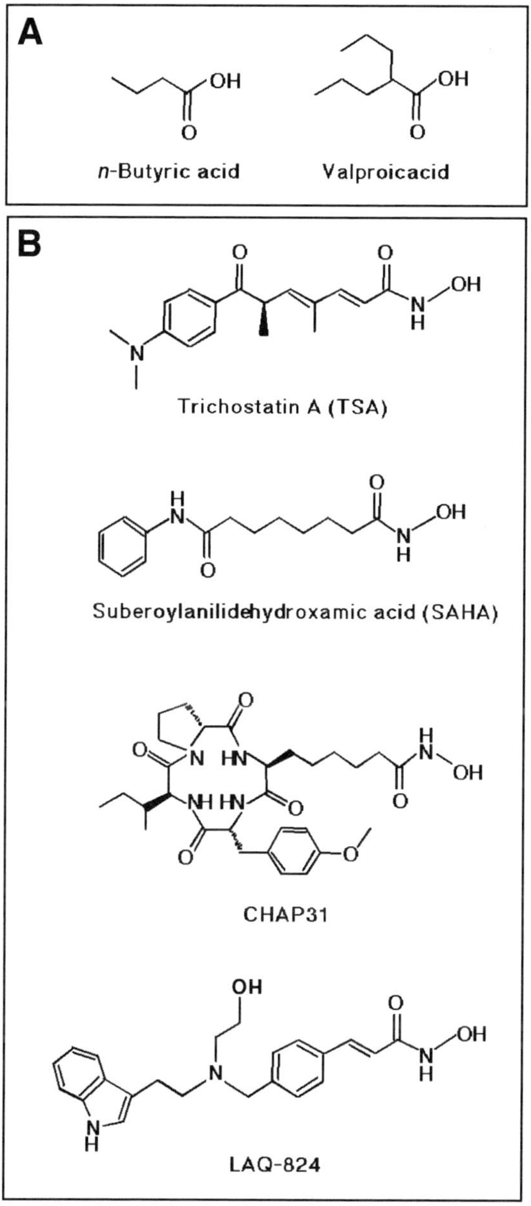

A

n-Butyric acid

Valproic acid

B

Trichostatin A (TSA)

Suberoylanilidehydroxamic acid (SAHA)

CHAP31

LAQ-824

originally isolated as an antifungal antibiotic, was the first specific HDAC inhibitor with a low nanomolar inhibition constant *(3)* (Fig. 1). TPX (Fig. 1), which had been discovered to induce morphological reversion of transformed

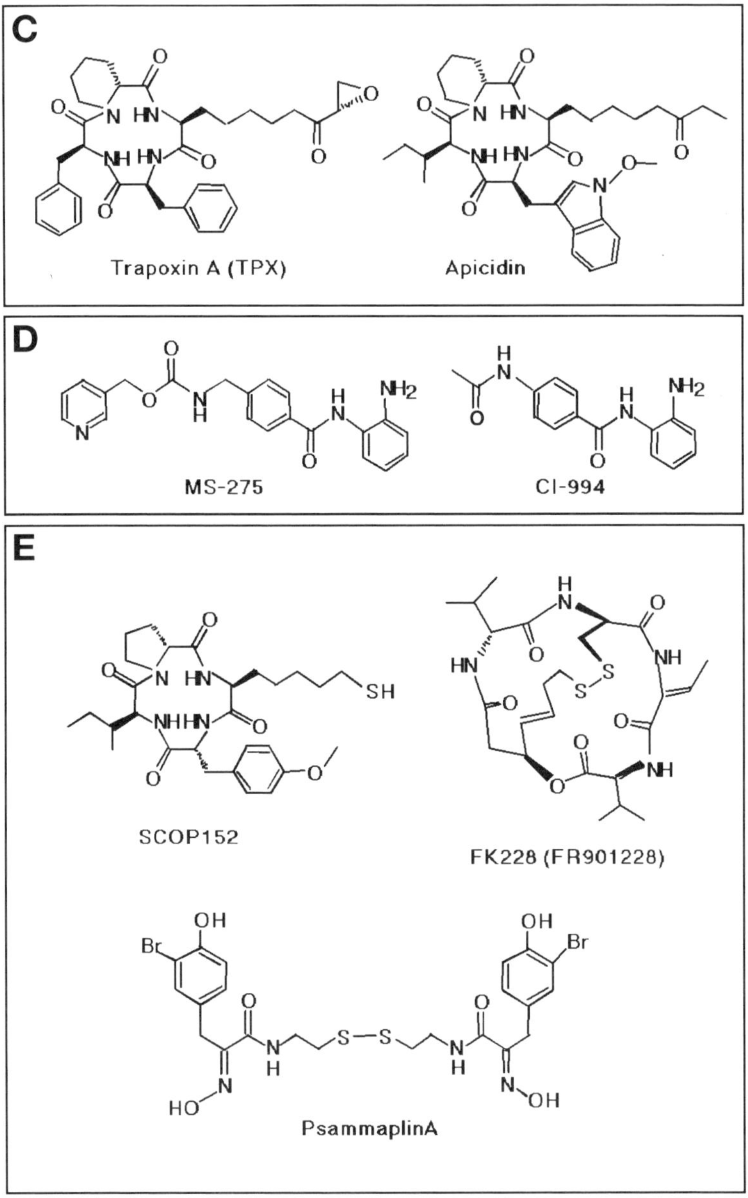

Fig. 1. Structure of class I/II HDAC inhibitors. (**A**) Carboxylates. (**B**) Hydroxamic acids. (**C**) Electrophilic ketones. (**D**) Anilides. (**E**) Thiols.

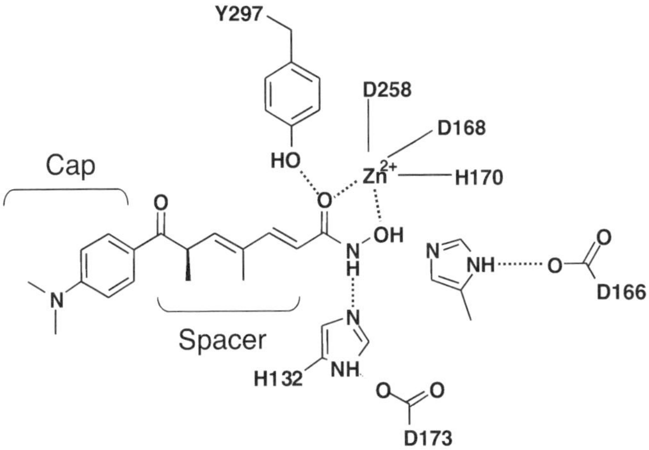

Fig. 2. A model for TSA interaction with the active site of HDAC. Zinc chelation occurs through carbonyl and hydroxyl groups of TSA to form a penta-coordinated zinc, which is essential for the inhibitory effect of TSA.

phenotype to normal in several oncogene-transformed cells, was also shown to inhibit HDAC *(4)*. In contrast to TSA, TPX was an irreversible inhibitor of HDACs. Cocrystallization of the bacterial histone deacetylase-like protein (HDLP) with TSA demonstrated that TSA mimics the substrate and that TSA binds by inserting its long aliphatic chain into the tube-like HDLP pocket and inhibits the enzyme activity by interacting with the zinc and active-site residues through its hydroxamic acid at one end of the aliphatic chain *(7)*. Hydroxamic acid, a functional group of the inhibitor, coordinates the zinc through its carbonyl and hydroxyl groups, resulting in the formation of a penta-coordinated zinc (Fig. 2).

The classes of compounds that have been identified as strong HDAC inhibitors have basic structures mimicking that of TSA, which possesses an aromatic group as a cap, an aliphatic chain for a spacer, and a hydroxamic acid as a functional group interacting with the active-site zinc (Fig. 2). The functional groups include carboxylates, hydroxamic acids, electrophilic ketones containing epoxyketones, anilides, and thiols (Fig. 1). The class I/II HDAC active site structure may have features of both metallo- and serine proteases, and the proposed catalytic mechanism for deacetylation is analogous to that of the zinc proteases such as thermolysin and matrix metalloproteinases (Fig. 3A). Since the zinc protease inhibitors have a zinc-chelating group such as a hydroxamic acid and thiol *(45)*, it is reasonable that these functional groups have great potential to inhibit HDAC activity (Fig. 3B).

In contrast to the zinc proteases, however, HDAC has a tube-like tunnel in the active-site pocket, which forms van der Waals interactions between

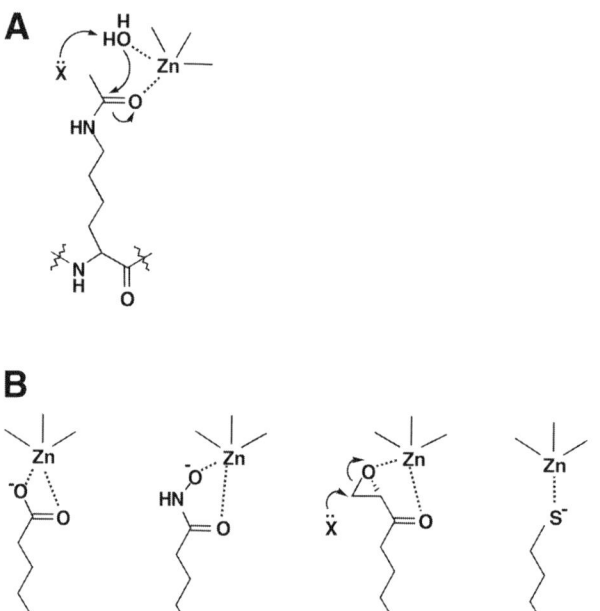

Fig. 3. Mechanism of catalytic activity of class I/II enzymes and inhibition by HDAC inhibitors. (**A**) Zinc-dependent acetamide cleavage reaction. (**B**) Chelation of the active site zinc by various functional groups.

the residues lining the pocket and the aliphatic chain of acetylated lysine. It is therefore likely that a long spacer of the inhibitor is necessary for access of the functional group to the active site zinc (Fig. 2). The aliphatic chain length of 5 that corresponds to the length between the carbonyl group and the α-carbon in acetylated lysine was proposed as the best spacer for inhibition *(46)*. The cap group may be necessary for packing the inhibitor at the rim of the tube-like active-site pocket (Fig. 2). Recently, some novel synthetic inhibitors have been developed based on this structure-activity relationship information.

Carboxylates

The carboxylate class *(47)*, which is defined as possessing a carboxylate in the metal binding moiety, has generally poor HDAC inhibitory activity in comparison with other inhibitors (Fig. 1A). Butyrate, a natural product generated in humans by both metabolism of fatty acids and bacterial fermentation of fiber in the colon, was the first identified HDAC inhibitor *(48)*. Related compounds such as phenyl butyrate and the anticonvulsant valproic acid *(49)* were later found to be HDAC inhibitors.

If the metal chelating functional group is a carboxylic acid, it seems that the activity is lower than the other functional groups such as hydroxamic acid. This may be owing to the weak coordination with zinc ions in comparison with other functional groups. It has been shown that butyrate possesses some selectivity, which poorly inhibits class IIb HDACs such as HDAC6 and -10 *(12)*. Pivaloyloxymethyl butyrate (AN-9) is an acyloxyalkyl ester prodrug of butyrate. Owing to better cell permeability in comparison with butyrate, AN-9 was shown to be greater than butyrate at inducing inhibition of cancer cell proliferation and malignant cell differentiation *(50,51)*.

Hydroxamic Acids

Hydroxamic acid is one of the well-studied ligands for the zinc present at the bottom of the narrow binding pocket of HDAC. TSA, which was originally isolated from a *Streptomyces* as an antifungal antibiotic against *Trichophyton (52)*, was rediscovered as a strong differentiation inducer in murine erythroleukemia (MEL) cells *(53)*. Another biological character of TSA was to induce cell cycle arrest at both the G1 and G2 phases *(54)*. During analysis of the target molecule for TSA, it was accidentally found that TSA induced hyperacetylation of core histones in cells. Furthermore, TSA blocked partially purified mouse HDAC activity with a low nanomolar inhibition constant in vitro, and HDAC activity from a mutant cell line resistant to TSA was resistant to TSA *(3)*. This genetic evidence clearly showed that HDAC is the molecular target for TSA.

The chemical structure of TSA is unique as a natural product in that it contains a hydroxamic acid at one end of the aliphatic chain. Suberoylanilide hydroxamic acid (SAHA) (Fig. 1B) was developed as a strong differentiation inducer during the designed synthesis of the hybrid polar compounds containing a hydroxamic acid and was found to be a potent inhibitor of partially purified HDACs *(55)*. SAHA has been shown to suppress cell growth in prostate cancer cell lines *(56)* and human breast cancer cells *(57)* and to inhibit the growth of the human prostate CWR22 xenograft in nude mice *(56)*. Furthermore, SAHA inhibited the incidence and growth of carcinogen-induced mammary tumors in rats without toxicity *(58)* and induced remission in a transgenic model mouse of therapy-resistant acute promyelocytic leukemia *(59)*. The phase I trial of SAHA has been completed, and the results showed that it could be administered safely and had antitumor activity in solid and hematologic tumors *(60)*. A phase II trial has been launched.

Pyroxamide (suberoyl-3-aminopyridineamide hydroxamic acid) is a new member of the hydroxamic acid-based hybrid polar compounds and was designed to increase solubility in aqueous solution compared with SAHA. Pyroxamide was shown to induce growth inhibition of tumor cells *(61)*. LAQ-824 is a novel cinnamyl hydroxamic acid derivative (Fig. 1B).

LAQ-824 selectively inhibited growth of cancer cells at submicromolar concentration, induced apoptosis in tumor cells only but not in normal cells, and exhibited antitumor activity in a xenograft animal model *(62)*. Of the cinnamyl hydroxamic acid derivatives, LAQ-824 exhibited a high maximum tolerated dose with low gross toxicity *(63)*. Both pyroxamide and LAQ-824 are currently under phase I trials. Cyclic hydroxamic acid-containing peptide (CHAP) is an analog of TPX, in which the epoxyketone is replaced with the hydroxamic acid (Fig. 1B). CHAP has the ability to inhibit HDAC1 at a low nanomolar concentration *(46,64)*. Based on the structure of TSA and SAHA associated with HDLP, a large number of inhibitors with the hydroxamic acids have been designed and synthesized.

Electrophilic Ketones

TPX is a cyclic tetrapeptide containing a unique amino acid, 2-amino-8-oxo-9, 10-epoxydecanoic acid (Aoe; Fig. 1C), and was originally identified as a fungal metabolite inducing morphological reversion of v-*sis*-transformed NIH-3T3 cells *(65)*. A number of structurally related cyclic tetrapeptides with Aoe have been isolated from the natural source, some of which were toxins produced by phytopathogens. Since the biological activity of TPX is similar to that of TSA, which can induce morphology reversion of the transformed cells, it was speculated that the target molecule for TPX is HDAC or its functionally related proteins. Indeed, TPX caused hyperacetylation of histones in a variety of mammalian cells. An in vitro experiment using partially purified HDAC revealed that TPX inhibited HDAC activity at low nanomolar concentrations. The epoxy ketone group in Aoe seems likely to play a role in forming a covalent bond between TPX and the active-site residues of enzymes, since the chemical reduction of the epoxide group impaired the inhibitory activity *(4)*. Taking advantage of the ability of TPX to bind covalently to HDAC, Taunton et al. *(5)* succeeded in isolating HDAC1 by means of a synthesized affinity probe using TPX.

Although the cyclic tetrapeptide compounds containing Aoe are potent inhibitors for HDAC in vitro, they exhibit very weak activity in animal models, probably owing to the chemical instability of the epoxy ketone group in blood. Apicidin (Fig. 1C), a cyclic tetrapeptide isolated from *Fusarium pallodoroseum* as a potent and broad-spectrum antiprotozoal agent, exerts its biological activity by reversibly inhibiting HDAC activity *(66)*. Apicidin contains an ethyl ketone moiety in its side chain instead of the epoxy ketone. The high potency of HDAC inhibitory activity of apicidin further confirmed the importance of the cyclic tetrapeptide scaffold for the inhibitor design. SAHA-based straight-chain trifluoromethyl ketones have also been reported as HDAC inhibitors *(67)*. Trifluoromethyl ketones are known to be readily hydrated, resulting in zinc chelation and inhibition of zinc proteases *(68)*. We have synthesized cyclic tetrapeptide containing trifluoromethyl ketones as the zinc binding functionality and these compounds exhibited excellent inhibitory activity *(69)*.

Anilides

The anilide class of inhibitors includes bezamides with a phenylene diamine as the functional group such as MS-275 (Fig. 1D), which is suggested to interact with the HDAC active-site zinc through the 2-substituted anilide moiety. It has been shown that MS-275 inhibits HDACs purified from human leukemia cells and induces accumulation of hyperacetylation at submicromolar concentrations *(70)*. In addition, MS-275 has been shown to inhibit cell growth of diverse solid tumor cell lines *(71)*. This class exhibits generally weak inhibitory activity against HDACs in comparison with the hydroxamic acids. However, MS-275 strongly inhibited growth in various types of human tumor xenografts *(70)*. CI-994 (Fig. 1D), originally identified as an angiogenesis inhibitor, has been shown to possess poor inhibitory activity against HDACs in vitro. CI-994 increased the amount of acetylated histones and delayed tumor growth in mouse xenograft models *(72)*. Phase II clinical investigations are in progress for both MS-275 and CI-994.

Thiols

FK228 (also known as FR901228 and depsipeptide; Fig. 1E) isolated as the bacterial metabolite is an atypical HDAC inhibitor as it does not contain a visible functional group that interacts with the zinc ion in the HDAC binding pocket, although FK228 has strong HDAC-inhibitory activity *(73)*. Recently, it has been shown that FK228 was activated by chemical reduction, yielding two free thiol groups, one of which is accessible to the catalytic zinc as a functional group. Blocking the thiol groups by methylation completely abolished the inhibitory activity. Since glutathione is present at millimolar concentrations in the cell, FK228 can be converted to its active and reduced form (RedFK) by cellular reducing activity. Consistent with this idea, mutations in the glutathione synthesis pathway conferred FK228 resistance on yeast cells *(74)*. FK228 exhibited a potent antitumor activity in xenograft models *(75)*. FK228 is currently being evaluated clinically in a phase II trial.

Psammaplins (Fig. 1E) isolated from the sponge *Pseudoceratina purpurea* are structurally unique inhibitors of HDAC *(76)*. These compounds contain a disulphide linkage, and therefore the inhibitory activity may be owing to chelation of the zinc ion with sulfhydryl in the active-site pocket. Studies on the mechanism of action of psammaplin and its synthetic derivatives also supported the possibility of a cellular disulphide cleavage-type

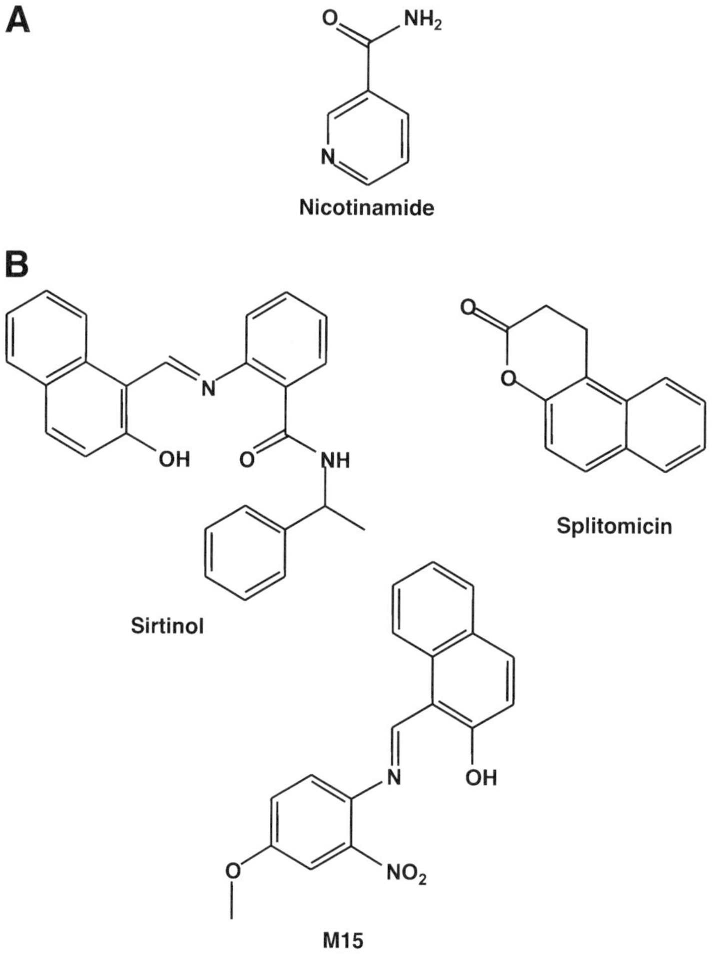

Fig. 4. Structure of class II HDAC inhibitors. (**A**) Nicotinamide. (**B**) β-Naphthol analogs.

mechanism of inhibition *(77,78)*. Recently, we synthesized a series of cyclic tetrapeptides containing a functional thiol group named sulfur-containing cyclic peptide (SCOP; Fig. 1E). SCOP inhibited HDAC1 and -4 at nanomolar concentrations but was weak in inhibiting HDAC6 and -8 *(79)*. By disulfide formation with SCOP itself or other mercaptans, SCOP can be converted to a "homodimer" or a "heterodimer", acting as a pro-drug like FK228. Once the homodimer is incorporated into the cells, it becomes reduced and activated by cellular reducing activity, giving two active molecules. In the case of hybrid-type inhibitors, other functions such as better solubility, drug delivery, and other enzyme inhibitory activity can be added into the partner compounds.

INHIBITORS OF CLASS III HDACs

The first compounds that were demonstrated to inhibit in vitro deacetylase activity of sirtuins were nonhydrolyzable NAD analogs such as Carba-NAD *(80)*. However, such compounds do not appear to be suitable for in vivo studies since they are not cell permeable and they inhibit other NAD-dependent enzymes. To solve these problems, high-throughput cell-based screens were conducted to identify cell-permeable small-molecule inhibitors of NAD-dependent deacetylase activity of sirtuin *(81,82)*. All small-molecule inhibitors identified by these screens were analogs of α-substituted β-naphthol, such as sirtinol, M15, and splitomicin (Fig. 4), and they inhibited transcriptional silencing by Sir2 in yeast. Sirtinol and M15 were shown to inhibit yeast Sir2 and human SIRT2 in vitro, whereas split-omicin demonstrated some selectivity against inhibition of deacetylase activity between yeast sirtuins. These compounds were used to elucidate cellular functions of sirtuin in plant or mammalian cells *(83–85)*.

NAD Analog

Based on the requirement of NAD for the deacetylation reaction by Sir2, an uncleavable NAD analog was designed as a Sir2 inhibitor. Carba-NAD is a carbocyclic analog of NAD in which a 2,3-di-hydroxycylopentane methanol replaces the β-D-ribonucleotide ring of the nicotinamide ribonu-cleoside moiety of NAD *(86)*. It inhibits HST2 deacetylase activity in a competitive manner in vitro *(80)*. This result is also consistent with the requirement for NAD cleavage during the enzymatic reaction.

Nicotinamide

Nicotinamide (Fig. 4A) is a byproduct of the Sir2 deacetylase reaction and is a natural noncompetitive inhibitor for Sir2. Nicotinamide abolishes silencing at the rDNA, telomeres, and mating-type loci and shortens life span, indicating that nicotinamide creates a phenocopy of the *sir2* muta-tion in yeast *(87)*. Nicotinamide also suppresses transcriptional repression of Hst1 *(88)*. Indeed, the deacetylase activity of several Sir2 family mem-bers, including yeast Sir2 and Hst2 *(29,87)* and human SIRT1, -2, and -3 *(36,42,89)*, can be inhibited by nicotinamide. Nicotinamide inhibits the enzyme activity by intercepting an ADP-ribosyl-enzyme-acetyl peptide intermediate with regeneration of NAD *(90)*. Since nicotinamide inhibi-tion is uniquely tied to the catalytic mechanism of the Sir2 deacetylation reaction, nicotinamide is most likely a general inhibitor for all Sir2 family members. Physiological concentrations of nicotinamide inhibit yeast Sir2 and human SIRT1 in vitro *(80,87)*. In addition, reduction of nicotinamide by Pnc1, which encodes a nicotinamidase that converts nicotinamide to nicotinic acid, enhanced Sir2-mediated silencing and longevity in yeast *(88)*. Thus, nicotinamide may function as an in vivo negative regulator for Sir2 *(91)*.

β-*Naphthol Analogs*

Small-molecule inhibitors were identified by cell-based chemical screening for compounds that suppress Sir2-mediated silencing using yeast strains in which either URA3 or TRP1 is inserted within Sir2-silenced loci such as the telomere or homeodomain regulator (HMR). All these inhibitors are structurally related analogs of α-substituted β-naphthol. Sirtinol and M15 (Fig. 4B) were first identified as small-molecule inhibitors for sirtuins by Schreiber and co-workers *(81)*. Sirtinol inhibits in vivo silencing activity of yeast Sir2 as well as in vitro deacetylase activity of recombinant yeast Sir2 and human SIRT2 but not HDAC1, indicating that sirtinol is a specific inhibitor for sirtuins. Since sirtinol and M15 share 2-hydroxy-1-naphthaldehyde within their structure, the 2-hydroxy-1-naphthaldehyde moiety could be responsible for the inhibitory activity of these compounds. Indeed, 2-hydroxy-1-naphthaldehyde alone can partially inhibit SIRT2 activity in vitro. Recently, sirtinol was used to identify SIR1 in *Arabidopsis*, a regulator of many auxin-inducible genes, by a genetic screen for mutants that were resistant to the effects of sirtinol *(83)*. Furthermore, sirtinol and M15 were used to delineate a role of Sir2 in regulating skeletal muscle differentiation *(84)*.

Splitomicin (Fig. 4B), identified by Simon and co-workers *(81)*, is structurally related to sirtinol. It can create a phenocopy of a *sir2* mutant in yeast and can inhibit in vitro deacetylase activity of Sir2 against a histone H4 peptide *(82)*. A screen for the alleles of *SIR2* that are resistant to the antisilencing effects of splitomicin revealed a small helical module of Sir2 that creates a putative substrate binding site *(92–94)* as a possible site where splitomicin acts *(82)*. Thus, splitomicin probably inhibits deacetylase activity of Sir2 by interfering with the access of an acetylated substrate to this region. Among Sir2 and four Sir2 homologs (Hst1–4) in *S. cerevisiae*, the effects of splitomicin on transcription correlated most highly with a *sir2* mutation, less with an *hst1* mutation, and not at all with other *sir2* homologs mutations *(95)*, suggesting that splitomicin is a selective inhibitor for Sir2 in *S. cerevisiae*.

In contrast to splitomicin, dehydrosplitomicin, an analog of splitomicin unsaturated at the 1,2-position of splitomicin, has been shown to repress Hst1-regulated genes but not to perturb the silencing by Sir2 *(95)*, indicating that an inhibitory activity of dehydrosplitomicin is selective for Hst1. The chimeric and mutagenetic approaches revealed that leucine-244 within the small helical module of Hst1, which corresponds to tyrosine-298 of Sir2, is an essential residue for the relative resistance of Hst1 toward split-omicin *(95)*. These observations suggest that splitomicin and dehydros-plitomicin may be useful tools for investigating individual roles of Sir2 and Hst1 in *S. cerevisiae*.

MECHANISM OF ANTITUMOR ACTIVITY

There is growing evidence that HDACs are important agents for cancer therapy, and HDAC inhibitors bear great potential as anticancer drugs. First, some of the class I/II HDACs have been shown to be involved in the proliferation of normal and cancer cells. Chicken HDAC3 was reported to be essential for cell proliferation in DT40 cells *(96)*. A knockout of HDAC1 in mouse embryonic stem cells resulted in embryonic lethality and severely impaired proliferation, which correlated with an increase in histone acetylation and expression of the cyclin-dependent kinase (CDK) inhibitors p21 and p27 *(97)*. HDAC1 and -3 small interfering RNA (siRNA) produced a concentration-dependent inhibition of HeLa cell pro-liferation, whereas HDAC4 and -7 siRNA showed no effect. HDAC3 siRNA caused histone hyperacetylation and increased the percent of apoptotic cells, suggesting that the class I HDACs such as HDAC1 and -3 are important in the regulation of proliferation and survival in cancer cells *(98)*.

Second, aberrant transcriptional repression by histone deacetylation is commonly observed in many cancers. In leukemia, chimeric fusion pro-teins produced by chromosomal translocation recruit class I/II HDAC-containing complexes *(99)*. The promyelocytic leukemia-retinoic acid receptor α(PML-RARα) fusion protein generated by 15;17 chromosomal translocation in acute promyelocytic leukemia (APL) cells strongly represses the gene expression required for myeloid differentiation by recruiting HDACs. However, since the protein is still able to bind the ligand retinoic acid, pharmacological concentrations of retinoic acid can induce the release of repression and therefore cause reinitiation of differ-entiation. Thus, most APL patients can be cured by all-*trans* retinoic acid treatment. In contrast, another fusion protein, promyelocytic leukemia zinc finger (PLZF)RARα, is unable to be activated, since PLZF also binds the corepressor/HDAC complex. In this case, combined treatment with HDAC inhibitors can overcome the transcriptional repression and induce blast differentiation *(100)*. In acute myeloid leukemia (AML) with 8;21 translocation, acute myeloid leukemia 1-eight-twenty-one (AML1-ETO) also aberrantly recruits HDACs to the target genes *(101,102)*. Aberrant transcriptional repression of tumor suppressor genes such as *INK4A* by DNA methylation has been shown to be one of the major causes for cancer development *(103)*. Methylated DNA binds factors like methyl CpG binding protein 2 (MeCP2) that can recruit DNA methyltransferase and HDACs to repress the genes and to propagate gene silencing. Synergistic reactivation of the methylated genes by methylation inhibitors such as 5-azadeoxycytidine and HDAC inhibitors is one of the important therapeutic strategies currently expected *(104)*.

Third, the possibility of HDACs as a target for anticancer treatment was validated by the effects of HDAC inhibitors. In contrast to other potential molecular targets for cancer therapy, HDAC is unique because its inhibitors had already been known and the importance for cancer therapy had been proposed based on the efficacy of the inhibitors before HDAC genes were cloned *(105)*. HDAC inhibitors induce differentiation in a variety of leukemias both in vitro and in vivo. They also seem to have great potential as drugs against solid tumors, probably owing to their ability to induce apoptosis. Indeed, some HDAC inhibitors such as AN-9 (phase II), CI-994 (phase II), FK228 (phase II), LAQ-824 (phase I), MS-275 (phase II), SAHA (phase II), and valproic acid (phase I) have already exhibited remarkable antitumor activity.

Despite extensive studies on HDAC inhibitors, the general mechanism by which they exhibit antitumor activity is still unclear. Three major possibilities are assumed as the basis for the selective toxicity of cancer cells to HDAC inhibitors (Fig. 5). First, it is widely speculated that the ability of HDAC inhibitors to modulate gene expression through histone hyperacetylation is the critical determinant for antitumor activity by inducing gene expression in the areas of cell cycle arrest, differentiation, apoptosis *(106)*, and inhibition of angiogenesis *(107)*. The second possibility is that hyperacetylation of nonhistone proteins such as p53 and α-tubulin modulates the activity of specific proteins. Following the discovery of p53 acetylation, a number of nonhistone proteins were identified as in vitro substrates for p300/CBP or PCAF, most of which are involved in transcriptional regulation. In the case of some but not all DNA-binding transcription factors, the acetylation site falls directly adjacent to the DNA-binding domain and acetylation results in stimulation of DNA binding. Subcellular localization, protein-protein interaction, and protein stability are also regulated by acetylation. Therefore, it is also likely that protein acetylation induced by HDAC inhibitors causes dramatic changes in the transformed state in cancer cells more specifically than histone acetylation, which may cause general changes in both normal and cancer cells.

A third possibility is independent of gene regulation but involves aberrant mitosis in the cell cycle of cancer cells. Mitotic checkpoint dysfunction is likely to be a common feature of cancers. It was reported that some HDAC inhibitors trigger a G2 phase cell cycle checkpoint response in normal human cells. On the other hand, this checkpoint is

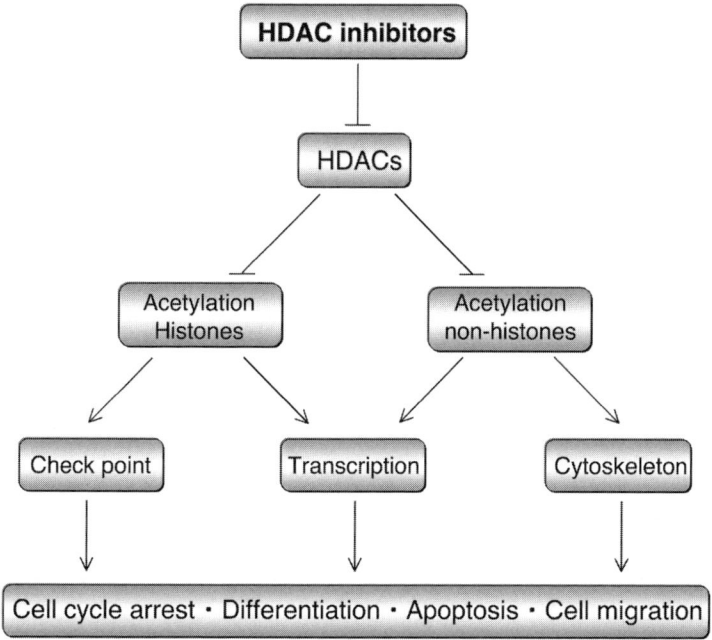

Fig. 5. Possible mechanisms by which HDAC inhibitors exert biological activities. Acetylation of histones and nonhistone proteins is induced by treatment with HDAC inhibitors. Two distinct pathways downstream of histone acetylation, which are dependent on and independent of changes in gene expression, have been postulated. Hyperacetylation of histones by HDAC inhibitors modulates expression of subsets of genes responsible for the cell cycle arrest, differentiation, and apoptosis. On the other hand, histone hyperacetylation also induces a G2 cell cycle checkpoint, and cancer cells, which lack cell cycle checkpoints, undergo aberrant mitosis, resulting in apoptotic cell death. Nonhistone proteins such as p53 and α-tubulin are also acetylated, and HDAC inhibitors can modulate their activity by accumulating the acetylation. For instance, an increase in the p53 acetylation by HDAC inhibitors stabilizes the protein and enhances its transcriptional activity. Hyperacetylation of α-tubulin by HDAC inhibitors inhibits cell motility, which may contribute to suppression of cancer cell invasion.

defective in tumor cells, which results in aberrant mitosis and eventual cell death *(108)*. More recently, HDAC activity was shown to be required for maintaining pericentric heterochromatin *(109)* and proper loading of the centromere-specific histone H3 variant CENP-A to the centromere region *(110)*. These results suggest that HDAC inhibitor-induced apoptosis is related to aberrant mitosis in cancer cells lacking cell cycle checkpoints.

HDAC INHIBITORS AS THERAPEUTICS AGAINST HUMAN DISEASES OTHER THAN CANCER

Polyglutamine diseases such as Huntington's disease are hereditary neurodegenerative disorders caused by the expansion of the polyglutamine repeat in the diseased gene. The pathogenesis of these diseases may be associated with transcriptional dysregulation and loss of function of transcriptional coactivators *(111)*. It has been shown that the expanded polyglutamine negatively regulates activity of histone acetyltransferases (HATs) such as CBP by either sequestering them in cytoplasmic and nuclear aggregates *(112,113)* or inhibiting their acetyltransferase activity, leading to a reduction in the amount of acetylated histones, which can be reverted by an HDAC inhibitor *(112)*. In addition, ectopic overexpression of CBP reduces polyglutamine-mediated cell death *(113,114)*.

These observations suggest that the acetylating activity plays important roles in regulating polyglutamine-induced neurodegeneration and that HDAC inhibitors are useful as therapeutic agents against these disorders. Indeed, some inhibitors of class I/II HDACs such as SAHA and butyrate have been shown to reduce neuronal death induced by the expanded polyglutamine in cultured cells *(115)* and in the *Drosophila* model of Huntington's disease *(112)*. Furthermore, SAHA and butyrate increased acetylated protein levels including histones and specificity protein 1 (Sp1) in the brain and improved motor performance in the transgenic mouse model of Huntington's disease *(116,117)*. In addition, it has been shown that HDAC6 plays a critical role in the aggresome formation that is associated with a number of neurodegenerative diseases including Parkinson's disease and amyotrophic lateral sclerosis *(118)*. Indeed, HDAC inhibitors were shown to prevent aggresome formation *(119)*. Thus, inhibitors of class I/II HDACs may provide clinical benefits in neurodegenerative diseases.

Forkhead transcription factors (Foxos) are homologous to the *C. elegans* dauer formation 16 (DAF-16) and act downstream of the insulin signaling pathway. It has been shown that haploinsufficiency of the *foxo1* gene restored insulin sensitivity and rescued the diabetic phenotype in insulin-resistant mice, whereas activation of Foxo1 in liver and pancreatic β-cells induced diabetes by an increase in hepatic glucose production *(120)*. Foxo1 interacts with peroxisome proliferator-activated receptor-γ coactivator 1α (PCG-1α) and controls insulin-regulated gluconeogenesis *(121)*. Recently, the activity of Foxos was shown to be regulated by reversible acetylation. Deacetylation by SIRT1 potentiates Foxo transactivation. Treatment with both nicotinamide and TSA has been shown to increase the amount of acetylated Foxos and mostly attenuates Foxo functions while it enhances Foxo-mediated apoptosis *(122–124)*. Furthermore, Scriptide, a hydroxamic acid-based HDAC inhibitor, was recently reported to stimulate 2-deoxyglucose uptake through an increase in the expression and translocation of glucose transporter 4 (Glut4) *(125)*. Thus, inhibitors of both class I/II and class III HDACs may become therapeutic agents against diabetes by modifying Foxo and/or Glut4 activities.

Identification and characterization of novel T-cell-inhibitory compounds are generally important for developing new strategies to suppress autoimmune diseases. Skov et al. *(126)* recently revealed that TSA inhibited proliferation and CD154 expression in CD4 T cells by a mechanism distinct from that of well-known drugs against autoimmune diseases such as cyclosporine and FK506. In addition, the cyclic tetrapeptide FR235222, a potent HDAC inhibitor, exhibited marked immunosuppressive effects *(127,128)*. These reports suggest the clinical use of HDAC inhibitors as novel therapeutic agents in the field of autoimmune diseases.

THE COMING GENERATION OF HDAC INHIBITORS

Target enzyme specificity of current HDAC inhibitors is poorly understood, mainly because of the difficulty in obtaining in vitro active recombinant enzymes and in vivo complex formation with other HDAC enzymes in cells. Nevertheless, TSA has been shown to inhibit HDAC1, -2, -4, and -6 to almost the same extent *(46)*. However, HDAC8 is relatively resistant to TSA *(129)*. SAHA and MS-275 are also poor inhibitors for HDAC8. HDAC6 was described to be insensitive to the cyclic tetrapeptide inhibitors with large cap groups including TPX, FK228, and MS-275 *(40)*. Short-chain fatty acids like butyrate also failed to inhibit HDAC6. By contrast, tubacin inhibits HDAC6 but not other enzymes *(41)*. These observations suggest that the current inhibitors have intrinsic selectivity to some extent. However, lessons from the great success of protein tyrosine kinase inhibitors as antitumor drugs emphasize the importance of developing inhibitors with high specificity for a certain enzyme with pathogenic function. Enzyme-specific HDAC inhibitors would be valuable both as tools for probing the biological functions of the enzymes and for therapeutic purposes. How can one design the enzyme-specific inhibitors? Whereas residues forming the active-site pocket are highly conserved, those of the enzyme surface are diversified. It is therefore likely that the difference in structure around the pocket entrance is responsible for the different sensitivity to the drugs, since the large-cap groups probably make extensive contacts at the rim of the pocket and in the shallow grooves surrounding the pocket entrance. Indeed, FK228, which contains a large cap, strongly inhibited HDAC1 and -2 but was relatively weak in inhibiting HDAC4 or -6 *(74)*. Thus, it should be possible to generate specific inhibitors for different HDACs by creating diverse cap groups with a terminal functional group.

CONCLUSIONS

In the 20th century, we learned a great deal about DNA, chromosomes, and the mechanisms of segregation of genetic information, which are concomitantly important areas of research for cancer treatment. Indeed, most of the current anticancer drugs target DNA or microtubules. To overcome the limitations of the current anticancer drugs, however, it is urgent that novel therapeutic agents be discovered and validated. Epigenetic events are alterations in gene expression without changes in DNA sequence, which are heritable through cell division. Dysfunction of epigenetic events such as DNA methylation and histone modifications may be a key driving force in the development of cancer *(103)*. Elucidation of epigenetic control will be one of the major tasks for cell biology in this century. We can confidently anticipate that aberrant epigenetic control by chromatin-modifying enzymes will be important for future therapy of human diseases including cancer. It is the hope that the application of HDAC inhibitors to human diseases, probably in combination with DNA methyltransferase inhibitors or current chemotherapeutics, will lead to broad clinical utility.

REFERENCES

1. Grunstein M. Histone acetylation in chromatin structure and transcription. Nature 1997;389:349–352.
2. Imai S, Armstrong CM, Kaeberlein M, Guarente L. Transcriptional silencing and longevity protein Sir2 is an NAD-dependent histone deacetylase. Nature 2000;403:795–800.
3. Yoshida M, Kijima M, Akita M, Beppu T. Potent and specific inhibition of mammalian histone deacetylase both in vivo and in vitro by trichostatin A. J Biol Chem 1990;265:17,174–17,179.
4. Kijima M, Yoshida M, Sugita K, Horinouchi S, Beppu T. Trapoxin, an antitumor cyclic tetrapeptide, is an irreversible inhibitor of mammalian histone deacetylase. J Biol Chem 1993;268:22,429–22,435.
5. Taunton J, Hassig CA, Schreiber SL. A mammalian histone deacetylase related to the yeast transcriptional regulator Rpd3p. Science 1996;272:408–411.
6. Khochbin S, Verdel A, Lemercier C, Seigneurin-Berny D. Functional significance of histone deacetylase diversity. Curr Opin Genet Dev 2001;11:162–166.
7. Finnin MS, Donigian JR, Cohen A, et al. Structures of a histone deacetylase homologue bound to the TSA and SAHA inhibitors. Nature 1999;401:188–193.
8. Verdin E, Dequiedt F, Kasler HG. Class II histone deacetylases: versatile regulators. Trends Genet 2003;19:286–293.
9. Grozinger CM, Hassig CA, Schreiber SL. Three proteins define a class of human histone deacetylases related to yeast Hda1p. Proc Natl Acad Sci U S A 1999;96: 4868–4873.
10. Verdel A, Khochbin S. Identification of a new family of higher eukaryotic histone deacetylases. Coordinate expression of differentiation-dependent chromatin modifiers. J Biol Chem 1999;274:2440–2445.
11. Verdel A, Curtet S, Brocard MP, et al. Active maintenance of mHDA2/mHDAC6 histone-deacetylase in the cytoplasm. Curr Biol 2000;10:747–749.

12. Guardiola AR, Yao TP. Molecular cloning and characterization of a novel histone deacetylase HDAC10. J Biol Chem 2002;277:3350–3356.

13. Miller TA, Witter DJ, Belvedere S. Histone deacetylase inhibitors. J Med Chem 2003;46:5097–5116.

14. Marks PA, Miller T, Richon VM. Histone deacetylases. Curr Opin Pharmacol 2003;3:344–351.

15. Meinke PT, Liberator P. Histone deacetylase: a target for antiproliferative and antiprotozoal agents. Curr Med Chem 2001;8:211–235.

16. North BJ, Verdin E. Sirtuins: Sir2-related NAD-dependent protein deacetylases. Genome Biol 2004;5:224.

17. Aparicio OM, Billington BL, Gottschling DE. Modifiers of position effect are shared between telomeric and silent mating-type loci in *S. cerevisiae*. Cell 1991;66:1279–1287.

18. Strahl-Bolsinger S, Hecht A, Luo K, Grunstein M. SIR2 and SIR4 interactions differ in core and extended telomeric heterochromatin in yeast. Genes Dev 1997;11:83–93.

19. Gottschling DE, Aparicio OM, Billington BL, Zakian VA. Position effect at *S. cerevisiae* telomeres: reversible repression of Pol II transcription. Cell 1990;63: 751–762.

20. Rine J, Herskowitz I. Four genes responsible for a position effect on expression from HML and HMR in *Saccharomyces cerevisiae*. Genetics 1987;116:9–22.

21. Smith JS, Boeke JD. An unusual form of transcriptional silencing in yeast ribosomal DNA. Genes Dev 1997;11:241–254.

22. Bryk M, Banerjee M, Murphy M, Knudsen KE, Garfinkel DJ, Curcio MJ. Transcriptional silencing of Ty1 elements in the RDN1 locus of yeast. Genes Dev 1997;11:255–269.

23. Fritze CE, Verschueren K, Strich R, Easton Esposito R. Direct evidence for SIR2 modulation of chromatin structure in yeast rDNA. EMBO J 1997;16:6495–6509.

24. Brachmann CB, Sherman JM, Devine SE, Cameron EE, Pillus L, Boeke JD. The SIR2 gene family, conserved from bacteria to humans, functions in silencing, cell cycle progression, and chromosome stability. Genes Dev 1995;9:2888–2902.

25. Kaeberlein M, McVey M, Guarente L. The SIR2/3/4 complex and SIR2 alone promote longevity in *Saccharomyces cerevisiae* by two different mechanisms. Genes Dev 1999;13:2570–2580.

26. Tissenbaum HA, Guarente L. Increased dosage of a sir-2 gene extends lifespan in *Caenorhabditis elegans*. Nature 2001;410:227–230.

27. Frye RA. Characterization of five human cDNAs with homology to the yeast SIR2 gene: Sir2-like proteins (sirtuins) metabolize NAD and may have protein ADP-ribosyltransferase activity. Biochem Biophys Res Commun 1999;260: 273–279.

28. Tanny JC, Dowd GJ, Huang J, Hilz H, Moazed D. An enzymatic activity in the yeast Sir2 protein that is essential for gene silencing. Cell 1999;99:735–745.

29. Landry J, Sutton A, Tafrov ST, et al. The silencing protein SIR2 and its homologs are NAD-dependent protein deacetylases. Proc Natl Acad Sci U S A 2000;97: 5807–5811.

30. Smith JS, Brachmann CB, Celic I, et al. A phylogenetically conserved NAD+-dependent protein deacetylase activity in the Sir2 protein family. Proc Natl Acad Sci U S A 2000;97:6658–6663.

31. Denu JM. Linking chromatin function with metabolic networks: Sir2 family of NAD(+)-dependent deacetylases. Trends Biochem Sci 2003;28:41–48.

32. Kouzarides T. Acetylation: a regulatory modification to rival phosphorylation? EMBO J 2000;19:1176–1179.

33. Sterner DE, Berger SL. Acetylation of histones and transcription-related factors. Microbiol Mol Biol Rev 2000;64:435–459.

34. Gu W, Roeder RG. Activation of p53 sequence-specific DNA binding by acetylation of the p53 C-terminal domain. Cell 1997;90:595–606.

35. Luo J, Su F, Chen D, Shiloh A, Gu W. Deacetylation of p53 modulates its effect on cell growth and apoptosis. Nature 2000;408:377–381.

36. Luo J, Nikolaev AY, Imai S, et al. Negative control of p53 by Sir2alpha promotes cell survival under stress. Cell 2001;107:137–148.

37. Vaziri H, Dessain SK, Ng Eaton E, et al. hSIR2(SIRT1) functions as an NAD-dependent p53 deacetylase. Cell 2001;107:149–159.

38. Ito A, Kawaguchi Y, Lai CH, et al. MDM2-HDAC1-mediated deacetylation of p53 is required for its degradation. EMBO J 2002;21:6236–6245.

39. Hubbert C, Guardiola A, Shao R, et al. HDAC6 is a microtubule-associated deacetylase. Nature 2002;417:455–458.

40. Matsuyama A, Shimazu T, Sumida Y, et al. In vivo destabilization of dynamic microtubules by HDAC6-mediated deacetylation. EMBO J 2002;21:6820–6831.

41. Haggarty SJ, Koeller KM, Wong JC, Grozinger CM, Schreiber SL. Domain-selective small-molecule inhibitor of histone deacetylase 6 (HDAC6)-mediated tubulin deacetylation. Proc Natl Acad Sci U S A 2003;100:4389–4394.

42. North BJ, Marshall BL, Borra MT, Denu JM, Verdin E. The human Sir2 ortholog, SIRT2, is an NAD+-dependent tubulin deacetylase. Mol Cell 2003; 11:437–444.

43. Xandid EPM, Peeves P, Davie JP. Sodium butyrate inhibits histone deacetylation in cultured cells. Cell 1978;14:105–113.

44. Xousens LS, Gallwitz D, Alberts BM. Different accessibilities in chromatin to histone acetylase. J Biol Chem 1979;254:1716–1723.

45. Nishino N, Powers JC. Design of potent reversible inhibitors for thermolysin. Peptides containing zinc coordinating ligands and their use in affinity chromatography. Biochemistry 1979;18:4340–4347.

46. Furumai R, Komatsu Y, Nishino N, Khochbin S, Yoshida M, Horinouchi S. Potent histone deacetylase inhibitors built from trichostatin A and cyclic tetrapeptide antibiotics including trapoxin. Proc Natl Acad Sci U S A 2001;98:87–92.

47. Chen JS, Faller DV, Spanjaard RA. Short-chain fatty acid inhibitors of histone deacetylases: promising anticancer therapeutics? Curr Cancer Drug Targets 2003;3:219–236.

48. Boffa LC, Vidali G, Mann RS, Allfrey VG. Suppression of histone deacetylation in vivo and in vitro by sodium butyrate. J Biol Chem 1978;253:3364–3366.

49. Phiel CJ, Zhang F, Huang EY, Guenther MG, Lazar MA, Klein PS. Histone deacetylase is a direct target of valproic acid, a potent anticonvulsant, mood stabilizer, and teratogen. J Biol Chem 2001;276:36,734–36,741.

50. Rephaeli A, Rabizadeh E, Aviram A, Shaklai M, Ruse M, Nudelman A. Derivatives of butyric acid as potential anti-neoplastic agents. Int J Cancer 1991;49:66–72.

51. Zimra Y, Wasserman L, Maron L, Shaklai M, Nudelman A, Rephaeli A. Butyric acid and pivaloyloxymethyl butyrate, AN-9, a novel butyric acid derivative, induce apoptosis in HL-60 cells. J Cancer Res Clin Oncol 1997;123:152–160.

52. Tsuji N, Kobayashi M, Nagashima K, Wakisaka Y, Koizumi K. A new antifungal antibiotic, trichostatin. J Antibiot (Tokyo) 1976;29:1–6.

53. Yoshida M, Nomura S, Beppu T. Effects of trichostatins on differentiation of murine erythroleukemia cells. Cancer Res 1987;47:3688–3691.

54. Yoshida M, Beppu T. Reversible arrest of proliferation of rat 3Y1 fibroblasts in both the G1 and G2 phases by trichostatin A. Exp Cell Res 1988;177:122–131.

55. Richon VM, Emiliani S, Verdin E, et al. A class of hybrid polar inducers of transformed cell differentiation inhibits histone deacetylases. Proc Natl Acad Sci U S A 1998;95:3003–3007.

56. Butler LM, Agus DB, Scher HI, et al. Suberoylanilide hydroxamic acid, an inhibitor of histone deacetylase, suppresses the growth of prostate cancer cells in vitro and in vivo. Cancer Res 2000;60:5165–5170.

57. Munster PN, Troso-Sandoval T, Rosen N, Rifkind R, Marks PA, Richon VM. The histone deacetylase inhibitor suberoylanilide hydroxamic acid induces differentiation of human breast cancer cells. Cancer Res 2001;61:8492–8497.

58. Cohen LA, Amin S, Marks PA, Rifkind RA, Desai D, Richon VM. Chemoprevention of carcinogen-induced mammary tumorigenesis by the hybrid polar cytodifferentiation agent, suberanilohydroxamic acid (SAHA). Anticancer Res 1999;19:4999–5005.

59. He LZ, Tolentino T, Grayson P, et al. Histone deacetylase inhibitors induce remission in transgenic models of therapy-resistant acute promyelocytic leukemia. J Clin Invest 2001;108:1321–1330.

60. Kelly WK, Richon VM, O'Connor O, et al. Phase I clinical trial of histone deacetylase inhibitor: suberoylanilide hydroxamic acid administered intravenously. Clin Cancer Res 2003;9:3578–3588.

61. Butler LM, Webb Y, Agus DB, et al. Inhibition of transformed cell growth and induction of cellular differentiation by pyroxamide, an inhibitor of histone deacetylase. Clin Cancer Res 2001;7:962–970.

62. Atadja P, Gao L, Kwon P, et al. Selective growth inhibition of tumor cells by a novel histone deacetylase inhibitor, NVP-LAQ824. Cancer Res 2004;64:689–695.

63. Remiszewski SW, Sambucetti LC, Bair KW, et al. N-hydroxy-3-phenyl-2-propenamides as novel inhibitors of human histone deacetylase with in vivo antitumor activity: discovery of (2E)-N-hydroxy-3-[4-[[(2-hydroxyethyl)[2-(1H-indol-3-yl)ethyl]amino]methyl]phenyl]-2-propenamide (NVP-LAQ824). J Med Chem 2003;46:4609–4624.

64. Komatsu Y, Tomizaki KY, Tsukamoto M, et al. Cyclic hydroxamic-acid-containing peptide 31, a potent synthetic histone deacetylase inhibitor with antitumor activity. Cancer Res 2001;61:4459–4466.

65. Itazaki H, Nagashima K, Sugita K, et al. Isolation and structural elucidation of new cyclotetrapeptides, trapoxins A and B, having detransformation activities as antitumor agents. J Antibiot (Tokyo) 1990;43:1524–1532.

66. Darkin-Rattray SJ, Gurnett AM, Myers RW, et al. Apicidin: a novel antiprotozoal agent that inhibits parasite histone deacetylase. Proc Natl Acad Sci U S A 1996;93:13,143–13,147.

67. Frey RR, Wada CK, Garland RB, et al. Trifluoromethyl ketones as inhibitors of histone deacetylase. Bioorg Med Chem Lett 2002;12:3443–3447.

68. Patel DV, Rielly-Gauvin K, Ryono DE, Free CA, Smith SA, Petrillo EW Jr. Activated ketone based inhibitors of human renin. J Med Chem 1993;36:2431–2447.

69. Jose B, Oniki Y, Kato T, Nishino N, Sumida Y, Yoshida M. Novel histone deacetylase inhibitors: cyclic tetrapeptide with trifluoromethyl and pentafluoroethyl ketones. Bioorg Med Chem Lett 2004;14:5343–5346.

70. Saito A, Yamashita T, Mariko Y, et al. A synthetic inhibitor of histone deacetylase, MS-27-275, with marked in vivo antitumor activity against human tumors. Proc Natl Acad Sci U S A 1999;96:4592–4597.

71. Jaboin J, Wild J, Hamidi H, et al. MS-27-275, an inhibitor of histone deacetylase, has marked in vitro and in vivo antitumor activity against pediatric solid tumors. Cancer Res 2002;62:6108–6115.

72. Cress WD, Seto E. Histone deacetylases, transcriptional control, and cancer. J Cell Physiol 2000;184:1–16.

73. Nakajima H, Kim YB, Terano H, Yoshida M, Horinouchi S. FR901228, a potent antitumor antibiotic, is a novel histone deacetylase inhibitor. Exp Cell Res 1998;241:126–133.

74. Furumai R, Matsuyama A, Kobashi N, et al. FK228 (depsipeptide) as a natural prodrug that inhibits class I histone deacetylases. Cancer Res 2002;62:4916–4921.

75. Ueda H, Manda T, Matsumoto S, et al. FR901228, a novel antitumor bicyclic depsipeptide produced by *Chromobacterium violaceum* No. 968. III. Antitumor activities on experimental tumors in mice. J Antibiot (Tokyo) 1994;47:315–323.

76. Pina IC, Gautschi JT, Wang GY, et al. Psammaplins from the sponge *Pseudoceratina purpurea*: inhibition of both histone deacetylase and DNA methyltransferase. J Org Chem 2003;68:3866–3873.

77. Nicolaou KC, Hughes R, Pfefferkorn JA, Barluenga S, Roecker AJ. Combinatorial synthesis through disulfide exchange: discovery of potent psammaplin A type antibacterial agents active against methicillin-resistant *Staphylococcus aureus* (MRSA). Chemistry 2001;7:4280–4295.

78. Nicolaou KC, Hughes R, Pfefferkorn JA, Barluenga S. Optimization and mechanistic studies of psammaplin A type antibacterial agents active against methicillin-resistant *Staphylococcus aureus* (MRSA). Chemistry 2001;7:4296–4310.

79. Nishino N, Jose B, Okamura S, et al. Cyclic tetrapeptides bearing sulfhydoryl group potently inhibit histone deacetylases. Org Lett 2003;5:5079–5082.

80. Landry J, Slama JT, Sternglanz R. Role of NAD(+) in the deacetylase activity of the SIR2-like proteins. Biochem Biophys Res Commun 2000;278:685–690.

81. Grozinger CM, Chao ED, Blackwell HE, Moazed D, Schreiber SL. Identification of a class of small molecule inhibitors of the sirtuin family of NAD-dependent deacetylases by phenotypic screening. J Biol Chem 2001;276:38,837–38,843.

82. Bedalov A, Gatbonton T, Irvine WP, Gottschling DE, Simon JA. Identification of a small molecule inhibitor of Sir2p. Proc Natl Acad Sci U S A 2001;98: 15,113–15,118.

83. Zhao Y, Dai X, Blackwell HE, Schreiber SL, Chory J. SIR1, an upstream component in auxin signaling identified by chemical genetics. Science 2003;301:1107–1110.

84. Fulco M, Schiltz RL, Iezzi S, et al. Sir2 regulates skeletal muscle differentiation as a potential sensor of the redox state. Mol Cell 2003;12:51–62.

85. Yeung F, Hoberg JE, Ramsey CS, et al. Modulation of NF-kappaB-dependent transcription and cell survival by the SIRT1 deacetylase. EMBO J 2004;23: 2369–2380.

86. Wall KA, Klis M, Kornet J, et al. Inhibition of the intrinsic NAD+ glycohydrolase activity of CD38 by carbocyclic NAD analogues. Biochem J 1998;335:631–636.

87. Bitterman KJ, Anderson RM, Cohen HY, Latorre-Esteves M, Sinclair DA. Inhibition of silencing and accelerated aging by nicotinamide, a putative negative regulator of yeast sir2 and human SIRT1. J Biol Chem 2002;277:45,099–45,107.

88. Gallo CM, Smith DL Jr, Smith JS. Nicotinamide clearance by Pnc1 directly regulates Sir2-mediated silencing and longevity. Mol Cell Biol 2004;24:1301–1312.

89. Onyango P, Celic I, McCaffery JM, Boeke JD, Feinberg AP. SIRT3, a human SIR2 homologue, is an NAD-dependent deacetylase localized to mitochondria. Proc Natl Acad Sci U S A 2002;99:13,653–13,658.

90. Jackson MD, Schmidt MT, Oppenheimer NJ, Denu JM. Mechanism of nicotinamide inhibition and transglycosidation by Sir2 histone/protein deacetylases. J Biol Chem 2003;278:50,985–50,998.

91. Denu JM. Linking chromatin function with metabolic networks: Sir2 family of NAD(+)-dependent deacetylases. Trends Biochem Sci 2003;28:41–48.

92. Finnin MS, Donigian JR, Pavletich NP. Structure of the histone deacetylase SIRT2. Nat Struct Biol 2001;8:621–625.

93. Min J, Landry J, Sternglanz R, Xu RM. Crystal structure of a SIR2 homolog-NAD complex. Cell 2001;105:269–279.

94. Avalos JL, Celic I, Muhammad S, Cosgrove MS, Boeke JD, Wolberger C. Structure of a Sir2 enzyme bound to an acetylated p53 peptide. Mol Cell 2002;10:523–535.

95. Hirao M, Posakony J, Nelson M, et al. Identification of selective inhibitors of NAD+-dependent deacetylases using phenotypic screens in yeast. J Biol Chem 2003;278:52,773–52,782.

96. Takami Y, Nakayama T. N-terminal region, C-terminal region, nuclear export signal, and deacetylation activity of histone deacetylase-3 are essential for the viability of the DT40 chicken B cell line. J Biol Chem 2000;275:16,191–16,201.

97. Lagger G, O'Carroll D, Rembold M, et al. Essential function of histone deacetylase 1 in proliferation control and CDK inhibitor repression. EMBO J 2002;21:2672–2681.

98. Glaser KB, Li J, Staver MJ, Wei RQ, Albert DH, Davidsen SK. Role of class I and class II histone deacetylases in carcinoma cells using siRNA. Biochem Biophys Res Commun 2003;310:529–536.

99. Torchia J, Glass C, Rosenfeld MG. Co-activators and co-repressors in the integration of transcriptional responses. Curr Opin Cell Biol 1998;10:373–383.

100. Petti MC, Fazi F, Gentile M, et al. Complete remission through blast cell differentiation in PLZF/RARalpha-positive acute promyelocytic leukemia: in vitro and in vivo studies. Blood 2002;100:1065–1067.

101. Ferrara FF, Fazi F, Bianchini A, et al. Histone deacetylase-targeted treatment restores retinoic acid signaling and differentiation in acute myeloid leukemia. Cancer Res 2001;61:2–7.

102. Wang J, Saunthararajah Y, Redner RL, Liu JM. Inhibitors of histone deacetylase relieve ETO-mediated repression and induce differentiation of AML1-ETO leukemia cells. Cancer Res 1999;59:2766–2769.

103. Jones PA, Baylin SB. The fundamental role of epigenetic events in cancer. Nat Rev Genet 2002;3:415–428.

104. Claus R, Lubbert M. Epigenetic targets in hematopoietic malignancies. Oncogene 2003;22:6489–6496.

105. Yoshida M, Horinouchi S, Beppu T. Trichostatin A and trapoxin: novel chemical probes for the role of histone acetylation in chromatin structure and function. Bioessays 1995;17:423–430.

106. Marks PA, Richon VM, Rifkind RA. Histone deacetylase inhibitors: inducers of differentiation or apoptosis of transformed cells. J Natl Cancer Inst 2000;92:1210–1216.

107. Kim MS, Kwon HJ, Lee YM, et al. Histone deacetylases induce angiogenesis by negative regulation of tumor suppressor genes. Nat Med 2001;7:437–443.

108. Qiu L, Burgess A, Fairlie DP, Leonard H, Parsons PG, Gabrielli BG. Histone deacetylase inhibitors trigger a G2 checkpoint in normal cells that is defective in tumor cells. Mol Biol Cell 2000;11:2069–2083.

109. Taddei A, Maison C, Roche D, Almouzni G. Reversible disruption of pericentric heterochromatin and centromere function by inhibiting deacetylases. Nat Cell Biol 2001;3:114–120.

110. Hayashi T, Fujita Y, Iwasaki O, Adachi Y, Takahashi K, Yanagida M. Mis16 and Mis18 are required for CENP-A loading and histone deacetylation at centromeres. Cell 2004;118:715–729.

111. Cha JH. Transcriptional dysregulation in Huntington's disease. Trends Neurosci 2000;23:387–392.

112. Steffan JS, Bodai L, Pallos J, et al. Histone deacetylase inhibitors arrest polyglutamine-dependent neurodegeneration in *Drosophila*. Nature 2001;413: 739–743.

113. Nucifora FC Jr, Sasaki M, Peters MF, et al. Interference by huntingtin and atrophin-1 with cbp-mediated transcription leading to cellular toxicity. Science 2001;291:2423–2428.

114. McCampbell A, Taylor JP, Taye AA, et al. CREB-binding protein sequestration by expanded polyglutamine. Hum Mol Genet 2000;9:2197–2202.

115. McCampbell A, Taye AA, Whitty L, Penney E, Steffan JS, Fischbeck KH. Histone deacetylase inhibitors reduce polyglutamine toxicity. Proc Natl Acad Sci U S A 2001;98:15,179–15,184.

116. Hockly E, Richon VM, Woodman B, et al. Suberoylanilide hydroxamic acid, a histone deacetylase inhibitor, ameliorates motor deficits in a mouse model of Huntington's disease. Proc Natl Acad Sci U S A 2003;100:2041–2046.

117. Ferrante RJ, Kubilus JK, Lee J, et al. Histone deacetylase inhibition by sodium butyrate chemotherapy ameliorates the neurodegenerative phenotype in Huntington's disease mice. J Neurosci 2003;23:9418–9427.

118. Kawaguchi Y, Kovacs JJ, McLaurin A, Vance JM, Ito A, Yao TP. The deacetylase HDAC6 regulates aggresome formation and cell viability in response to mis-folded protein stress. Cell 2003;115:727–738.

119. Corcoran LJ, Mitchison TJ, Liu Q. A novel action of histone deacetylase inhibitors in a protein aggresome disease model. Curr Biol 2004;14:488–492.

120. Nakae J, Biggs WH 3rd, Kitamura T, et al. Regulation of insulin action and pan-creatic beta-cell function by mutated alleles of the gene encoding forkhead tran-scription factor Foxo1. Nat Genet 2002;32:245–253.

121. Puigserver P, Rhee J, Donovan J, et al. Insulin-regulated hepatic gluconeogenesis through FOXO1-PGC-1alpha interaction. Nature 2003;423:550–555.

122. Brunet A, Sweeney LB, Sturgill JF, et al. Stress-dependent regulation of FOXO transcription factors by the SIRT1 deacetylase. Science 2004;303:2011–2015.

123. Daitoku H, Hatta M, Matsuzaki H, et al. Silent information regulator 2 potenti-ates Foxo1-mediated transcription through its deacetylase activity. Proc Natl Acad Sci U S A 2004;101:10,042–10,047.

124. Motta MC, Divecha N, Lemieux M, et al. Mammalian SIRT1 represses forkhead transcription factors. Cell 2004;116:551–563.

125. Takigawa-Imamura H, Sekine T, Murata M, Takayama K, Nakazawa K, Nakagawa J. Stimulation of glucose uptake in muscle cells by prolonged treat-ment with scriptide, a histone deacetylase inhibitor. Biosci Biotechnol Biochem 2003;67:1499–1506.

126. Skov S, Rieneck K, Bovin LF, et al. Histone deacetylase inhibitors: a new class of immunosuppressors targeting a novel signal pathway essential for CD154 expression. Blood 2003;101:1430–1438.

127. Mori H, Abe F, Furukawa S, Sakai F, Hino M, Fujii T. FR235222, a fungal metabolite, is a novel immunosuppressant that inhibits mammalian histone deacetylase (HDAC) II. Biological activities in animal models. J Antibiot (Tokyo) 2003;56:80–86.

128. Mori H, Urano Y, Abe F, et al. FR235222, a fungal metabolite, is a novel immuno- suppressant that inhibits mammalian histone deacetylase (HDAC). I. Taxonomy, fermentation, isolation and biological activities. J Antibiot (Tokyo) 2003;56:72–79.

129. Vannini A, Volpari C, Filocamo G, et al. Crystal structure of a eukaryotic zinc- dependent histone deacetylase, human HDAC8, complexed with a hydroxamic acid inhibitor. Proc Natl Acad Sci U S A 2004;101:15,064–15,069.

13 Cell Cycle Targets of Histone Deacetylase Inhibitors

Brian Gabrielli, *PhD*

CONTENTS

SUMMARY

Histone deacetylase inhibitors (HDIs) can potentially affect a broad spectrum of cellular events by stabilizing the acetylation of an increasing number of proteins. One of the most notable outcomes is the effect on cell cycle progression almost universally observed following treatment with this class of drugs. These effects are either G1 or G2/M phase cell cycle arrests, and mitosis is also adversely affected. Histone hyperacetylation and consequent transcriptional changes contribute directly to the G1 phase arrest, but the

From: *Cancer Drug Discovery and Development*
Histone Deacetylases: Transcriptional Regulation and Other Cellular Functions
Edited by: E. Verdin © Humana Press Inc., Totowa, NJ

Acronyms and Abbreviations	
ATM	Ataxia telangiectasia mutated
INK4	Inhibitor of cdk4
CTP	Cytidine triphosphate
ATM/ATR	ATR is ATM and RAD3 related
Gadd45	Growth arrest and DNA damage-inducible
CENP-A	Centromere protein A
SUV39H1	Suppressor of variegation 39 Human 1

hyperacetylated targets for the G2 phase arrest and mitotic defects are yet to be absolutely identified. These cell cycle effects are the basis of the antiproliferative activity and tumor cell selectivity of these drugs, properties that potentially make them highly effective anticancer drugs.

Key Words: G2/M, centromere, kinetochore, G1, p21$^{WAF1/CIP1}$, checkpoint.

HDI-INDUCED G1 PHASE ARREST

G1/S-Phase Progression

Progression through the cell cycle is controlled by the ordered activation of family of protein kinases known as the cyclin dependent kinases (cdks). Cdk activity is regulated in a complex manner, including association with a regulatory cyclin subunit, phosphorylation of both the cdk and cyclin subunits, and association with inhibitory protein subunits, the cdk inhibitors. Individual cdks associate with a limited repertoire of cyclins at specific stages of the cell cycle, and the activation and inactivation of the specific cyclin/cdk control progression into, through, and exit from each cell cycle stage. Cell cycle progression through G1 into replicative S phase requires the sequential activation of cyclin D/cdk4 or cdk6, and cyclin E/cdk2, although cyclin E/cdk2 can perform both functions in cells that lack cyclin D/cdk4 activity *(1)*. These two cdk complexes phosphorylate retinoblastoma protein (Rb) to allow for the full activity of the Rb-bound E2F, a transcription factor required for expression of an array of genes required for progression into and though S phase (Fig. 1; reviewed in ref. 2). Cyclin E/cdk2 and cyclin A/cdk2 also have essential roles in the initiation and maintenance of DNA replication *(3–5)*.

HDI Induction of p21$^{WAF1/CIP1}$ and Other cdk Inhibitors

Histone deacetylase inhibitor (HDI) treatment of most cultured cell lines causes G1-phase cell cycle arrest. The G1 arrest is associated with

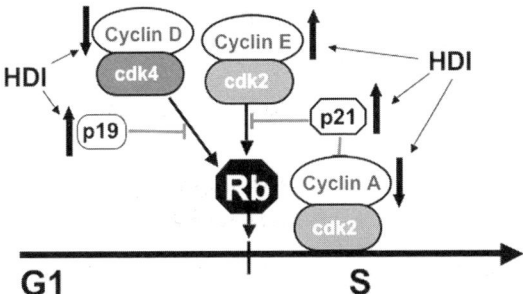

Fig. 1. G1/S transition is regulated by cyclin-dependent kinase (cdk)4/cyclin D and cdk2/cyclin E kinase activities, whereas cdk2/cyclin A is required for S-phase progression. Histone deacetylase inhibitor (HDI) treatment upregulates the expression of the cdk2 inhibitor p21$^{WAF1/CIP1}$ and the cdk4 inhibitor p19^{INK4D} while downregulating cyclin D and cyclin A levels, thereby blocking retinoblastoma protein (Rb) phosphorylation and promoting G1 phase arrest. Cyclin E levels are upregulated, but the increased p21$^{WAF1/CIP1}$ expression can block activity of this complex.

hypophosphorylation of Rb, loss of S-phase population and DNA synthetic activity, and inhibition or loss of the G1 phase cdk/cyclin complexes responsible for Rb phosphorylation (6–8). The arrest appears to be a direct consequence of HDI-induced up- or downregulation of a number of genes that control G1/S-phase progression. The most prominent of the upregulated genes encodes the cdk inhibitor p21$^{WAF1/CIP1}$. HDI treatment increases acetylation of chromatin in the promotor region of the p21$^{WAF1/CIP1}$ gene, increasing access to a specificity protein (Sp)1/Sp3 site that is correlated with increased gene transcription (6,9–11), although other modifications to the transcriptional machinery also appear to be required for full transcriptional activation to occur (12,13). p21$^{WAF1/CIP1}$ upregulation is independent of the tumor suppressor p53, which can transactivate p21$^{WAF1/CIP1}$ expression in response to a wide range of external stimuli including DNA damage (2).

In the DNA damage response, p53 is downstream of the cell cycle checkpoint signaling complex containing ATM (14,15). HDI treatment does not produce DNA strand breaks, but there does appear to be a role for ATM, independent of p53, in the HDI-induced upregulation of p21$^{WAF1/CIP1}$ expression, as inactivating mutation or inhibition of ATM severely reduces HDI-induced p21$^{WAF1/CIP1}$ expression (16). Increased p21 levels bind and inhibit cyclin E and A/cdk2 complexes, which are responsible for phosphorylation and inactivation of Rb and are essential for progression into and through S phase, thereby producing a G1/S phase arrest. Deletion of the p21$^{WAF1/CIP1}$ gene or failure of HDI treatment to

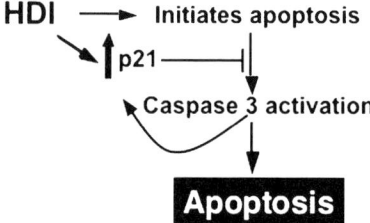

Fig. 2. Histone deacetylase inhibitor (HDI) treatment can initiate an apoptotic response in cancer cells, but the increased expression of p21[WAF1/CIP1] can inhibit this by inhibiting the activation of caspase 3. However, caspase 3 can also cleave and inactivate p21[WAF1/CIP1]; therefore the kinetics of caspase 3 activation and p21[WAF1/CIP1] expression will determine the degree of apoptosis initiated after drug treatment.

upregulate p21[WAF1/CIP1] expression, possibly owing to silencing of the CDKN1A locus encoding p21[WAF1/CIP1], correlates with a lack of a G1-phase arrest following HDI treatment *(8,17,18)*. There are also reports of other cdk inhibitors (such as the cdk4- and cdk6-specific p15[INK4B] and p19[INK4D] and the p21[WAF1/CIP1]-related p57[KIP2]) being upregulated in various cell lines with HDI treatment *(19–22)* (Fig. 2).

These cdk inhibitors may contribute to a G1-phase arrest in some cell lines by inhibiting either cdk4/cyclin D complexes by the INK4 family proteins, or cdk2/cyclin E and cdk2/cyclin A complexes by the p21[WAF1/CIP1]-related proteins *(23)*. The INK4 proteins can also cause redistribution of p21[WAF1/CIP1] family proteins off cdk4 complexes, where they have little inhibitory activity in vivo, onto cdk2 complexes of which they are potent inhibitors, thereby reinforcing the G1 arrest *(24)*. The upregulation of p21[WAF1/CIP1] is widely observed in both normal and tumor cell lines *(7,18)*, but it is not clear how common upregulation of the other cdk inhibitor genes is following HDI treatment.

Other G1 Phase Targets

Upregulation of p21[WAF1/CIP1] and other cdk inhibitors may not be solely responsible for the G1 arrest observed. Loss of expression of cyclin D and cyclin A is also commonly observed following HDI treatment and probably contributes to the loss of cdk2 and cdk4 kinase activities and the hypophosphorylated Rb *(6–8,25,26)*. Surprisingly, HDI treatment also increases cyclin E expression, although this is not associated with increased cdk2 activity, probably because increased p21[WAF1/CIP1] levels inhibit this kinase activity *(6,8,25)* (Fig. 1). Genes involved in DNA synthesis such as CTP synthase, thymidylate synthetase, and thymidine kinase have been reported as targets for HDI-induced downregulation *(21,27)*.

Loss of these enzymes would have a similar effect to treatment with antimetabolites such as hydroxyurea, blocking S-phase progression and thereby also contributing to the G1/S arrest. Thus, many mechanisms may combine to impose the observed HDI-induced G1-phase arrest.

All the genes involved in the arrest display transcriptional changes in response to HDI treatment, although the particular genes that are up- and downregulated and the arrest mechanisms utilized may depend on the cell line and HDI used. It has been clearly demonstrated that although the overall cell cycle responses to treatment with HDIs are common to most cell lines with all HDIs *(7,28)*, there are significant differences in the genes affected by different HDIs in the same cell lines (and even different structures within the same class of HDIs) and in the genes affected by the same HDI in different cell lines *(27)*. One constant appears to be p21$^{WAF1/CIP1}$ upregulation, which is clearly a major contributor to the G1 arrest observed in most cell lines. Interesting, HDI treatment during S phase did not appear to affect the time taken to transit S phase, suggesting that drug treatment had little direct effect on DNA replication *(7)*.

p21$^{WAF1/CIP1}$ INHIBITS APOPTOSIS

HDIs possess antiproliferative activity through their ability to cause cell cycle arrest; they also promote cell death in many tumor cell lines, which in many cases displays the characteristics of apoptosis *(7,18,29–31)*. The upregulated expression of p21$^{WAF1/CIP1}$ and the associated G1 arrest requires relatively low, nontoxic doses of drug, whereas higher doses are associated with significant levels of cell death *(11,18)*. At the high, cytotoxic doses of HDIs, the upregulated p21$^{WAF1/CIP1}$ levels have the paradoxical effect of inhibiting apoptosis induced by the drugs. A small subset of cell lines that are hypersensitive to killing by HDI, requiring up to 10-fold lower concentrations of drug to achieve high levels of apoptosis, fail to induce p21$^{WAF1/CIP1}$ protein expression *(18)*, and knockout of p21$^{WAF1/CIP1}$ expression by either antisense or homologous deletion increases the sensitivity of tumors to killing by HDIs *(18,32)*.

Other studies have also shown that a range of combination treatments with HDIs increased the potency of HDI treatment by blocking HDI-induced p21$^{WAF1/CIP1}$ expression *(33–37)*. The hypersensitivity to HDIs was reversed by treatment with caspase inhibitors to inhibit apoptosis *(18)*, suggesting that the increased p21$^{WAF1/CIP1}$ levels reduce HDI cytotoxicity by blocking apoptosis. p21$^{WAF1/CIP1}$ can directly bind procaspase 3 and inhibit its cleavage *(38)*, thereby blocking activation of a major executioner caspase and full expression of the apoptotic phenotype. However, p21$^{WAF1/CIP1}$ is also a substrate of caspase 3, and cleavage of p21$^{WAF1/CIP1}$ destroys its caspase 3 inhibitory activity *(39)*; thus the kinetics of p21$^{WAF1/CIP1}$ expression and caspase 3 activation determine the relative sensitivity of cells to HDI treatment *(18)* (Fig. 2).

The INK4 family cdk4 inhibitor p16 has also been reported to block HDI-induced apoptosis in a leukemic cell line *(29,31)*, but we have recently demonstrated that other cell lines with either stable or inducible p16 expression remained sensitive to HDI-induced cell death *(40)*.

G2 PHASE CHECKPOINT DETERMINES SENSITIVITY TO HDI-INDUCED CYTOTOXICITY

An HDI-Sensitive G2 Checkpoint

One of the most distinctive characteristics of HDIs is their in vitro, and apparently in vivo, selective cytotoxicity; they are toxic to a wide range of immortalized, virally transformed and tumor cells, but normal, nonimmortalized primary cell cultures and a small number of tumor cell lines are resistant to killing by even very high doses of these drugs *(7,18,41)*. The basis of the selectivity is an HDI-sensitive G2-phase cell cycle checkpoint. G1-phase arrest was detected in most cell lines following HDI treatment, but G2-phase arrest has been detected in a comparatively restricted number of cell lines *(7)*. G2 arrest is only observed at higher doses of HDI than required for G1 arrest *(8,11,18)*. Treatment of most cell lines with these high doses of HDI results in cell death, normally via an apoptotic mechanism, but the cell lines that arrest in G2 phase are resistant to the cytotoxic effects of these drugs *(7,11,42)*. A few reports have claimed G2/M arrest in tumor cell lines that are clearly sensitive to killing by HDIs *(29,43)*, although in each case G2 arrest was defined only by a single-time-point fluorescence-activated cell sorting analysis showing an accumulation of cells with 4n DNA content. These are probably cells that enter mitosis and fail cytokinesis, producing multinuclear cells with 4n content rather than G2-phase-arrested cells *(7)*.

Mechanism of the HDI-Sensitive Checkpoint and G2-Phase Arrest

G2-phase arrest occurs via a unique HDI-sensitive G2 checkpoint mechanism that is independent of other G2 checkpoints responding to DNA-damaging agents *(7)*. However, the HDI-sensitive checkpoint does utilize the common, caffeine-sensitive ATM/ATR checkpoint signaling pathway, possibly via Chk2 *(42)*. The checkpoint arrest operates through a blockade of cdc2/cyclin B activation, and prolonged arrest also results in downregulation of cyclin B1 protein levels, possibly to ensure that entry into mitosis is blocked until after removal of the drug, when cells can recommence cycling *(7,44)*. The activity of this critical mitotic kinase is unaffected by HDI treatment in cells with a defective checkpoint, although, interestingly, the levels of an activator of cdc2/cyclin B, cdc25C, are reduced after 24 h of drug treatment. The expression of Gadd45, a growth arrest and DNA damage inducible gene that can cause G2/M arrest by inhibiting cdc2/cyclin B activity *(45)*, has been found to be upregulated following HDI treatment and may also participate in the G2 arrest observed *(46)*.

The G2 Checkpoint Protects Against HDI-Induced Cell Death

Correlative evidence from a large panel of cell lines tested demonstrated that the presence of a G2-phase checkpoint arrest at 24 h after high-dose HDI treatment was always associated with resistance to killing by these drugs *(7)*. Furthermore, reintroducing a G2 checkpoint arrest in HDI-sensitive cells rescues the cells from HDI-induced apoptosis, whereas knockout of the ATM/ATR-dependent G2 checkpoint mechanism by expression of the Epstein-Barr virus EBNA 3 family of proteins converts an HDI-resistant cell line to an HDI-sensitive cell line *(7,42)*. Thus, the functional status of the HDI-sensitive G2 checkpoint determines the tumor-selective cytotoxicity of these drugs. Normal tissue-derived primary cell lines are resistant to killing by even high doses of HDI, which is directly attributable to the functional G2 checkpoint. This checkpoint is defective in most of the immortalized, virally transformed, and tumor cell lines tested, and thus the lines are sensitive to killing by these drugs.

HDI TREATMENT DISRUPTS MITOSIS
AND THE MITOTIC CHECKPOINT

HDI Treatment Causes Aberrant Mitosis

A number of studies have demonstrated that under HDI treatment, cells undergo an aberrant mitosis, with the condensed chromosomes often failing to congress to the metaphase plate although a relatively normal microtubule spindle has formed, and also failing to segregate chromosomes properly, resulting in multinuclear cells *(7,28,47–49)*. These cell lines must be defective for the HDI-sensitive G2 checkpoint by definition, as cells with this checkpoint intact would not progress into mitosis. The basis of the mitotic defect is unclear. Mitotic histone H3 Ser-10 phosphorylation is unaffected by HDI treatment *(49)*, although binding of the heterochromatin protein HP1 to the centromeric regions is reduced *(47,49)*. This will be discussed in more detail below, in the section entitled Molecular Mechanism Triggering the HDI-Sensitive G2 Checkpoint and Disruption of the Mitotic Checkpoint.

The outcome of mitotic defects is dependent on the dose and timing of HDI treatment. Treatment with relatively low doses of HDIs, levels that cause little cytotoxicity, cause cells to delay in mitosis *(28,48,49)*, presumably under the influence of the mitotic checkpoint that detects such mitotic defects and blocks anaphase promoting complex/cyclosome (APC/C) function and mitotic exit until the defects are rectified *(50)*. The timing of drug addition is also critical. The drug must be present at least through S phase to produce the aberrant mitotic phenotype; addition of even high doses of drug in early G2 phase, which induces a similar extent of histone hyperacetylation by mitosis as drug addition in S phase, failed to produce aberrant mitosis, whereas exposure to high doses of HDI during S phase only, which results in reduction in histone hyperacetylation prior to mitosis to levels that were above untreated controls, still produced high levels of aberrant mitosis *(28)*.

High-Dose HDI Treatment Disrupts Mitotic Spindle Checkpoint Function

Treatment with high doses of HDIs throughout S and G2 phases causes cells to enter mitosis after a 1- to 2-h delay in G2 phase; then more than 90% of cells undergo mitotic failure. In contrast to low-dose treatment, it appears that the aberrant mitosis is either not triggered or bypasses the mitotic spindle checkpoint-dependent arrest, with the result that cells exit mitosis, often without partitioning their chromosomes. Certainly few anaphase figures are observed, although many of the normal markers of mitotic exit, cyclin B destruction, and loss of mitosis-specific MPM-2 immunoreactivity are observed. The result of this mitotic catastrophe is rapid initiation of apoptosis within hours of mitotic exit *(28)*.

Thus, following treatment with even low doses of HDIs during S phase, cells with a defective HDI-sensitive G2 checkpoint progress into an aberrant mitosis. At low drug doses or conditions of reduced hyperacetylation, the mitotic spindle checkpoint delays the cells in mitosis until normal partitioning of the replicated chromosomes can be achieved. However, the presence of massively hyperacetylated chromatin causes either failure or bypass of the mitotic checkpoint, premature exit from mitosis, and rapidly initiated apoptosis. This is an example of synthetic lethality, whereby loss of a single checkpoint results in reduced viability but when a second, compensatory checkpoint is lost in addition, cells lose viability rapidly. In this case, loss of the G2 checkpoint is an intrinsic property of the tumor cells, and knockout of the normally compensatory mitotic checkpoint by HDI action results in widespread apoptosis. Cells with an intact G2 checkpoint response do not enter mitosis and are thus protected from the cytotoxic effects of the drugs (Fig. 3).

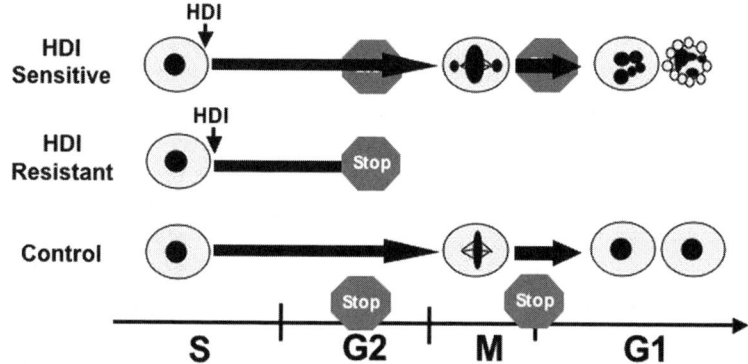

Fig. 3. During normal progression through S phase into mitosis, checkpoints in G2 and mitosis remain latent unless specific stresses activate them to block further progression. Histone deacetylase inhibitor (HDI)-resistant cells have an intact HDI-sensitive G2 checkpoint that blocks progression into mitosis. These remain arrested in G2 phase until removal of the drug, when they can recommence normal progression. In cells sensitive to killing by HDIs, this G2 checkpoint is defective, and the cells undergo an aberrant mitosis. This would normally be detected by the mitotic spindle checkpoint, but the drugs either knock out or bypass this arrest and prematurely exit mitosis, resulting in either multinuclear cells that are likely to have limited proliferative potential or rapid onset of apoptosis.

MOLECULAR MECHANISM TRIGGERING THE HDI-SENSITIVE G2 CHECKPOINT AND DISRUPTION OF THE MITOTIC CHECKPOINT

The unanswered question is how HDI treatment triggers the G2 checkpoint response and whether this is related to the disruption or bypass of the subsequent mitotic checkpoint. It is clear that transcriptional changes, many perhaps directly attributable to HDI-dependent changes in the acetylation state of promotor regions and/or transcription factor acetylation and activity, underlie the G1 phase arrest, with the upregulation of inhibitors such as p19^{INK4D} and p21$^{WAF1/CIP1}$ and down-regulation of promoters of G1/S progression such as cyclin D. The G1 arrest probably accounts for the cytostatic activity of HDIs, but this requires only relatively low drug doses, which do not promote significant cell death. Up regulation of p21$^{WAF1/CIP1}$ expression is detected at these low doses *(18)*, indicating that many of the HDI-dependent transcriptional changes may be elicited by low drug concentrations. High doses of HDI are required for G2 checkpoint arrest in resistant cells and cytotoxicity in sensitive cells.

An explanation for this dosage effect could be that the HDACs regulating transcriptional targets that effect G2/M are less sensitive to HDI treatment. Another possibility is that the HDIs are inhibiting HDACs affecting targets that differ in the stability of their acetylation. Chromatin domains that are normally hypoacetylated may require higher HDI concentrations to block deacetylation effectively, possibly owing to high concentrations of HDACs in the vicinity of these domains to ensure the normal hypoacetylated state. Lower drug concentrations are sufficient to maintain the hyperacetylated state of targets that normally continuously alter their acetylation state. The heterochromatin is normally hypoacetylated and is only transiently acetylated during deposition of histones onto newly replicated DNA during S phase. This contrasts with the continuously changing acetylation state of the actively transcribed euchromatin, which is readily affected by low doses of HDI *(51–53)*.

A number of lines of evidence support the hypothesis that the hyperacetylation of heterochromatin underlies the cytotoxicity of HDI treatment by promoting aberrant mitosis and knockout of spindle checkpoint function in drug-sensitive cells, causing the G2 checkpoint response in drug-resistant cells. First, the aberrant mitotic phenotype in drug-sensitive cells is dependent on HDI treatment during S phase *(28)*. Deposition of chromatin onto newly synthesized DNA during S phase requires site-specific acetylation of histones, which are then rapidly deacetylated in the heterochromatin regions *(52,53)*. Thus transient S-phase acetylation of the normally hypoacetylated heterochromatin provides the rationale for S-phase HDI treatment stabilizing heterochromatin acetylation. Second, the aberrant mitosis phenotype, with formation of a relatively normal microtubule spindle but failure of chromosome congression to the metaphase plate, is a phenocopy of mutations of kinetochore and centromeric proteins *(54–57)*. The identity of the phenotypes produced by HDI treatment and centromere/kinetochore protein mutations indicates that drug treatment disrupts normal centromere/kinetochore function. The most obvious effect of the drugs is hyperacetylation of the normally hypoacetylated centromeric heterochromatin, possibly disrupting its higher order structure.

HDI treatment does not affect either the expression or the localization of centromere-specific proteins such as the histone H3-like CENP-A *(7,47)*, nor does it affect mitotic H3 Ser10 phosphorylation, which is also required, or the fidelity of mitotic chromosome segregation *(49,58)*; HDI treatment does result in loss of heterochromatin protein 1 (HP1) binding to the heterochromatin *(47,59)*. HP1 appears to be required for the higher order structure of the centromeric heterochromatin, and deletion of SUV39H1 (the methyltransferase responsible for histone H3 Lys-9 methylation, which acts as the binding site for HP1) or mutation of H3 Lys-9 also result in aberrant mitosis *(60–62)*. Thus HDI treatment appears to instigate aberrant mitosis and to disrupt kinetochore function by hyper-acetylating the centromeric heterochromatin and blocking HP1 binding. The presence of centromere-specific HDACs has been described in both yeast and mammals associated with the Sin3 corepressor (63,64). Together these provide compelling evidence that the centromeric heterochromatin is the likely target of the HDI-stablized acetylation that causes the mitotic effects of these drugs.

The existence of numerous checkpoint pathways that ensure the integrity of genomic DNA emphasizes the paramount importance the cell places on ensuring genomic integrity. The genome contains all possible genes and other noncoding regulatory sequences that the whole organism requires for normal growth and development. The large number of modifications that chromatin histone can undergo and the diverse biological outcomes of these modifications imply that changes to the heterochromatin could radically affect the biology of the cell (65,66). Thus, whereas the DNA codes for all possible genes and thereby biologies of a cell, the heterochromatin defines the potential transcriptome in each cell, thereby determining cell fate and function. It would be inevitable that such a critical function would be protected by checkpoint responses to ensure the fidelity of this process. The checkpoint would be particularly critical in G2/M progression, in which the specialized centromeric heterochromatin has an essential function in ensuring the fidelity of partitioning of the replicated genome. Thus there is good evidence that HDI treatment may target histone deacetylation to produce its clinically important tumor-selective cytotoxicity. However, the mechanism may not necessarily involve changes in transcription but may rather involve changes in heterochromatin structure and function.

ACKNOWLEDGMENTS

Thanks to Drs. Heather Beamish and Andrew Burgess for critical reading of the manuscript. This work was supported by funding from the National Health and Medical Research Council of Australia.

REFERENCES

1. Gray-Bablin J, Zalvide J, Fox MP, Knickerbocker CJ, DeCaprio JA, Keyomarsi K. Cyclin E, a redundant cyclin in breast cancer. Proc Natl Acad Sci U S A 1996;93:15,215–15,220.
2. Sherr CJ. The Pezcoller lecture: cancer cell cycles revisited. Cancer Res 2000;60:3689–3695.
3. Ohtsubo M, Theodoras AM, Schumacher J, Roberts JM, Pagano M. Human cyclin E, a nuclear protein essential for the G1-to-S phase transition. Mol Cell Biol 1995;15:2612–2624.

4. Pagano M, Pepperkok R, Verde F, Ansorge W, Draetta G. Cyclin A is required at two points in the human cell cycle. EMBO J 1992;11:961–971.

5. Strausfeld UP, Howell M, Descombes P, et al. Both cyclin A and cyclin E have S-phase promoting (SPF) activity in *Xenopus* egg extracts. J Cell Sci 1996;109:1555–1563.

6. Sambucetti LC, Fischer DD, Zabludoff S, et al. Histone deacetylase inhibition selectively alters the activity and expression of cell cycle proteins leading to specific chromatin acetylation and antiproliferative effects. J Biol Chem 1999;274:34,940–34,947.

7. Qiu L, Burgess A, Fairlie DP, Leonard H, Parsons PG, Gabrielli BG. Histone deacetylase inhibitors trigger a G2 checkpoint in normal cells that is defective in tumor cells. Mol Biol Cell 2000;11:2069–2083.

8. Sandor V, Senderowicz A, Mertins S, et al. P21-dependent g(1)arrest with down-regulation of cyclin D1 and upregulation of cyclin E by the histone deacetylase inhibitor FR901228. Br J Cancer 2000;83:817–825.

9. Huang L, Sowa Y, Sakai T, Pardee AB. Activation of the p21WAF1/CIP1 promoter independent of p53 by the histone deacetylase inhibitor suberoylanilide hydroxamic acid (SAHA) through the Sp1 sites. Oncogene 2000;19:5712–5719.

10. Xiao H, Hasegawa T, Isobe K. p300 collaborates with Sp1 and Sp3 in p21(waf1/cip1) promoter activation induced by histone deacetylase inhibitor. J Biol Chem 2000;275:1371–1376.

11. Richon VM, Sandhoff TW, Rifkind RA, Marks PA. Histone deacetylase inhibitor selectively induces p21WAF1 expression and gene-associated histone acetylation. Proc Natl Acad Sci U S A 2000;97:10,014–10,019.

12. Kim YK, Han JW, Woo YN, et al. Expression of p21(WAF1/Cip1) through Sp1 sites by histone deacetylase inhibitor apicidin requires PI 3-kinase-PKC epsilon signaling pathway. Oncogene 2003;22:6023–6031.

13. Gui CY, Ngo L, Xu WS, Richon VM, Marks PA. Histone deacetylase (HDAC) inhibitor activation of p21WAF1 involves changes in promoter-associated proteins, including HDAC1. Proc Natl Acad Sci U S A 2004;101:1241–1246.

14. Canman CE, Lim DS, Cimprich KA, et al. Activation of the ATM kinase by ionizing radiation and phosphorylation of p53. Science 1998;281:1677–1679.

15. Khanna KK, Keating KE, Kozlov S, et al. ATM associates with and phosphorylates p53: mapping the region of interaction. Nat Genet 1998;20:398–400.

16. Ju R, Muller MT. Histone deacetylase inhibitors activate p21(WAF1) expression via ATM. Cancer Res 2003;63:2891–2897.

17. Archer SY, Meng S, Shei A, Hodin RA. p21(WAF1) is required for butyrate-mediated growth inhibition of human colon cancer cells. Proc Natl Acad Sci U S A 1998;95:6791–6796.

18. Burgess AJ, Pavey S, Warrener R, et al. Up-regulation of p21(WAF1/CIP1) by histone deacetylase inhibitors reduces their cytotoxicity. Mol Pharmacol 2001;60:828–837.

19. Hitomi T, Matsuzaki Y, Yokota T, Takaoka Y, Sakai T. p15(INK4b) in HDAC inhibitor-induced growth arrest. FEBS Lett 2003;554:347–350.

20. Sato N, Fukushima N, Maitra A, et al. Discovery of novel targets for aberrant methylation in pancreatic carcinoma using high-throughput microarrays. Histone acetylation-mediated regulation of genes in leukaemic cells. Gene expression profiling of multiple histone deacetylase (HDAC) inhibitors: defining a common

gene set produced by HDAC inhibition in T24 and MDA carcinoma cell lines. Cancer Res 2003;63:3735–3742.

21. Mitsiades CS, Mitsiades NS, McMullan CJ, et al. Transcriptional signature of histone deacetylase inhibition in multiple myeloma: biological and clinical implications. Proc Natl Acad Sci U S A 2004;101:540–545.

22. Yokota T, Matsuzaki Y, Miyazawa K, Zindy F, Roussel MF, Sakai T. Histone deacetylase inhibitors activate INK4d gene through Sp1 site in its promoter. Oncogene 2004;26:26.

23. Sherr CJ, Roberts JM. Inhibitors of mammalian G1 cyclin-dependent kinases. Genes Dev 1995;9:1149–1163.

24. McConnell BB, Gregory FJ, Stott FJ, Hara E, Peters G. Induced expression of p16(INK4a) inhibits both CDK4- and CDK2-associated kinase activity by reassortment of cyclin-CDK-inhibitor complexes. Mol Cell Biol 1999;19:1981–1989.

25. Kim YB, Lee KH, Sugita K, Yoshida M, Horinouchi S. Oxamflatin is a novel antitumor compound that inhibits mammalian histone deacetylase. Oncogene 1999;18:2461–2470.

26. Wharton W, Savell J, Cress WD, Seto E, Pledger WJ. Inhibition of mitogenesis in Balb/c-3T3 cells by trichostatin A. Multiple alterations in the induction and activation of cyclin-cyclin-dependent kinase complexes. J Biol Chem 2000;275: 33,981–33,987.

27. Glaser KB, Staver MJ, Waring JF, Stender J, Ulrich RG, Davidsen SK. Gene expression profiling of multiple histone deacetylase (HDAC) inhibitors: defining a common gene set produced by HDAC inhibition in T24 and MDA carcinoma cell lines. Mol Cancer Ther 2003;2:151–163.

28. Warrener R, Beamish H, Burgess A, et al. Tumor cell-selective cytotoxicity by targeting cell cycle checkpoints. FASEB J 2003;17:1550–1552.

29. Bernhard D, Ausserlechner MJ, Tonko M, et al. Apoptosis induced by the histone deacetylase inhibitor sodium butyrate in human leukemic lymphoblasts. FASEB J 1999;13:1991–2001.

30. Ruefli AA, Ausserlechner MJ, Bernhard D, et al. The histone deacetylase inhibitor and chemotherapeutic agent suberoylanilide hydroxamic acid (SAHA) induces a cell-death pathway characterized by cleavage of Bid and production of reactive oxygen species. Proc Natl Acad Sci U S A 2001;98:10,833–10,838.

31. Peart MJ, Tainton KM, Ruefli AA, et al. Novel mechanisms of apoptosis induced by histone deacetylase inhibitors. Cancer Res 2003;63:4460–4471.

32. Vrana JA, Decker RH, Johnson CR, et al. Induction of apoptosis in U937 human leukemia cells by suberoylanilide hydroxamic acid (SAHA) proceeds through pathways that are regulated by Bcl-2/Bcl-XL, c-Jun, and p21CIP1, but independent of p53. Oncogene 1999;18:7016–7025.

33. Rosato RR, Wang Z, Gopalkrishnan RV, Fisher PB, Grant S. Evidence of a functional role for the cyclin-dependent kinase-inhibitor p21WAF1/CIP1/MDA6 in promoting differentiation and preventing mitochondrial dysfunction and apoptosis induced by sodium butyrate in human myelomonocytic leukemia cells (U937). Int J Oncol 2001;19:181–191.

34. Rahmani M, Yu C, Dai Y, et al. Coadministration of the heat shock protein 90 antagonist 17-allylamino-17-demethoxygeldanamycin with suberoylanilide hydroxamic acid or sodium butyrate synergistically induces apoptosis in human leukemia cells. Cancer Res 2003;63:8420–8427.

35. Rosato RR, Almenara JA, Yu C, Grant S. Evidence of a functional role for p21WAF1/CIP1 down-regulation in synergistic antileukemic interactions between

the histone deacetylase inhibitor sodium butyrate and flavopiridol. Mol Pharmacol 2004;65:571–581.

36. Rahmani M, Yu C, Reese E, et al. Inhibition of PI-3 kinase sensitizes human leukemic cells to histone deacetylase inhibitor-mediated apoptosis through p44/42 MAP kinase inactivation and abrogation of p21(CIP1/WAF1) induction rather than AKT inhibition. Oncogene 2003;22:6231–6242.

37. Rosato RR, Almenara JA, Grant S. The histone deacetylase inhibitor MS-275 promotes differentiation or apoptosis in human leukemia cells through a process regulated by generation of reactive oxygen species and induction of p21CIP1/WAF1 1. Cancer Res 2003;63:3637–3645.

38. Suzuki A, Tsutomi Y, Yamamoto N, Shibutani T, Akahane K. Mitochondrial regulation of cell death: mitochondria are essential for procaspase 3-p21 complex formation to resist Fas-mediated cell death. Mol Cell Biol 1999;19:3842–3847.

39. Park JA, Kim KW, Kim SI, Lee SK. Caspase 3 specifically cleaves p21WAF1/CIP1 in the earlier stage of apoptosis in SK-HEP-1 human hepatoma cells. Eur J Biochem 1998;257:242–248.

40. Burgess A, Ruefli A, Beamish H, et al. Histone deacetylase inhibitors specifically kill nonproliferating tumour cells. Oncogene 2004;23:6693–6701.

41. Qiu L, Kelso MJ, Hansen C, West ML, Fairlie DP, Parsons PG. Anti-tumour activity in vitro and in vivo of selective differentiating agents containing hydroxamate. Br J Cancer 1999;80:1252–1258.

42. Krauer KG, Burgess A, Buck M, Flanagan J, Sculley TB, Gabrielli B. The EBNA-3 gene family proteins disrupt the G2/M checkpoint. Oncogene 2004;23: 1342–1353.

43. Mitsiades N, Mitsiades CS, Richardson PG, et al. Molecular sequelae of histone deacetylase inhibition in human malignant B cells. Blood 2003;101: 4055–4062.

44. Lallemand F, Courilleau D, Buquet-Fagot C, Atfi A, Montagne MN, Mester J. Sodium butyrate induces G2 arrest in the human breast cancer cells MDA-MB-231 and renders them competent for DNA rereplication. Exp Cell Res 1999;247:432–440.

45. Jin S, Antinore MJ, Lung FD, et al. The GADD45 inhibition of Cdc2 kinase correlates with GADD45-mediated growth suppression. J Biol Chem 2000;275: 16,602–16,608.

46. Hirose T, Sowa Y, Takahashi S, et al. p53-independent induction of Gadd45 by histone deacetylase inhibitor: coordinate regulation by transcription factors Oct-1 and NF-Y. Oncogene 2003;22:7762–7773.

47. Taddei A, Maison C, Roche D, Almouzni G. Reversible disruption of pericentric heterochromatin and centromere function by inhibiting deacetylases. Nat Cell Biol 2001;3:114–120.

48. Shin HJ, Baek KH, Jeon AH, et al. Inhibition of histone deacetylase activity increases chromosomal instability by the aberrant regulation of mitotic checkpoint activation. Oncogene 2003;22:3853–3858.

49. Cimini D, Mattiuzzo M, Torosantucci L, Degrassi F. Histone hyperacetylation in mitosis prevents sister chromatid separation and produces chromosome segregation defects. Mol Biol Cell 2003;14:3821–3833.

50. Musacchio A, Hardwick KG. The spindle checkpoint: structural insights into dynamic signalling. Nat Rev Mol Cell Biol 2002;3:731–741.

51. Sobel RE, Cook RG, Perry CA, Annunziato AT, Allis CD. Conservation of deposition-related acetylation sites in newly synthesized histones H3 and H4. Proc Natl Acad Sci U S A 1995;92:1237–1241.

52. Taddei A, Roche D, Sibarita JB, Turner BM, Almouzni G. Duplication and maintenance of heterochromatin domains. J Cell Biol 1999;147:1153–1166.

53. Mello JA, Almouzni G. The ins and outs of nucleosome assembly. Curr Opin Genet Dev 2001;11:136–141.

54. Mackay AM, Ainsztein AM, Eckley DM, Earnshaw WC. A dominant mutant of inner centromere protein (INCENP), a chromosomal protein, disrupts prometaphase congression and cytokinesis. J Cell Biol 1998;140:991–1002.

55. Nishihashi A, Haraguchi T, Hiraoka Y, et al. CENP-I is essential for centromere function in vertebrate cells. Dev Cell 2002;2:463–476.

56. Schaar BT, Chan GK, Maddox P, Salmon ED, Yen TJ. CENP-E function at kinetochores is essential for chromosome alignment. J Cell Biol 1997;139:1373–1382.

57. Taylor SS, McKeon F. Kinetochore localization of murine Bub1 is required for normal mitotic timing and checkpoint response to spindle damage. Cell 1997;89:727–735.

58. Prigent C, Dimitrov S. Phosphorylation of serine 10 in histone H3, what for? J Cell Sci 2003;116:3677–3685.

59. Ekwall K, Olsson T, Turner BM, Cranston G, Allshire RC. Transient inhibition of histone deacetylation alters the structural and functional imprint at fission yeast centromeres. Cell 1997;91:1021–1032.

60. Rea S, Eisenhaber F, O'Carroll D, et al. Regulation of chromatin structure by site-specific histone H3 methyltransferases. Nature 2000;406:593–599.

61. Bannister AJ, Zegerman P, Partridge JF, et al. Selective recognition of methylated lysine 9 on histone H3 by the HP1 chromo domain. Nature 2001;410:120–124.

62. Mellone BG, Ball L, Suka N, Grunstein MR, Partridge JF, Allshire RC. Centromere silencing and function in fission yeast is governed by the amino terminus of histone H3. Curr Biol 2003;13:1748–1757.

63. David G, Turner GM, Yao Y, Protopopov A, DePinho RA. mSin3-associated protein, mSds3, is essential for pericentric heterochromatin formation and chromosome segregation in mammalian cells. Genes Dev 2003;17:2396–2405.

64. Silverstein RA, Richardson W, Levin H, Allshire R, Ekwall K. A new role for the transcriptional corepressor SIN3; regulation of centromeres. Curr Biol 2003;13:68–72.

65. Dillon N, Festenstein R, Cheung WL, Briggs SD, Allis CD. Unravelling heterochromatin: competition between positive and negative factors regulates accessibility. Acetylation and chromosomal functions. Trends Genet 2002;18:252–258.

66. Jenuwein T, Allis CD. Translating the histone code. Science 2001;293:1074–1080.

14 HDAC Inhibitors

An Emerging Anticancer
Therapeutic Strategy

Paul Kwon, Meier Hsu,
Dalia Cohen, PhD,
and Peter Atadja, PhD

CONTENTS

SUMMARY
HISTONES AND THE REMODELING OF CHROMATIN
    STRUCTURE
HISTONE ACETYLATION, GENE REGULATION,
    AND CANCER
HDAC INHIBITORS
ANTICANCER EFFECTS OF HDAC INHIBITORS
CURRENT ISSUES AND FUTURE OUTLOOK
REFERENCES

SUMMARY

Coordinated and tight transcriptional regulation of genetic information is vital for maintenance of normal cell growth and differentiation. Cancer is typified by inappropriate gene expression—aberrant expression of genes associated with increased cellular proliferation and survival (e.g., oncogenes), as well as alterations in genes encoding tumor suppressor proteins. Therefore, targeting the gene expression machinery to restore its normalcy promises to be a useful anticancer therapeutic strategy. In the past, targeting

From: *Cancer Drug Discovery and Development*
Histone Deacetylases: Transcriptional Regulation and Other Cellular Functions
Edited by: E. Verdin © Humana Press Inc., Totowa, NJ

the DNA binding multiprotein transcription factors with reasonable potency and specificity has been challenging owing to difficulties in disrupting protein-protein and protein-DNA interactions. However, recent studies showed that epigenetic modifications by enzymes play key roles in regulating gene expression, providing an opportunity to target such enzymes with small molecules for therapeutic purposes. Histone deacetylases (HDACs) can regulate gene expression by deacetylating histones, leading to repressed chromatin structure. In addition, HDACs can target nonhistone substrates, including several oncoproteins and tumor suppressors. Thus abnormal HDAC activity may lead to aberrant gene expression as well as perturbation in critical pathways. HDAC inhibitors have demonstrated efficacy in a variety of solid and hematological malignancies in early clinical trials. The current review focuses on the emerging utility of histone deacetylase inhibition as an anticancer therapeutic strategy.

Key Words: HDAC, HDAC inhibitor, histone, acetylation, deacetylation, cancer, therapy, small molecule.

HISTONES AND THE REMODELING OF CHROMATIN STRUCTURE

In eukaryotic cells, DNA is packaged into chromatin. The packaging unit in the chromatin is the nucleosome. The nucleosome is made up of a core histone tetramer consisting of a histone H3/H4 dimer and a histone H2A/H2B dimer, which wraps approx 145 bp of DNA. A histone H1/DNA complex links nucleosomes to form the primary structure of chromatin; secondary internucleosomal and other DNA-protein interactions form higher order chromosomal structures. Chromatin structure may be regulated either locally or globally. Whereas local effects occur at the level of single genes, global effects may occur over larger domains or entire chromosomes. The higher ordered supranucleosomal structures of chromatin form, on the one hand, the heterochromatic domains, which are largely inaccessible to transcription factors, and on the other hand, the euchromatin domains, which are more transcriptionally active.

Chromatin structure is modulated by various mechanisms including enzymes that modify histones posttranslationally. In the past, histones were viewed as inert packaging material, but recent findings have shown that posttranslational modifications of their lysine tails, which protrude through the nucleosome, affect chromatin structure in a manner that imparts gene expression, epigenetic silencing, or centromeric functions *(1)*. The major modifications of the core histones include acetylation of lysine, methylation of arginine, ubiquitination of lysine, and phosphorylation of serine, and threonine residues. More recent studies indicate that combinations of posttranslational histone modifications on single

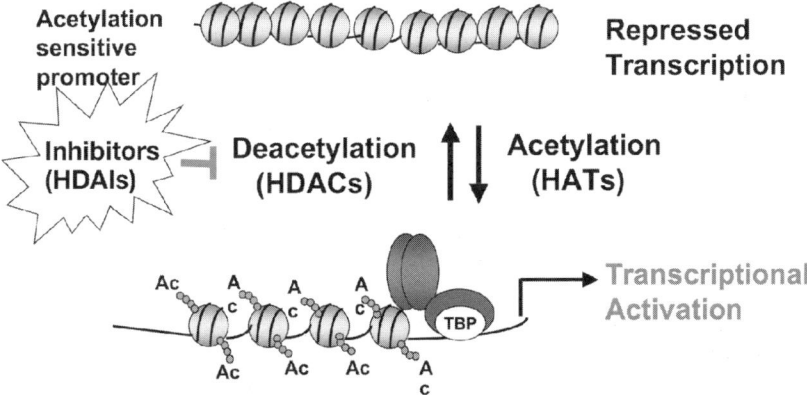

Fig. 1. Modulation of chromatin structure by histone acetylation affects transcription of genes. HAT, histone acetyltransferase; HDAC, histone deacetylase; HDAI, HDAC inhibitor.

nucleosomes or nucleosomal domains establish local and global chromatin patterns that provide a framework for activation or silencing of gene expression. The histone code hypothesis postulates that multiple histone modifications, acting in a combinatorial or sequential fashion on one or multiple histone tails, specify unique downstream functions *(2,3)*. Thus chromatin is currently thought of, on the one hand, as an integrator of multiple extracellular and intracellular signals, which it receives through enzymatic epigenetic factors, and on the other, as a transducer of these signals through the control of gene expression *(3)*.

HISTONE ACETYLATION, GENE REGULATION, AND CANCER

One of the most abundant chromatin modifications is reversible acetylation of histones. In euchromatin, transcriptionally active regions are often associated with hyperacetylated histones, whereas transcriptionally silent heterochromatin regions are frequently hypoacetylated *(1)*. Generally, histone acetyltransferases (HATs) are thought of as transcriptional activators, whereas histone deacetylases (HDACs) are regarded as transcriptional repressors (Fig. 1). To date 18 isoforms of HDACs have been identified and are subdivided into three classes based on homology. Of the three, the class III HDACs, which are mammalian homologs of the yeast silent information regulator 2 (sir2) protein family, are the most diverse and require NAD for catalytic activity.

Aberrant histone acetylation is implicated in several solid tumor types and hematological malignancies. Genes encoding HAT proteins, such as cyclic AMP-responsive element binding protein (CBP) and p300 are amplified, translocated, or mutated in many cancers *(4,5)*. For example, Rubinstein-Tabi syndrome, a genetic predisposition to cancer, is associated with mutations in the CBP gene that inactivates the HAT activity of the CBP protein *(6,7)*. In addition, Muraoka et al. *(8)* detected somatic missense mutations of p300 in colorectal and gastric carcinomas. These mutations were coupled to deletion of the second allele of the gene, resulting in complete inactivation of p300. In other mutations, loss of heterozygosity, translocations, or overexpression of HAT encoding genes have been reported in various solid tumors and in hematological malignancies *(9–12)*.

The role of HDACs in cancer was first demonstrated in hematological malignancies. In acute promyeloctyic leukemia (APL), the tumor-associated fusion proteins partner with a corepressor complex containing HDAC activity *(13,14)*. These chromosomal translocations involve the retinoic acid receptor-α (RAR-α) gene fused to one of several gene loci producing the promyelocytic leukemia (PML), PML-RAR-α t(15;17), and promyelocytic leukemia zinc finger (PLZF), PLZF-RAR-α t(11;17), translocations *(15)*. During normal hematopoiesis, physiological amounts of retinoic acid induce the release of HDAC complexes from RAR-α followed by binding of coactivator complexes with HAT activity that favors expression of differentiation-related genes. In t(15;17) APL, the PML-RAR-α fusion protein has an abnormally high affinity for HDAC corepressors; thus pharmacological amounts of retinoic acid are required to induce expression of differentiation-specific genes. Furthermore, the PLZF-RAR-α fusion protein produced by the t(11;17) translocation, unlike the PML-RAR-α translocation, fails to release corepressors under the influence of retinoic acid, leading to a retinoid-resistant form of the disease *(16)*. In this scenario, a combination of retinoic acid with HDAC inhibitors is required for transcriptional activation of the differentiation genes. Similarly, the t(8;21) chromosomal translocation fusion protein, AML1-ETO, characteristic of the acute myelogenous leukemia (AML) M2 subtype, has been shown to interact physically with class I HDACs and can be inactivated by the HDAC inhibitors trichostatin A (TSA) and phenylbutyrate *(17–19)*.

Another example of HDAC involvement in disease may be depicted by the TAL1/SCL gene. This gene, which is the most frequent gain-of-function mutation in T-cell acute lymphoblastic leukemia (T-ALL), has been shown to associate with a member of the class I HDACs as well as the corepressor mSin3A, thereby restricting its function in erythroid differentiation *(20)*.

In solid tumors, HDAC1 is overexpressed in human prostate and gastric tumor tissues compared with levels in their adjacent normal tissues. Patra et al. *(21)* detected greater expression of HDAC1 mRNA in several prostate cancer cell lines including PC3, TSUPr1, and DuPro as well as in

ND1, a human primary prostate cancer line. This increased HDAC1 level carried over to patient samples, in which archived prostate cancer specimens showed elevated HDAC1 expression compared with adjacent normal tissue. Another group investigating HDAC1 overexpression reported that 61% of primary gastric cancer biopsies contained markedly elevated levels of HDAC1 *(22)*. More recently, HDAC2 overexpression has also been linked to disease. Loss of the adenomatosis polyposis coli (APC) tumor suppressor in human colorectal carcinomas was coupled with high HDAC2 expression *(23)*. These findings support the targeting of HDACs as a viable therapeutic approach in cancer treatment, and currently there are several efforts to develop HDAC inhibitors as anticancer agents.

HDAC INHIBITORS

Sodium butyrate was one of the first HDAC inhibitors discovered when Riggs et al. *(24)* reported increased histone acetylation in Hela and Friend erythroleukemia cells following treatment. Subsequent studies revealed suppression of histone deacetylation in vivo and in vitro. Other short-chain fatty acids such as phenylbutyrate and valproic acid were reported as HDAC inhibitors with antitumor effects. Phenylbutyrate, although clinically approved for treating certain hematological disorders, has poor potency as an HDAC inhibitor owing to numerous side effects and poor pharmaceutical properties, making it unattractive for development as an anticancer agent *(26,27)*.

Various other structurally diverse HDAC inhibitors have been described. The hydroxamic acid derivatives, which are highly potent as HDAC inhibitors, comprise the largest structural class. Examples include TSA, suberoylanilide hydroxamic acid (SAHA), NVP-LAQ824, NVP-LBH589, pyroxamide, and oxamflatin. Crystallographic studies with TSA and SAHA indicate that these compounds inhibit HDACs by interacting with the catalytic site of the enzyme and chelating the divalent zinc cation, which is necessary for histone deacetylation *(28)*. The hydroxamic acids such as TSA, NVP-LAQ824, NVP-LBH589, and SAHA inhibit HDACs at nanomolar concentrations and produce potent antitumor activity in vivo. However, hydroxamic acid analogs inhibit both class I and II HDAC isoforms in a nonselective manner.

A number of natural product cyclic tetrapeptides have also been identified as HDAC inhibitors. Examples include trapoxin, HC-toxin, chlamydocin, FK-228, and apidicin. The cyclic tetrapeptides are also potent nanomolar inhibitors of HDACs and possess in vitro antiproliferative activity. However, there are insufficient in vivo antitumor efficacy data, most likely resulting from the metabolic instability of these molecules *(29)*. Interestingly, the cyclic tetrapeptides appear to have some isoform

Table 1
Examples of Some HDAC Inhibitors in Development

Compound name	Structure	Structural class
SAHA		Hydroxamic acid
CI-994		Benzamide
FK228 (depsipeptide)		Macrocycle
Sodium phenylbutyrate		Carboxylate
NVP-LAQ824		
NVP-LBH589		Hydroxamic acid
Valproic acid		Carboxylate
MS-27-275		Benzamide
Pyroxamide		Hydroxamic acid

selectivity. Trapoxin and apicidin selectively inhibit class I HDACs but are inactive against some class II HDACs such as HDAC6. The cyclic depsipeptide FK-228 is a nanomolar HDAC inhibitor with selectivity against class I enzymes *(30)*. The mechanism of action of HDAC inhibition is thought to involve intracellular reduction of a disulfide bond, resulting in a thiol that interacts with the zinc cation at the active site. Unlike the other cyclic peptides, FK-228 has shown in vivo antitumor efficacy both in animal models and in clinical trials.

A third class of HDAC inhibitors has a benzamide group; of this group, MS-27-275 inhibits HDACs at micromolar concentrations *(31)*. The mechanism of HDAC inhibition is thought to involve interaction of the two substituted amides with the zinc cation at the active site of the enzyme. Despite the relatively low potency of HDAC inhibition by the benzamide derivatives compared with the hydroxamates and the cyclic peptides, MS-27-275 produced marked in vivo tumor efficacy in animal models *(32)*. Table 1 gives a list of the different HDAC inhibitors currently under development for cancer therapy.

ANTICANCER EFFECTS OF HDAC INHIBITORS

Chromatin and Transcription Effects

As compounds that directly affect transcription of genes, it was originally feared that HDAC inhibitors would be toxic owing to nonspecific pleiotropic effects on gene expression. These concerns were somewhat abated with microarray experiments showing that treatment of cells with HDAC inhibitors modulated the expression of about 1% of the total genes *(33)*. This finding suggests that HDACs are recruited to specific promoters and that activation of these promoters may be sensitive to HDAC inhibitors.

In a recent microarray experiment profiling three HDAC inhibitors, SAHA, TSA, and MS-27-275, Glaser et al. *(34)* verified similar expression patterns for genes that are involved in cell cycle, apoptosis, and DNA synthesis. In addition, of the 6800 genes evaluated on the microarray, fewer than 10% were either positively or negatively regulated, supporting the earlier findings. Furthermore, expression profiling of three different cell lines with four inhibitors, NVP-LAL902, MS-27-275, trapoxin, and NVP-LAQ824, revealed a core set of genes that are either up- or downregulated and could be classified by function. These genes are thought to play a role in cell cycling, apoptosis, signal transduction, metabolism, transcription, cytoskeletal structure, and adhesion (Fig. 2; *see* Color Plate 9 following p. 180). It now appears that HDAC inhibitors modulate expression profiles of specific genes and that by utilizing microarray analysis it may be feasible to identify functional and subtle differences in inhibition that affect efficacy.

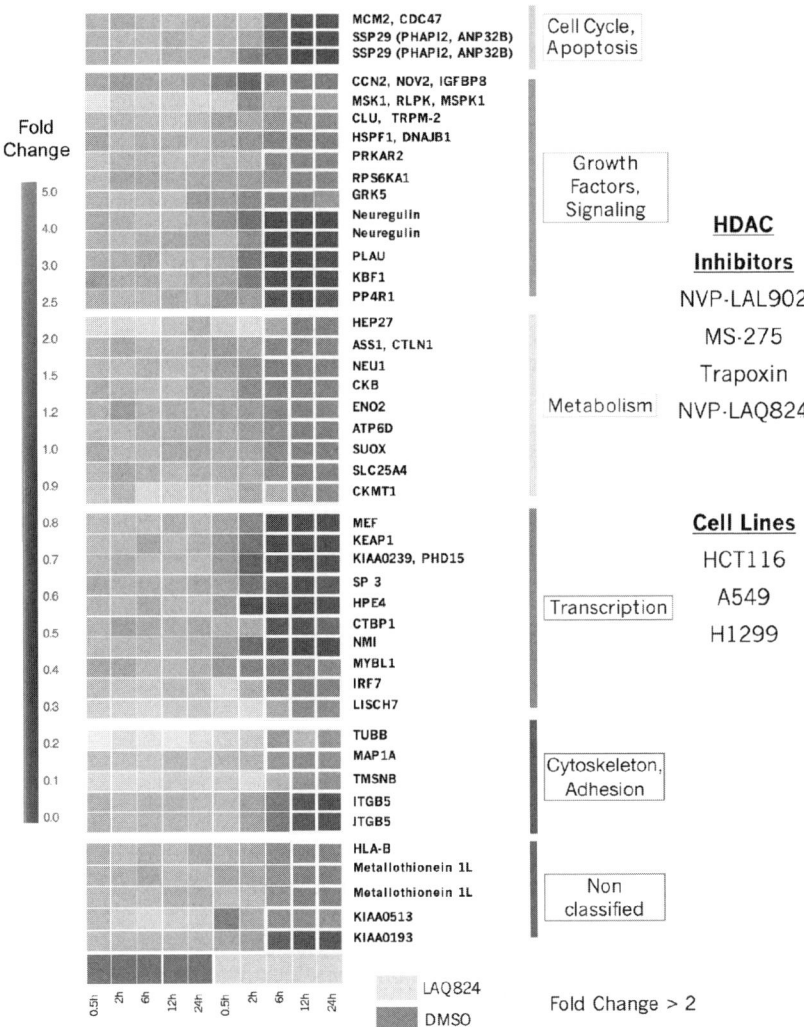

Fig. 2. Genes/pathways modulated by histone deacetylase (HDAC) inhibitors. *See* Color Plate 9 following p. 180.

The recent discovery of nonhistone acetylated proteins has generated great interest, adding an additional level of complexity to protein regulation. Nonhistone acetylases modify lysine residues of transcription factors p53, E2F1, T-cell factor (TCF), GATA1, nuclear factor-κB (NF-κB), and hypoxia-inducible factor-1α (HIF-1α), whose functions are affected in the following ways: binding to DNA, protein-protein interaction, cellular localization, and proteasomal degradation *(35–42)*. Understanding the downstream events following reversible acetylation of these factors may give additional insight into mechanisms involved in proliferation, differentiation, apoptosis, and angiogenesis as well as help identify novel therapeutic approaches to combat cancer.

The consequences of persistent acetylation of proteins vary greatly depending on the specific factor. Transcription factors such as p53, E2F1, and GATA1 are currently thought to rely on acetylation to promote binding to target DNA. Inhibition of deacetylases that have enzymatic activity against the acetylated form of p53 increases p21 levels to obstruct cell cycle progression, whereas activity against the deacetylation of E2F1 may promote retinoblastoma protein (Rb)-mediated differentiation *(35,36,38,41)*. Additionally, HDAC inhibition permits the continued acetylated state of proteins, such as TCF in *Drosophila* and ACTR, disrupting protein-protein interaction with its partner armadillo and nuclear receptors, respectively *(37,43)*. Furthermore, there is now evidence that shows the importance of reversible acetylation in regulating factor localization and signaling. Chen et al. *(40)* show evidence that acetylated NF-κB possesses prosurvival transcription proficiency. They propose that inhibitor κB (IκB), NF-κB's inhibitory partner, fails to bind to the acetylated form of NF-κB, blocking IκB-mediated transport of the complex out of the nucleus.

Nontranscription Effects

HDAC inhibition affects protein stability through several mechanisms including promotion of apoptosis, cell cycle arrest, and prevention of tumor-mediated angiogenesis. Recent evidence shows that HDAC inhibitors increase the acetylation status of heat shock protein 90 (Hsp90) whereby the chaperone activity of the acetylated form is inactivated, leading to destabilization of its client proteins including Her-2/neu, AKT, c-Raf-1, mutant p53, and Bcr-Abl *(41,44,45)*. Nimmanapalli et al. *(44)* revealed activity of NVP-LAQ824 in chronic myelogenous leukemia-blast crisis (CML-BC) cells, maintaining acetylation of Hsp90 and directing proteasomal degradation of wild-type Bcr-Abl as well as imatinib-refractory mutant Bcr-Abl. This Hsp90-mediated proteasomal degradation of Bcr-Abl in conjunction with degradation of c-Raf-1, Src, and AKT appears to promote CMC-BL cell apoptosis. In studies involving breast cancer, exposure of cells to NVP-LAQ824 increased acetylated Hsp90, leading to inefficient binding of ATP. This event destabilizes the Her2/neu oncoprotein and facilitates polyubiquitination and proteasomal degradation, promoting antitumorigenesis and apoptosis *(45)*.

Other studies suggest that the p53 tumor suppressor is regulated by multiple levels of protein acetylation. The transcriptionally efficient p53 protein appears to be acetylated, and the levels of cellular p53 appear to be regulated by the chaperon activity of Hsp90 *(41)*. Interestingly, this report identifies a mutant p53 that is depleted upon treatment with a HDAC inhibitor, whereas the wild-type p53 is unchanged. Lastly, HIF-1α, a transcription factor thought to be involved in angiogenesis, appears to be destabilized by acetylation. Investigators identified a novel acetyl transferase (ARD1) that specifically acetylates HIF-1α, driving its fate down the ubiquitin-mediated degradation pathway *(42)*. Interpretation of these results suggests a role for deacetylase inhibitors in blocking tumor cell-driven angiogenesis.

Cellular Effects

Inhibition of HDACs has profound effects on cellular mechanisms that affect the cells' ability to proliferate, differentiate, and/or die. Although the precise mechanisms that control cellular fate are not completely understood, several lines of evidence suggest that aberrant recruitment of HDACs and the resulting chromatin modifications may lead to the changes in gene expression seen in transformed cells: (1) silencing of tumor suppressor genes at the chromatin level *(46–52)*; (2) interaction of HDAC-containing complexes with proteins involved in tumorigenesis *(53–55)*; (3) reports of HDAC inhibitors having significant antiproliferative effects, such as promoting differentiation, cell cycle arrest, or apoptosis *(56–61)*; and (4) alterations in key mediators of G1 cell cycle arrest and differentiation such as induction of p21, reduction of Rb phosphorylation, and inhibition of cyclin-dependent kinase 2 (cdk2) activity *(56,62–66)*.

One intriguing feature of the antiproliferative effects of HDAC inhibitors is that they induce apoptosis in tumor cell lines while causing normal cells to undergo reversible cell cycle arrest *(32,67,68)*. When normal diploid fibroblasts and normal lung epithelial cells were treated with NVP-LAQ824, they arrested at the G1-S and G2-M phases. Contrary to the situation in normal cells, treatment of HCT116 (colon carcinoma), A549 (lung carcinoma), or SV40/hTERT (transformed lung epithelial) cell lines with much lower concentrations of NVP-LAQ824 resulted in death by apoptosis (Fig. 3; *see* Color Plate 10 following p. 180) *(67)*. Interestingly, NVP-LAQ824 induced p21 expression and Rb hypophosphorylation in both normal and tumor cells, but only normal cells underwent growth arrest. This suggests that the downstream effects of hypophosphorylated Rb, which result in cell cycle arrest in normal cells, may not be operational in the tumor cells, leading to aberrant G1-S progression. Similarly, checkpoints that allow normal cells to arrest at the G2-M phase may be lacking in the tumor cells, leading to abnormal progression and cell death. In fact, there is evidence that the eventual death of tumor cells may be attributed to their loss of mitotic checkpoint mechanisms, leading to their inability to arrest stably *(69)*.

DMSO   **NVP-LAQ824**

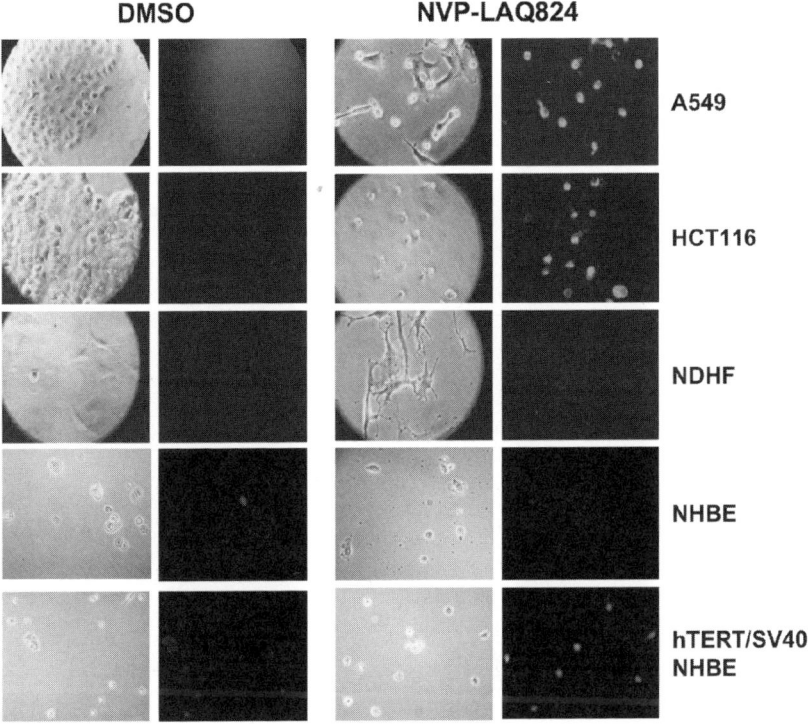

Fig. 3. NVP-LAQ824 induces apoptosis in transformed but not in normal cells DMSO, dimethyl sulfoxide. *See* Color Plate 10 following p. 180.

Differences have been observed between the antiproliferative effects of different HDAC inhibitors. For example, treatment of tumor cells with MS-27-275 and SAHA causes both G1-S and G2-M arrest, but continued exposure for more than 24 h triggers progression to apoptosis. In contrast, treatment of the same cells with NVP-LAQ824 induces only a G2-M block followed by apoptosis. The mechanism behind this disparity is unknown, but it presents an interesting opportunity to investigate regulation of G1-S checkpoint mechanisms using the different inhibitors.

In Vivo Pharmacology

In vivo preclinical experiments using small-molecule inhibitors of HDACs such as MS-27-275, SAHA, FR-22, NVP-LAQ824, and NVP-LBH589 exhibited efficacy against several human tumor xenografts in athymic mice *(15,32,65,67)*. When NVP-LAQ824 was given intravenously to athymic nude mice bearing HCT116 (colon), A549 (non-small cell lung carcinoma [NSCLC]), H1299- NSCLC, MDA-MB-435 (breast), SW620

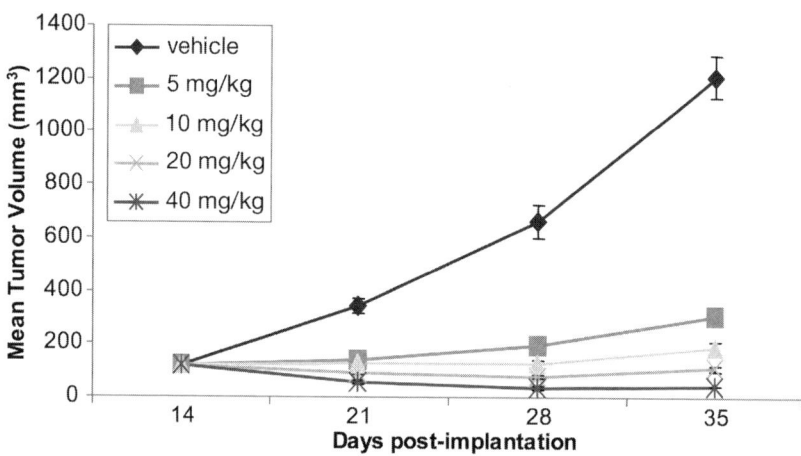

Fig. 4. NVP-LBH589 causes regression in HCT116 xenografts. *See* Color Plate 11 following p. 180.

(colorectal adenocarcinoma), A431 (epidermoid carcinoma), or T24 (urinary carcinoma) xenograft tumors, potent antitumor efficacy was observed with high tolerability *(70)*. Furthermore, NVP-LBH589, which is structurally similar to NVP-LAQ824, produced profound tumor regression in a number of tumor models (Fig. 4; *see* Color Plate 11 following p. 180). Moreover, antitumor efficacy was observed in subcutaneous, orthotopic, and metastasis models, and peritoneal or oral administration of the inhibitor proved equally efficacious.

In xenograft experiments, NVP-LAQ824-treated mice bearing tumors were harvested and analyzed for the acetylation state of histones. Histone acetylation levels increased as early as 30 min post dose and persisted for at least 24 h after a single dose. Induction of histone acetylation in the xenograft tumors indicates that the compound's antitumor activity probably operates through the predicted mechanism of histone deacetylase inhibition. Additionally, pharmacokinetic analysis of NVP-LAQ824 administered to tumor-bearing mice revealed high plasma and tumor levels of the compound. However, in plasma, levels dropped precipitously while in tumors, levels persisted for several hours. These results may suggest that even less frequent dosing schedules of the drug may produce the desired antitumor effect.

Clinical Experience With HDAC Inhibitors

Early clinical studies indicate that different classes of HDAC inhibitors are well tolerated in the clinic, and some anticancer activity has been observed. The first evidence of clinical efficacy with an HDAC inhibitor was observed when an APL patient who had experienced multiple relapses was treated with retinoic acid alone or in combination with phenylbutyrate.

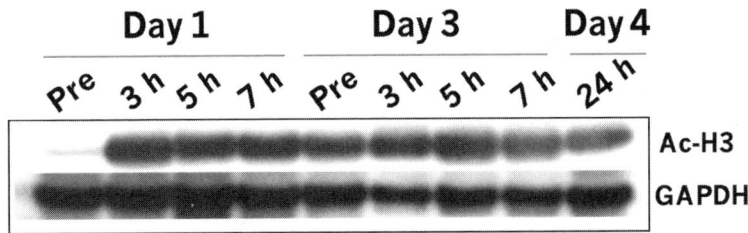

Fig. 5. NVP-LAQ824 upregulates histone H3 acetylation levels in acute myelocytic leukemia (AML) patients.

In this study, the APL patient proved clinically resistant to all-trans-retinoic acid (ATRA). However, a combination of ATRA with phenylbutyrate produced complete clinical and cytogenetic remission *(16)*. Over the last 2 yr, other HDAC inhibitors including FK-228, SAHA, NVP-LAQ824, NVP-LBH589, CI-994, MS-27-275, and valproic acid have entered clinical investigation for solid and hematological malignancies. In all cases, the studies demonstrate increased histone acetylation in surrogate tissues such as peripheral mononucleocytes following administration of the inhibitor, signifying that the drugs inhibit the desired mechanism (Fig. 5).

An indication for which HDAC inhibitors have shown the most clinical benefit as monotherapy is cutaneous T-cell lymphoma (CTCL), in which SAHA and FK-228 produced dramatic response rates *(71–73)*. The specific mechanisms responsible for the sensitivity of CTCL to HDAC inhibitors is, however, not currently understood. Other tumor types in which responses or stable disease have been reported include mesothelioma, head and neck cancer, diffused lymphoma (SAHA), AML (SAHA and NVP-LAQ824), NSCLC (Pivanex), and melanoma (MS-27-275).

Although the HDAC inhibitors that are currently undergoing clinical studies have been generally well tolerated, some dose-limiting toxicities and other adverse events have been reported. These include myelosuppression (thrombocytopenia), fatigue, somnolence, confusion, hepatotoxicity, and abnormal electrocardiographic effects such as T-wave and ST-wave changes and QTc prolongation.

CURRENT ISSUES AND FUTURE OUTLOOK

The preclinical and clinical experience with HDAC inhibitors raises several questions pertaining to their successful development in the clinic. These issues include: (1) which HDAC isoforms need to be inhibited for antitumor activity; (2) which mechanisms of action are responsible for their anticancer activity; (3) which biomarkers will be most informative to allow pharmacokinetic/pharmacodynamic modeling, dose selection, and schedule design; (4) how patients will be stratified for clinical trials to yield the most information and patient benefit; (5) which combinations of existing antitumor agents and HDAC inhibitors will be most useful; (6) whether patients will develop resistance to HDAC inhibitors; and (7) how to avoid toxicity and safety problems specifically associated with HDAC inhibitors. Successfully tackling the foregoing challenges will enable us to fulfill the tremendous therapeutic potential that HDAC inhibitors currently present as anticancer agents.

REFERENCES

1. Struhl K. Histone acetylation and transcriptional regulatory mechanisms. Genes Dev 1998;12:599–606.
2. Strahl BD, Allis CD. The language of covalent histone modifications. Nature 2000;403:41–45.
3. Schreiber SL, Bernstein BE. Signaling network model of chromatin. Cell 2002;111:771–778.
4. Giles RH, Peters DJ, Breuning MH. Conjunction dysfunction: CBP/p300 in human disease. Trends Genet 1998;14:178–183.
5. Gayther SA, Batley SJ, Linger L, et al. Mutations truncating the EP300 acetylase in human cancers. Nat Genet 2000;24:300–303.
6. Petrij F, Giles RH, Dauwerse HG, et al. Rubinstein-Taybi syndrome caused by mutations in the transcriptional co-activator CBP. Nature 1995;376:348–351.
7. Murata T, Kurokawa R, Krones A, et al. Defect of histone acetyltransferase activity of the nuclear transcriptional coactivator CBP n Rubinstein-Taybi syndrome. Hum Mol Genet 2001;10:1071–1076.
8. Muraoka M, Konishi M, Kikuchi-Yanoshita R, et al. p300 gene alterations in colorectal and gastric carcinomas. Oncogene 1996;12:1565–1569.
9. Rowley JD, Reshmi S, Sobulo O, et al. All patients with the T(11;16)(q23;p13.3) that involves MLL and CBP have treatment-related hematologic disorders. Blood 1997;90:535–541.
10. Borrow J, Stanton VP Jr, Andresen JM, et al. The translocation t(8;16)(p11;p13) of acute myeloid leukaemia fuses a putative acetyltransferase to the CREB-binding protein. Nat Genet 1996;14:33–41.
11. Ida K, Kitabayashi I, Taki T, et al. Adenoviral E1A-associated protein p300 is involved in acute myeloid leukemia with t(11;22)(q23;q13). Blood 1997;90:4699–4704.
12. Anzick SL, Kononen J, Walker RL, et al. AIB1, a steroid receptor coactivator amplified in breast and ovarian cancer. Science 1997;277:965–968.
13. Grignani F, De Matteis S, Nervi C, et al. Fusion proteins of the retinoic acid receptor-alpha recruit histone deacetylase in promyelocytic leukaemia. Nature 1998;391:815–818.
14. David G, Alland L, Hong SH, Wong CW, DePinho RA, Dejean A. Histone deacetylase associated with mSin3A mediates repression by the acute promyelocytic leukemia-associated PLZF protein. Oncogene 1998;16:2549–2556.
15. Marks P, Rifkind RA, Richon VM, Breslow R, Miller T, Kelly WK. Histone deacetylases and cancer: causes and therapies. Nat Rev Cancer 2001;1:194–202.
16. Lin RJ, Nagy L, Inoue S, Shao W, Miller WH Jr, Evans RM. Role of the histone deacetylase complex in acute promyelocytic leukaemia. Nature 1998;391:811–814.

17. Amann JM, Nip J, Strom DK, et al. ETO, a target of t(8;21) in acute leukemia, makes distinct contacts with multiple histone deacetylases and binds mSin3A through its oligomerization domain. Mol Cell Biol 2001;21:6470–6483.

18. Wang J, Saunthararajah Y, Redner RL, Liu JM. Inhibitors of histone deacetylase relieve ETO-mediated repression and induce differentiation of AML1-ETO leukemia cells. Cancer Res 1999;59:2766–2769.

19. Lutterbach B, Westendorf JJ, Linggi B, et al. ETO, a target of t(8;21) in acute leukemia, interacts with the N-CoR and mSin3 corepressors. Mol Cell Biol 1998;18:7176–7184.

20. Huang S, Brandt SJ. mSin3A regulates murine erythroleukemia cell differentiation through association with the TAL1 (or SCL) transcription factor. Mol Cell Biol 2000;20:2248–2259.

21. Patra SK, Patra A, Dahiya R. Histone deacetylase and DNA methyltransferase in human prostate cancer. Biochem Biophys Res Commun 2001;287:705–713.

22. Choi JH, Kwon HJ, Yoon BI, et al. Expression profile of histone deacetylase 1 in gastric cancer tissues. Jpn J Cancer Res 2001;92:1300–1304.

23. Zhu P, Martin E, Mengwasser J, Schlag P, Janssen KP, Gottlicher M. Induction of HDAC2 expression upon loss of APC in colorectal tumorigenesis. Cancer Cell 2004;5:455–463.

24. Riggs MG, Whittaker RG, Neumann JR, Ingram VM. n-Butyrate causes histone modification in HeLa and Friend erythroleukaemia cells. Nature 1977;268: 462–464.

25. Boffa LC, Vidali G, Mann RS, Allfrey VG. Suppression of histone deacetylation in vivo and in vitro by sodium butyrate. J Biol Chem 1978;253:3364–3366.

26. Gore SD, Carducci MA. Modifying histones to tame cancer: clinical development of sodium phenylbutyrate and other histone deacetylase inhibitors. Expert Opin Investig Drugs 2000;9:2923–2934.

27. Santini V, Gozzini A, Scappini B, Grossi A, Rossi Ferrini P. Searching for the magic bullet against cancer: the butyrate saga. Leuk Lymphoma 2001;42:275–289.

28. Finnin MS, Donigian JR, Cohen A, et al. Structures of a histone deacetylase homologue bound to the TSA and SAHA inhibitors. Nature 1999;401:188–193.

29. Remiszewski SW, Sambucetti LC, Bair KW, et al. N-hydroxy-3-phenyl-2-propenamides as novel inhibitors of human histone deacetylase with in vivo antitumor activity: discovery of (2E)-N-hydroxy-3-[4-[[(2-hydroxyethyl)[2-(1H-indol-3-yl) ethyl]amino]methyl]phenyl]-2-propenamide (NVP-LAQ824). J Med Chem 2003; 46:4609–4624.

30. Nakajima H, Kim YB, Terano H, Yoshida M, Horinouchi S. FR901228, a potent antitumor antibiotic, is a novel histone deacetylase inhibitor. Exp Cell Res 1998;241:126–133.

31. Suzuki T, Ando T, Tsuchiya K, et al. Synthesis and histone deacetylase inhibitory activity of new benzamide derivatives. J Med Chem 1999;42:3001–3003.

32. Saito A, Yamashita T, Mariko Y, et al. A synthetic inhibitor of histone deacetylase, MS-27-275, with marked in vivo antitumor activity against human tumors. Proc Natl Acad Sci U S A 1999;96:4592–4597.

33. Van Lint C, Emiliani S, Verdin E. The expression of a small fraction of cellular genes is changed in response to histone hyperacetylation. Gene Expr 1996;5:245–253.

34. Glaser KB, Staver MJ, Waring JF, Stender J, Ulrich RG, Davidsen SK. Gene expression profiling of multiple histone deacetylase (HDAC) inhibitors: defining a common gene set produced by HDAC inhibition in T24 and MDA carcinoma cell lines. Mol Cancer Ther 2003;2:151–163.

35. Gu W, Roeder RG. Activation of p53 sequence-specific DNA binding by acetylation of the p53 C-terminal domain. Cell 1997;90:595–606.

36. Boyes J, Byfield P, Nakatani Y, Ogryzko V. Regulation of activity of the transcription factor GATA-1 by acetylation. Nature 1998;396:594–598.

37. Waltzer L, Bienz M. Drosophila CBP represses the transcription factor TCF to antagonize Wingless signaling. Nature 1998;395:521–525.

38. Martinez-Balbas MA, Bauer UM, Nielsen SJ, Brehm A, Kouzarides T. Regulation of E2F1 activity by acetylation. EMBO J 2000;19:662–671.

39. Marzio G, Wagener C, Gutierrez MI, Cartwright P, Helin K, Giacca M. E2F family members are differentially regulated by reversible acetylation. J Biol Chem 2000;275:10,887–10,892.

40. Chen LF, Fischle W, Verdin E, Greene WC. Duration of nuclear NF-KB action regulated by reversible acetylation. Science 2001;293:1653–1657.

41. Yu X, Guo ZS, Marcu MG, et al. Modulation of p53, ErbB1, ErbB2, and Raf-1 expression in lung cancer cells by depsipeptide FR901228. J Natl Cancer Inst 2002;94:504–513.

42. Jeong JW, Bae MK, Ahn MY, et al. Regulation and destabilization of HIF-1alpha by ARD1-mediated acetylation. Cell 2002;111:709–720.

43. Chen G, Fernandez J, Mische S, Courey AJ. A functional interaction between the histone deacetylase Rpd3 and the corepressor groucho in *Drosophila* development. Genes Dev 1999;13:2218–2230.

44. Nimmanapalli R, Fuino L, Bali P, et al. Histone deacetylase inhibitor LAQ824 both lowers expression and promotes proteasomal degradation of Bcr-Abl and induces apoptosis of imatinib mesylate-sensitive or -refractory chronic myelogenous leukemia-blast crisis cells. Cancer Res 2003;63:5126–5135.

45. Fuino L, Bali P, Wittmann S, et al. Histone deacetylase inhibitor LAQ824 down-regulates Her-2 and sensitizes human breast cancer cells to trastuzumab, taxotere, gemcitabine, and epothilone B. Mol Cancer Ther 2003;2:971–984.

46. Corn PG, Kuerbitz SJ, van Noesel MM, et al. Transcriptional silencing of the p73 gene in acute lymphoblastic leukemia and Burkitt's lymphoma is associated with 5' CpG island methylation. Cancer Res 1999;59:3352–3356.

47. Domann FE, Rice JC, Hendrix MJ, Futscher BW. Epigenetic silencing of maspin gene expression in human breast cancers. Int J Cancer 2000;85:805–810.

48. Sharpless NE, Bardeesy N, Lee KH, et al. Loss of p16Ink4a with retention of p19Arf predisposes mice to tumorigenesis. Nature 2001;413:86–91.

49. Schagdarsurengin U, Gimm O, Hoang-Vu C, Dralle H, Pfeifer GP, Dammann R. Frequent epigenetic silencing of the CpG island promoter of RASSF1A in thyroid carcinoma. Cancer Res 2002;62:3698–3701.

50. van Engeland M, Roemen GM, Brink M, et al. K-ras mutations and RASSF1A promoter methylation in colorectal cancer. Oncogene 2002;21:3792–3795.

51. Gasco M, Sullivan A, Repellin C, et al. Coincident inactivation of 14-3-3sigma and p16INK4a is an early event in vulval squamous neoplasia. Oncogene 2002; 21:1876–1881.

52. Yanagawa N, Tamura G, Oizumi H, Takahashi N, Shimazaki Y, Motoyama T. Frequent epigenetic silencing of the p16 gene in non-small cell lung cancers of tobacco smokers. Jpn J Cancer Res 2002;93:1107–1113.

53. Shinagawa T, Nomura T, Colmenares C, Ohira M, Nakagawara A, Ishii S. Increased susceptibility to tumorigenesis of ski-deficient heterozygous mice. Oncogene 2001;20:8100–8108.

54. Boivin AJ, Momparler LF, Hurtubise A, Momparler RL. Antineoplastic action of 5-aza-2′-deoxycytidine and phenylbutyrate on human lung carcinoma cells. Anticancer Drugs 2002;13:869–874.

55. Won J, Yim J, Kim TK. Sp1 and Sp3 recruit histone deacetylase to repress transcription of human telomerase reverse transcriptase (hTERT) promoter in normal human somatic cells. J Biol Chem 2002;277:38,230–38,238.

56. Han JW, Ahn SH, Park SH, et al. Apicidin, a histone deacetylase inhibitor, inhibits proliferation of tumor cells via induction of p21WAF1/Cip1 and gelsolin. Cancer Res 2000;60:6068–6074.

57. Marks PA, Richon VM, Rifkind RA. Histone deacetylase inhibitors: inducers of differentiation or apoptosis of transformed cells. J Natl Cancer Inst 2000;92: 1210–1216.

58. Furumai R, Komatsu Y, Nishino N, Khochbin S, Yoshida M, Horinouchi S. Potent histone deacetylase inhibitors built from trichostatin A and cyclic tetrapeptide antibiotics including trapoxin. Proc Natl Acad Sci U S A 2001;98:87–92.

59. Greenberg VL, Williams JM, Cogswell JP, Mendenhall M, Zimmer SG. Histone deacetylase inhibitors promote apoptosis and differential cell cycle arrest in anaplastic thyroid cancer cells. Thyroid 2001;11:315–325.

60. Fournel M, Trachy-Bourget MC, Yan PT, et al. Sulfonamide anilides, a novel class of histone deacetylase inhibitors, are antiproliferative against human tumors. Cancer Res 2002;62:4325–4330.

61. Jaboin J, Wild J, Hamidi H, et al. MS-27-275, an inhibitor of histone deacetylase, has marked in vitro and in vivo antitumor activity against pediatric solid tumors. Cancer Res 2002;62:6108–6115.

62. Sambucetti LC, Fischer DD, Zabludoff S, et al. Histone deacetylase inhibition selectively alters the activity and expression of cell cycle proteins leading to specific chromatin acetylation and antiproliferative effects. J Biol Chem 1999; 274:34,940–34,947.

63. Kim YB, Ki SW, Yoshida M, Horinouchi S. Mechanism of cell cycle arrest caused by histone deacetylase inhibitors in human carcinoma cells. J Antibiot (Tokyo) 2000;53:1191–1200.

64. Suzuki T, Yokozaki H, Kuniyasu H, et al. Effect of trichostatin A on cell growth and expression of cell cycle- and apoptosis-related molecules in human gastric and oral carcinoma cell lines. Int J Cancer 2000;88:992–997.

65. Richon VM, Zhou X, Rifkind RA, Marks PA. Histone deacetylase inhibitors: development of suberoylanilide hydroxamic acid (saha) for the treatment of cancers. Blood Cells Mol Dis 2001;27:260–264.

66. Strait KA, Dabbas B, Hammond EH, Warnick CT, Iistrup SJ, Ford CD. Cell cycle blockade and differentiation of ovarian cancer cells by the histone deacetylase inhibitor trichostatin A are associated with changes in p21, Rb, and Id proteins. Mol Cancer Ther 2002;1:1181–1190.

67. Atadja P, Gao L, Kwon P, et al. Selective growth inhibition of tumor cells by a novel histone deacetylase inhibitor, NVP-LAQ824. Cancer Res 2004;64:689–695.

68. Munster PN, Troso-Sandoval T, Rosen N, Rifkind R, Marks PA, Richon VM. The histone deacetylase inhibitor suberoylanilide hydroxamic acid induces differentiation of human breast cancer cells. Cancer Res 2001;61:8492–8497.

69. Glick RD, Swendeman SL, Coffey DC, et al. Hybrid polar histone deacetylase inhibitor induces apoptosis and CD95/CD95 ligand expression in human neuroblastoma. Cancer Res 1999;59:4392–4399.

70. Remiszewski SW. The discovery of NVP-LAQ824: from concept to clinic. Curr Med Chem 2003;10:2393–2402.
71. Piekarz R, Bates S. A review of depsipeptide and other histone deacetylase inhibitors in clinical trials. Curr Pharm Des 2004;10:2289–2298.
72. Piekarz RL, Robey R, Sandor V, et al. Inhibitor of histone deacetylation, depsipeptide (FR901228), in the treatment of peripheral and cutaneous T-cell lymphoma: a case report. Blood 2001;98:2865–2868.
73. Kelly WK, Richon VM, O'Connor O, et al. Phase I clinical trial of histone deacetylase inhibitor: suberoylanilide hydroxamic acid administered intra-venously. Clin Cancer Res 2003;9:3578–3588.

Index